Juridification in Bioethics

Governance of Human Pluripotent Cell Research

Juridification
in
Bioethics

Governance of Human Pluripotent Cell Research

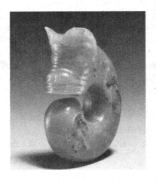

Calvin Wai-Loon Ho
National University of Singapore

Imperial College Press

ICP

Published by

Imperial College Press
57 Shelton Street
Covent Garden
London WC2H 9HE

Distributed by

World Scientific Publishing Co. Pte. Ltd.

5 Toh Tuck Link, Singapore 596224

USA office: 27 Warren Street, Suite 401-402, Hackensack, NJ 07601

UK office: 57 Shelton Street, Covent Garden, London WC2H 9HE

Library of Congress Cataloging-in-Publication Data
Names: Ho, W. Calvin, author.
Title: Juridification in bioethics : governance of human pluripotent cell research /
    Calvin Wai-Loon Ho, NUS, Singapore.
Description: New Jersey : Imperial College Press, 2016. |
    Includes bibliographical references and index.
Identifiers: LCCN 2016031970| ISBN 9781911299615 (hardcover : alk. paper) |
    ISBN 1911299611 (hardcover : alk. paper) | ISBN 9781911299622 (pbk. : alk. paper) |
    ISBN 191129962X (pbk. : alk. paper)
Subjects: LCSH: Bioethics. | Medical ethics. | Stem cells--Research.
Classification: LCC QH332 .H668 2016 | DDC 174.2--dc23
LC record available at https://lccn.loc.gov/2016031970

British Library Cataloguing-in-Publication Data
A catalogue record for this book is available from the British Library.

Printed in Singapore

Foreword

Against a backdrop of research scandals and abuses in the 1960's and 1970's, bioethics emerged as a framework to guide the responsible advancement of biomedical sciences and related technologies. Although scientific and social value are the fundamental justification for undertaking research, researchers, sponsors, research ethics committees and health authorities have a moral obligation to ensure that all research is carried out in ways that uphold human rights, and respect, protect, and are fair to study participants and the communities in which the research is conducted. Therefore, basic principles such as informed consent have been enshrined in landmark documents, including the ethical guidelines of the Council for International Organizations of Medical Societies (CIOMS) on health related research involving humans.

CIOMS was jointly established by WHO and UNESCO in 1949 as an international, non-governmental, and non-profit organization. Through membership, it represents a substantial proportion of the biomedical scientific community. First published in 1982, the CIOMS guidelines have been a source of reference for countries in defining national policies on the ethics of human biomedical research. At this time, these guidelines are being revised and updated, following an extensive public consultation. The revised guidelines are expected to be published early in 2017. Recurring themes on the social value of research and on the acceptability of particular formulation of risk-benefit ratios continue to underscore the importance of the principle of respect for persons. A similar finding is presented in this book, *Juridification in Bioethics*. As a longitudinal ethnographic study, this book explains how and why mutual respect and reciprocity must remain the bedrock for the development of bioethics as public policy and as governance practice. It further illustrates how, through the rationalities and instrumentality of law, bioethical questions about social value and uncertain risks in research are also concerns of public reason and of reasonable pluralism in society. Ultimately, the legitimacy of bioethical responses may well depend on – in the words of John Rawls – whether they satisfy the criteria of reciprocity and belong to the public reason of 'peoples' who are tolerant, decent and fair-minded, yet diverse in beliefs and socio-cultural practices.

Bioethics must remain an open, inclusive and multidisciplinary forum, enabling individuals and society to co-create scientific and technological developments on local and global scales. Just as the discursive power of law has been drawn upon to achieve bioethical goals, bioethics must sustain the law as a purposive social enterprise that facilitates social life through communication, coordination and mutual understanding. It is through such a mutually enriching and invigorating synergy that both are most likely to accomplish the shared vision of just ends.

Johannes JM van Delden
Professor of Medical Ethics
Julius Center, University Medical Center, Utrecht
The Netherlands
President of CIOMS

Preface

夷道若纇，上德若谷。老子《道德经》第四十一章

The smooth way seems knotty, Superior virtue seems like a valley.

Laozi

Daodejing, Chapter 41

The development of the natural sciences and technology, and the great ideologies on the organisation of political and economic systems, are two factors that have above all others shaped human history in the twentieth century. These are the opening words of Isaiah Berlin in *The Crooked Timber of Humanity*. On a modest scale, the study presented in this book relates to these two themes in that it is concerned with the advancement of human pluripotent stem cell science and technology, and also with systems of governance that have emerged alongside. Rather than viewing them as two distinct factors, my study of juridification in bioethics as public policy and governance practice presents them as intertwined and comingled.

This book presents an ethnographic study of law on the periphery. More precisely, it focuses on the role and contribution of law, in terms of its norms, concepts, rationalities, techniques, practices and language, to the policy construction of artefacts like the embryo, animal chimeras and cytoplasmic hybrids in human pluripotent stem cell research through the work of bioethical bodies like the Bioethics Advisory Committee (BAC) in Singapore. My methodology is inspired by actor-network theory (ANT) as applied in the field of science and technology studies (STS). A key objective of this research is to understand the relevance of law in the production of epistemic claims on pre-social and social life, and an explication of the mechanisms entailed. This book also proposes a broadening of juridification to mean the co-production of such claims by law, alongside other modalities of power, within bioethics as a power-complex or knowledge-order. In other words, my hope is to instaurate juridification as a means to open up law, and its various constituents and implements, by making them proper objects of inquiry in bioethics. This analytical approach better enables us to appreciate the complex relations of law, technology, culture and society, as well as bioethics as an emergent civic epistemology.

I am greatly indebted to very many people over the course of this more than a decade long research. The ethnographic component of this research was mainly conducted while I was a doctoral student at Cornell University. My supervisor, Professor Annelise Riles saw the value of this research before I did. Without her foresight and guidance, this research would not have been possible. I have benefitted immensely from the different knowledge fields that the members of my thesis advisory committee have initiated me to: from Professor Riles, I have acquired an understanding of legal anthropology; I learnt from Professor Mitchell Lasser a whole new meaning to comparative research, as well as different ways of drawing value from it; and Professor Stephen Hilgartner has been my crucial portal to the epistemologically rich and analytically powerful world of STS. Other faculty members of the Law School and the Department of STS have also been a source of invaluable guidance and inspiration, and here, I express my gratitude to Professors Eduardo Peñalver, Rachel Prentice, Peter Dear, and Trevor Pinch, Assistant Dean for Graduate Legal Studies Charles D. Cramton and Ms Dawne Peacock. Beyond Cornell,

I have greatly benefited from the knowledge and insights gained through the privilege of having interacted or worked with many colleagues in academia, including Professors Tracey Chan, Terry Kaan, Reidar Lie, Jonathan Montgomery, Bernard Rudden, Marilyn Strathern, Daniel Wilker, Zhai Xiaomei, as well as fellow scholars and colleagues at Ethox Centre at the University of Oxford, the Nuffield Council on Bioethics in London (UK), Hastings Center in Garrison (New York, USA), and Fondation Brocher in Hermance (Switzerland). I am grateful to Professor Johannes van Delden, with whom I have had the honour of collaborating with on a number of bioethical projects, for kindly providing the Foreword.

My fieldwork in Singapore would not have been possible without the support of the immediate past Chairman of the Bioethics Advisory Committee (BAC), Professor Lim Pin, and my former colleagues at the Secretariat, namely Dr Sylvia Lim, Professor John Elliott, Ms Charmaine Chan, Ms Atishah Ali, Mr Alvin Chew, Ms Linda Tan and Mrs Shailaja Suresh. I cannot sufficiently express my gratitude for their kindness, encouragement and support. I especially thank Sylvia, for our many conversations and collaborations since the founding of the BAC. The past and present members of the BAC, its working groups and its International Panel of Experts (particularly Professor Martin Bobrow, Professor Bartha Knoppers, Professor Bernard Lo, Dr Thomas Murray, and Professor (Baroness) Onora O'Neill) have also been exceptionally generous and kind in sharing their views and experiences. I record my deep thanks to all of them. Aside from the BAC, I am much indebted to Dr Fran Sharples (US National Academy of Sciences), Dr Geoffrey Lomax (California Institute of Regenerative Medicine), Dr Helen Munn (UK Academy of Medical Sciences), Professor Peder Agger (Danish Council of Ethics), Ms Anne Lykkeskov (Danish Council of Ethics), Ms Lise Wied Kirkegaard (Danish Council of Ethics), Dr Abha Saxena (World Health Organization), Dr Andreas Reis (World Health Organization) and Dr Marie-Charlotte Bouësseau (World Health Organization) for their views and insights. I also extend my gratitude and thanks to all whom I interviewed, for our conversations and documents that they shared with me. This publication is certainly not the endpoint, and I very much look forward to our continuing engagements.

I cannot adequately describe how immensely captivating and rewarding the field of bioethics has been for me. It is not an exaggeration to say that this study can only articulates a small fragment of the epistemic vibrance that is endogenous to the field. I am immensely grateful to Professors Alastair Campbell, John Wong and (Dean) Yeoh Khay Guan for their foresightedness and for the opportunity to be part of the Centre for Biomedical Ethics, at the Yong Loo Lin School of Medicine, National University of Singapore (NUS), and to Professor Simon Chesterman for the opportunity to remain engaged with the Law School. Consistent and active interactions with fellow colleagues at NUS, and with our students, have been a truly enriching experience. I also take this opportunity to thank Ms Lim Sook Cheng, Ms Yolande Koh and their respective teams at Imperial College Press for their great patience and support of this project, and to the peer reviewers of this book for their helpful and instructive comments. While far from perfect, I hope this book has done justice to the guidance that I have received through the course of its many and varied permutations.

Finally, I extend my deepest thanks to my family, and to Ms Rachel Teo and Mr Karel Caals. The publication of this book would not have been possible without your invaluable support and assistance.

Calvin Wai-Loon Ho

NUS, Singapore

July 2016

About the Author

Calvin is assistant professor at the Centre for Biomedical Ethics of the Yong Loo Lin School of Medicine, National University of Singapore (NUS). He is co-head of the World Health Organization Collaborating Centre on Bioethics in Singapore, and co-head of the Accountability Policy Task Team of the Global Alliance for Genomics & Health. Calvin is also an Ethics Board member of Médecins Sans Frontières, as well as a member on the advisory committees for transplantation and on genetic testing of the Singapore Ministry of Health and serves as an assistant director with the Singapore Legal Aid Bureau.

Calvin holds a doctorate in juridical science from Cornell University, and was also trained in law at NUS and University of Cambridge. In addition, he holds degrees in sociology and economics from LSE and SOAS (University of London), and has been a research associate with the Ethox Centre, Nuffield Department of Population Health, University of Oxford. He has published on global health law and ethics, research ethics and policy, health policy and governance, and is the co-editor of *Bioethics in Singapore: An Ethical Microcosm* (2010) and *Genetic Privacy: An Evaluation of the Ethical and Legal Landscape* (2013).

Abbreviations

AMS	Academy of Medical Sciences (UK)
ANT	Actor-Network-Theory
AR Directives	Licensing Terms and Conditions for Assisted Reproduction Centres, MOH, 2011
ART	Artificial Reproductive Technologies
A*STAR	Agency for Science Technology and Research (Singapore)
AVA	Agri-Food and Veterinary Authority (Singapore)
BAC	Bioethics Advisory Committee (Singapore)
CIOMS	Council for International Organizations of Medical Sciences
CIRM	California Institute for Regenerative Medicine
DCE	Danish Council of Ethics
DHHS	Department of Health and Human Services (US)
EC	European Commission
ECJ	European Court of Justice
RCD Report	Reproductive Cell Donation Report of the EC published in 2006
ED	Egg Donation
ED Report	Egg Donation Report of the BAC published in 2008
ELSI	Ethical, Legal and Social Implications
EPA	Environment Protection Agency (US)
ESCRO	Embryonic Stem Cell Research Oversight (US)

EU	European Union
GEC	German Ethics Council (Deutscher Ethikrat)
HAC	Human-Animal Combinations
HA Report	HAC Report of the BAC published in 2010
HBRA	Human Biomedical Research Act 2015 (Singapore)
HCOPA	Human Cloning and Other Prohibited Practices Act (Singapore)
hESC	Human Embryonic Stem Cell(s)
HECR	Human Embryo and Chimera Research Working Group (of the BAC)
HFEA	Human Fertilisation and Embryology Authority (UK)
HFE Act	Human Fertilisation and Embryology Act 2008 (UK)
HSCR	Human Stem Cell Research Sub-Committee of the BAC (Singapore)
IACUC	Institutional Animal Care and Use Committee
IFFS	International Federation of Fertility Societies
IOM	Institute of Medicine (US)
iPSC	Induced Pluripotent Stem Cell(s)
IRB	Institutional Review Board
IRGC	International Risk Governance Council
ISSCR	International Society for Stem Cell Research
IVF	In Vitro Fertilization
MOH	Ministry of Health (Singapore)
NACLAR	National Advisory Committee on Laboratory Animal Research (Singapore)
NAE	National Academy of Engineers (US)
NAS	National Academy of Sciences (US)
NBAC	National Bioethics Advisory Commission (US)
NIH	National Institutes of Health (US)
NRC	National Research Council (US)
NUS	National University of Singapore
OECD	Organisation for Economic Co-operation and Development

OHSS	Ovarian Hyper-stimulation Syndrome
SCLS	Steering Committee on Life Sciences, Singapore Cabinet
SCNT	Somatic Cell Nuclear Transfer
SC Report	Stem Cell Report of the BAC published in 2002
SCRO	Stem Cell Research Oversight
STS	Science and Technology Studies
UK	United Kingdom
UNESCO	United Nations Educational, Scientific and Cultural Organization
UN(GA)	United Nations (General Assembly)
US/USA	United States of America
WHO	World Health Organization

Contents

1

Juridification in Bioethics

1.1 Why Study Juridification?

At the turn of the century, policymakers in Singapore earmarked biomedical (or life) sciences as a driver for economic growth. The technological edge that it hopes to develop is expected to enhance the competitiveness of its thriving pharmaceutical and healthcare industries. Positive externalities from the investment are expected to include strengthening Singapore's standing as a regional research and education hub. Among the various initiatives adopted in furtherance of this goal was the establishment of the Bioethics Advisory Committee (BAC) in December 2000. A key responsibility of the BAC has been to assist the government in establishing an appropriate governance framework for human biomedical research. In 2002, the BAC published its first set of ethical recommendations concerning human cloning and embryonic stem cell research (the SC Report).[1] This report contributed to the enactment of legislation on cloning.[2] In 2006, shortage of human eggs needed for research,

---

[1] Bioethics Advisory Committee, *Ethical, Legal and Social Issues in Human Stem Cell Research, Reproductive and Therapeutic Cloning.* Singapore: Bioethics Advisory Committee, June 2002.

[2] *Human Cloning and Other Prohibited Practices Act* (Cap. 131B), Revised 2005.

1

along with related technological developments (particularly induced pluripotent stem cell (iPSC) technology) necessitated a review of its recommendations. Following a period of research, deliberation and consultation, the BAC published a new set of ethical guidelines on donation of human eggs for research in 2008 (the ED Report),[3] which was followed by the issuance of a revised set of directives on ARTs by the MOH (AR Directives).[4] The BAC published a separate set of guidelines on human-animal combinations in 2010 (i.e. the HA Report).[5] In 2015, the BAC consolidated the principles and recommendations in all three reports into a set of guidelines on human biomedical research, and a corresponding legislation has been enacted by the government shortly after.[6]

This book presents a study of the role and contribution of law – in terms of its norms, concepts, rationalities, techniques, practices and language – to bioethics as public policy and as governance practice.[7] I describe this phenomenon as juridification, and hence offer a much broader conception than only thinking of it as "a process (or processes) by which the state intervenes in areas of social life ... in ways which limit the autonomy of individuals or groups to determine their own affairs."[8] Teubner's formulation of juridification relates primarily to

---

3   Bioethics Advisory Committee, *Donation of Human Eggs for Research*. Singapore: Bioethics Advisory Committee, November 2008.

4   Ministry of Health, *Licensing Terms and Conditions for Assisted Reproduction Centres*, 2011.

5   Bioethics Advisory Committee, *Human-Animal Combinations in Stem Cell Research*. Singapore: Bioethics Advisory Committee, September 2010.

6   *Human Biomedical Research Act* of 2015.

7   Bartha Knoppers highlights the aims of bioethics policymaking as requiring these: "avoid being legalistic; be context-specific; speak plainly; address the diversity of issues, disciplines and cultures involved; facilitate harmonization, compliance and oversight; include all relevant stakeholders; be aspirational; be practical and yet, at the same time, be principled." Bartha M Knoppers, Does policy grow on trees? *BMC Medical Ethics* (2014) 15:87.

8   Jon Clark and Lord Wedderburn, Juridification – a Universal Trend? In Gunther Teubner (ed.), *Juridification of Social Spheres: A Comparative Analysis in the Areas of Labor, Corporate Antitrust and Social Welfare Law*. Berlin: Walter de Gruyter & Co, 1987, pp 163-190, at 165.

a concern with the proliferation of (especially regulatory) law, and may be traced to Max Weber's 'materialisation of formal laws'.[9] As we shall see, this is but one of several interpretations of 'juridification'. For Teubner, this term is essentially shorthand for the expansion of formal legal rationalisation, which is but one of many forms of legal rationality.[10] My goal is to reinstate a broader conception of 'juridification', as encompassing the competing forces of formal rationality and substantive rationality.[11] This richer account of 'juridification' has already been implicit in Weberian thought,[12] and one that was already very much engaged with Kantian conception of the *Rechtstaat* (constitutional state)[13] and Hegelian inquiry into conditions for morality, freedom and justice.[14] By this conception, juridification is not necessarily limiting of liberty interests, but also constitutive of them. The notion of 'co-production' in STS may be a term that provides a more apt depiction of legal contribution to bioethics and policy development in the context of my research, and 'juridification' is intended to show how the law has had an

---

9   Gunther Teubner, Juridification – Concepts, Aspects, Limits, Solutions. In Gunther Teubner (ed.), *Juridification of Social Spheres: A Comparative Analysis in the Areas of Labor, Corporate Antitrust and Social Welfare Law*. Berlin: Walter de Gruyter & Co, 1987, pp 3-48, at 4-5. In the most general terms, Teubner indicates that juridification is about the relation between state and society, and the balance between their relative influence on the way human beings conduct their lives.

10 See for instance: Tom R Hickman, The Reasonableness Principle: Reassessing its Place in the Public Sphere, *Cambridge Law Journal* (2004) 63, 1: 166-198.

11 A similarly broad approach to juridification has been adopted by Javier Couso and others: Javier Couso, Alexandra Huneeus and Rachel Sieder, *Cultures of Legality: Judicialization and Political Activism in Latin America*. Cambridge: Cambridge University Press, 2010.

12 Max Weber (Guenther Roth and Claus Wittich, eds.), *Economy and Society: An Outline of Interpretive Sociology* (in two volumes). Berkeley, Los Angeles and London: University of California Press, [1922] 1978. See especially, Volume 2, at 641-900.

13 Immanuel Kant (tr. M Campbell Smith), *Perpetual Peace: a philosophical essay*. London: G Allen & Unwin, [1795] 1917.

14 Georg W F Hegel (Thomas Malcolm Knox, ed.), *Hegel's Philosophy of Right*. Oxford: Oxford University Press, [1820] 2015. For a recent application of Hegelian thought on ethicality, legality and morality, see: Shannon Hoff, *The Laws of the Spirit: A Hegelian Theory of Justice*. Buffalo: SUNY Press, 2014.

indispensable role. In this study, I explain the ways that meanings, functions and constructions of legal rationalities, concepts, language and techniques have been taken up within a 'bioethics-as-public-policy' framework and in the governance of biomedical research. Through working in the field of bioethics, I ask: What is 'legal' about bioethics? What are the ideas and artefacts that bioethics encompasses, and how are they related to law? How do ideas move from one knowledge system to another? In particular, what is the role of law in bioethics?

As the BAC has been the leading actor in the institutionalisation of bioethics in Singapore, it was the primary subject of my ethnographic study from October 2007 to December 2012. Bioethics encompasses many varied aspects and processes of life, from synthetic biology to climate change. In a formal sense, the contribution of the BAC to this discourse has been through its policy/governance-oriented deliberations on the ethical, legal and social implications of advancements in the biomedical sciences. During the time that my research was carried out, the BAC was formulating recommendations for chimeras and hybrids – biological constructs that are now indispensable to many types of biomedical research. Hence my research is also about the historical and situational context within which regulations relating to chimeras and hybrids, along with other artefacts in human pluripotent stem cell research, have emerged in Singapore. Given the relatively lengthy duration of the study, my involvement has been as a member of its Secretariat, rather than an impartial and indifferent participant-observer, or as some might say, 'a fly on the wall'. As a legal researcher with the Secretariat, my responsibility has been to facilitate the work of the BAC through the application of legal expertise. Just as Annelise Riles has studied the practices surrounding the governance of the global financial markets through one motif (i.e. the 'collateral'),[15] I adopt and adapt

---

15 Annelise Riles, *Collateral Knowledge: Legal Reasoning in the Global Financial Markets*. Chicago and London: University of Chicago Press, 2011, at 224.

her approach in studying technical or 'knowledge practices' that constitute the governance of biomedical research in Singapore, and attempt to explicate some of the often taken-for-granted 'facts' that policymakers and regulators apply when preparing and putting forward guidelines and recommendations, for instance. I also find that artefacts like human embryos, oocytes (eggs) and human-animal combinations (principally hybrids and chimeras) constitute useful motifs in studying bioethics as a policy and governance framework for biomedical research for a number of reasons. First, they are directly related to what policymakers and regulators understand (their *mentalité*) to be the nature of 'bioethical' issues, as well as the means by which they could and should be responded to. Second, the very controversial character of the research highlights the role or function of law in engaging with the contentions. It is further instructive as to how policymakers and regulators have reacted to a controversy, and their actions could illustrate how they think about law and governance more generally. Third, these artefacts present one of the most contentious set of issues arising from human biomedical research. They are 'boundary objects', which enable the study of how different knowledge fields interact.[16]

I argue that studying how law connects with these artefacts can provide useful insights on how the law works vis-à-vis novel scientific and technological developments, and its contribution to the broader discourse of bioethics. By asking, as Annelise Riles does, 'what are chimeras (or embryos, or hybrids), really, in biomedical research?',[17]

---

[16] Susan Leigh Star, This is Not a Boundary Object: Reflections on the Origin of a Concept, *Science, Technology, & Human Values* (2010) 35, 5: 601-617.

[17] Riles suggests that "if one approaches regulatory debates from the standpoint of the deceptively naïve question, 'what is collateral, really, in the derivatives markets?' one begins to grasp a view of regulation as something very different ..." in Annelise Riles. *Collateral Knowledge: Legal Reasoning in the Global Financial Markets*. Chicago and London: University of Chicago Press, 2011, at 10. Lessig's observation that the law in its traditional sense – as an order backed by threat – is one of many tools that constrain behaviour, as well as law's impact on these

one can begin to appreciate how these constructs illustrate the legalisation of hybrid life.[18] It further allows us to question:[19] "Who is in control? Who is responsible for what? Could anyone take control? And to what end?"

Bioethics is concerned with more than scientific research. It is an assemblage of many forms of expertise and many kinds of technology in different domains.[20] Developments in Singapore reflect a broader trend of similar developments in leading scientific jurisdictions. Arguably, these developments are linked to those occurring in transnational and international discursive spaces. Notably, regional groupings, such as the EU, and international organisations and associations have also been agents of change. By studying the current changes in law and bioethics in Singapore, one can better appreciate the substance and direction of similar developments elsewhere.[21] The

---

other tools, is helpful: Lawrence Lessig, The Law of the Horse: What Cyberlaw Might Teach, *Harvard Law Review* (1999) 113: 501, at 502.

18 Annelise Riles. A New Agenda for the Cultural Study of Law: Taking on the Technicalities, *Buffalo Law Review* (2005) 53: 973-1033. Riles observes (at 973) the need to increase our "understanding of the very thing that defines our field, of what makes law as opposed to literature or economics or cognitive science: the technicalities of legal thought." She adds that as lawyers, the notion that law is more than just rules have not stopped "lawyers from loving their tools for their own sake ... from having a certain aesthetic appreciation for their uses. What defines the technical as a sphere of social practice, in other words, is lawyers' commitments to an aesthetic of instrumentality, not simply to an instrumentalist politics or project" (at 1026).

19 Sally Falk Moore. *Law and Anthropology: A Reader*. Cornwall: Blackwell Publishing, 2005, at 3.

20 Annelise Riles. *Collateral Knowledge: Legal Reasoning in the Global Financial Markets*. Chicago and London: University of Chicago Press, 2011, at 11. Just as markets are made up of more than finance, the varied expertise that makes up the BAC is illustrative of a similar plurality in bioethics.

21 I see this as parallel to Lasser's argument that serious attention will have to be paid to developments at the level of national legal systems, if only to gain a better understanding of the dynamics between developments on the domestic and supranational levels: Mitchel de S.-O.-l'E Lasser, *Judicial Transformations: The Rights Revolution in the Courts of Europe*. Oxford and New York: Oxford University Press, 2009, at 13-14.

converse is also true. Changes in Singapore can be better understood through studying parallel or related developments elsewhere. Studying developments in Singapore is important for other reasons. Susan Silbey and Patricia Ewick show the power of law in the minds of common people.[22] Indeed, this study lends support to their finding that the law has a vivid existence outside of the 'enchanted rationality' of legal scholars, judges and lawyers.[23] It takes varied forms in different cultural schemas or images and invokes different normative claims, justifications and values.[24] Yet in all of these accounts, there is a certain stability of meaning – even if fragmentary. How is this achieved? This study suggests that outside the 'enchanted realm', commoners understand both law and bioethics normatively.[25] In most respects, bioethics will be viewed no differently from law. I attempt to provide accounts of the mechanics by which these normative accounts of law (as legality) and bioethics (as ethical) are associated and stabilised. By examining the interaction and movement of ideas between law and other knowledge systems as diverse as ethics, medicine and the sciences (both physical and social) within the broader framework of bioethics, the character and role of legal norms become more explicit.[26] In examining legal norms, I also attempt to explicate the techniques and practices that are applied in a public policy environment. Some of them are closely associated with legal norms and rationalities, whereas others have a broader normative basis. These techniques and practices are "means, not ends – they are not tethered to any particular policy outcome or

---

22 Susan S Silbey and Patricia Ewick, The Double Life of Reason and Law, *University of Miami Law Review* (2003) 57: 497-512.
23 *Ibid* at 503.
24 *Ibid* at 506.
25 This should come as no surprise as Hans Kelsen has postulated that the law is in essence a system of norms. See Hans Kelsen (tr. M Knight). *Pure Theory of Law*, Berkeley and Los Angeles: University of California Press, 1967 (2nd edition).
26 Annelise Riles. Representing In-Between: Law, Anthropology, and the Rhetoric of Interdisciplinarity, *University of Illinois Law Review* (1994) 597-650.

political point of view", which may be described as "placeholders, documents, theories, dreams, fictions, analogies, and many others".[27] The core aspects of juridification are identified in its epistemology, its aesthetics, its materiality, and its sociality,[28] rather than by developing a formalistic and limited conception of juridification only as expansion of sovereign power. This study shows that legal norms, rationalities, language, techniques and practices have served as means of abstraction, objectification and fabrication; creating scripts or narratives; enabling comparison, conceptualisation and reconciliation with risks; and creating (or otherwise privileging certain) mindsets over others. In the context of public policy and governance, juridification further represents a hybridisation process by which a public sphere and an emergent civic epistemology are constituted.

1.2 What is Bioethics?

Robert Baker provides an insightful analysis of five English-language monographs that have been published on the history of bioethics: David Rothman's *Strangers at the Bedside*,[29] Albert Jonsen's *The Birth of Bioethics*,[30] Tina Stevens's *Bioethics in America*,[31] Renée Fox and Judith Swazey's *Observing Bioethics*[32] and John Evans's *The History and Future of Bioethics*.[33] He observes that there is substantial agreement among these scholars about the What, When, Where, Who

---

27 Annelise Riles. *Collateral Knowledge: Legal Reasoning in the Global Financial Markets*. Chicago and London: University of Chicago Press, 2011, at 228-229.
28 *Ibid*, at 230.
29 David J Rothman, *Strangers at the bedside: a history of how law and bioethics transformed medical decision making*. New York: BasicBooks, 1991.
30 Albert R Jonsen, *The Birth of Bioethics*. New York: Oxford University Press, 2003.
31 Tina M L Stevens, *Bioethics in America*. Baltimore: Johns Hopkins University Press, 2000.
32 Renée C Fox and Judith P Swazey (with Judith C Watkins), *Observing Bioethics*. Oxford and New York: Oxford University Press, 2008.
33 John H Evans, *The History and Future of Bioethics: a Sociological View*. Oxford and New York: Oxford University Press, 2012.

and How bioethics was conceived and born in the USA. A broad overview of Baker's analysis may be set out as follows:

(1) **What Happened**: A group of non-medical actors (what Rothman terms as 'strangers' to medicine) transformed medical decision-making. These actors were principally bureaucrats, ex-theologians, lawyers, legislators, philosophers and social scientists.

(2) **Where and When**: It occurred in America in the 1970's, although there is general agreement that important institutional changes that opened up access to medical decision-making occurred before the birth of bioethics (i.e. from the 1960's onwards).

(3) **Why was Bioethics Born**: Various reasons have been provided including the challenges presented by new medical technologies and the demand for appropriate oversight in the light of research scandals, and the relative ease of translating bioethical principles into bureaucratic regulation. In re-phrasing the question as:[34] 'Why did American medicine lose jurisdiction over "medical ethics"?', Baker's response suggests that it was due to the self-imposed restriction by American medical establishments (such as the American Medical Association) against making authoritative statements on medical ethics. Such a stance reflected the *laissez-faire* approach that was adopted from 1903 through to the 1970's where individual doctors were entrusted with ethical decision-making for their patients. Consequently, these medical establishments also did not have the power to negotiate on issues relating to end-of-life care and allocation of scarce resources with the US government. These issues had to be left to the

---

[34] Robert Baker, *Before Bioethics: A History of American Medical Ethics from the Colonial Period to the Bioethics Revolution*. New York: Oxford University Press, 2013, at 275-276.

'outsiders' composed of "a hodgepodge of ex-theologians, lawyers, philosophers, social scientists, and humanistic nurses, physicians, and researchers" who were empowered by American bureaucrats (and joined with governments and private foundations) to address issues that were presented by research ethics scandals and morally disruptive technologies.[35] Bioethics came to represent the workable solutions that were put forward. In contrast, European medical establishments did not abandon their jurisdiction over medical ethics. For this reason, bioethicists in Europe have had a less central role in addressing similar issues that have arisen in the US.

(4) **Who and How**: There is broad consensus among the key reference works that the 1978 Belmont Report (to be discussed later on in this book) was a watershed moment, and the socio-political conditions were such that it was heavily influenced by the Civil Rights Act of 1964, introduced to Congress by Senator Ted Kennedy, and who subsequently convened hearings to investigate the scandal of the Tuskegee Syphilis Study when it was publicised in 1972.[36] The Kennedy hearings culminated in the National Research Act of 1974. There is also general unanimity that American bioethics was conceived and born in an era of egalitarian reform. The egalitarian values of individual rights and choice are reflected in the Belmont principles of respect for persons, beneficence and justice. As this study similarly shows, the Belmont principles and other developments contributed to the emergence of a bioethics *lingua franca*.

In essence, the inter-disciplinary nature of bioethics as it emerged in the socio-political context of the US was more accidental than deliberate. The *laissez faire* approach that was adopted by the

---

35   *Ibid*, at 278-279.
36   *Ibid*, at 287.

American Medical Association inhibited its ability to govern professional conduct through ethical or other regulatory means. To fill this vacuum, "a coalition of bureaucrats, foundations, concerned humanistic physicians, and researchers joined with philosophers, lawyers, ex-theologians, and social scientists to create and valorise an alternative voice of moral authority that came to be known as 'bioethics'."[37]

The Belmont Report applies *principlism*, better known as the 'Georgetown Mantra'. It promotes a version of analytical philosophy that is principles-based, and has many points of intersection with American law, especially within a 'bioethics-as-public-policy' framework.[38] Alex Capron observes that the legal process by which certain bioethical issues have been addressed by US courts has much in common with philosophical principlism, primarily because the former is also largely a contextual process based on key principles (articulated in the language of rights typically framed in constitutional terms) rather than empirical facts.[39] George Annas goes further in arguing that the principles of American bioethics, including autonomy and justice, are drawn from American law.[40] Principlism is also the trait that has rendered bioethics amenable to bureaucratisation and to its uptake by both the medical and biomedical research communities. To be sure, principlism is not the only analytical approach in bioethics.[41] However, it is this particular approach that

---

[37] *Ibid*, at 317.

[38] Renée C Fox and Judith P Swazey, *Observing Bioethics*. New York: Oxford University Press, 2008, at 171-172.

[39] Alex M Capron, What contributions have social science and the law made to the development of policy on bioethics? (1999) *Daedalus* 128 (4): 295-325.

[40] George J Annas. *American bioethics: Crossing human rights and health law boundaries*. Oxford and New York: Oxford University Press, 2005, at xiv. In a similar vein, Carl Elliott considers law to be the *lingua franca* of bioethics. See: Carl Elliott, *A philosophical disease: Bioethics, culture and identity*. New York: Routledge, 1999, at xxviii.

[41] As Marcus Düwell observes, bioethics as an academic discipline encompasses a rather different set of issues and methods. See Marcus Düwell, *Bioethics: Methods, Theories, Domains*. London and New York: Routledge, 2013, at 21-22.

has enabled bioethics to contribute to progress in public policy and to governance practices. While we have broadly labelled this approach as principlism, it is often unclear if the bioethical contribution to public policy is ethical in nature or legal. Perhaps where the emphasis is not in finding the right response to first-order theoretical problems (such as the intrinsic nature of a human embryo), the distinction between ethics and law is unlikely to be great and not especially important within the context of public policy.[42]

What seems clear is the broad recognition that bioethics is and should remain an inter-(and multi-)disciplinary communal practice, rather than a discipline that is defined by a dominant discourse and/or methodology.[43] Even if the nature of bioethics is difficult to pin down, its practitioners working in the domains of public policy and governance have drawn on law, in terms of both its normative substance and modes of reasoning, its language of rights and also its more processual applications, in ways that are intended to advance the common good (variously constructed) and the goals of political liberalism. It may be helpful to recapitulate at this point that the civil rights movement has been profoundly influential on American

---

[42] Frances M Kamm, *Bioethical Prescriptions: To Create, End, Choose, and Improve Lives*. Oxford and New York: Oxford University Press, 2013, at 551-567.

[43] Onora O'Neill, *Autonomy and Trust in Bioethics*. Cambridge: Cambridge University Press, 2008, at 1; Sarah Chan, A Bioethics for All Seasons, *Journal of Medical Ethics* (2015) 14: 17-21; Lisa M Lee and Frances A McCarty, Growth in U.S. Postsecondary Bioethics Degrees, *Hastings Center Report* (2016) 46, 2: 19-21. Lee and McCarty observes (at 20): "In less than fifty years, bioethics has progressed from a side interest of philosophers and physicians to a multidisciplinary field comprising experts in medicine, philosophy, science, psychology, law, and public health, among others. Together, bioethicists from a wide range of disciplines have produced a robust, peer-reviewed literature and hundreds of books on topics as diverse as nanoethics, genethics, neuroethics, public health ethics, clinical ethics consultations, and methods for conducting empirical ethics"; Marcus Düwell observes that bioethical judgments are mixed judgments in that their cogency is justified by very diverse disciplines: Marcus Düwell, *Bioethics: Methods, Theories, Domains*. London and New York: Routledge, 2013, at 9.

bioethics; hence its emphasis on autonomy and rights should not be surprising. From the 1980's onwards, bioethics has taken root in a diverse range of countries, due in part to the intermediation of international organisations like UNESCO and WHO,[44] and international organisations like the International Association of Bioethics.[45] In these forums, the norms of international law and conventions are often indistinguishable from global ethical norms. To be sure, it is not the claim here that bioethics – even as a policy concern – is the same everywhere. Clearly, political cultures, as well as historical and social conditions, affect not only the choice of 'bioethical' issues, but also the way that they are addressed in different countries.[46] Here, it is argued that a generic form of bioethics has taken root in the public policy framework of many countries around the world.[47] This generic form of bioethics is outlined as an emergent civic epistemology later on in this book.

---

[44] On the International Bioethics Committee of UNESCO, see: Roberto Andorno, Global bioethics at UNESCO: in defence of the Universal Declaration on Bioethics and Human Rights, *Journal of Medical Ethics* (2007) 33, 3: 150-154. Bioethics as a health policy concern is promoted by WHO through a biennial international meeting that it supports. For a description of an aspect of its work, see: Calvin Ho, Andreas Reis and Abha Saxena, Vulnerability in International Policy Discussion on Research involving Children, *Asian Bioethics Review* (2015) 7, 2: 230-249.

[45] For a detailed description of an international meeting organised under the auspices of the International Association of Bioethics, see: Manuel H R de Chávez Guerrero (ed.), *12th World Congress of Bioethics: Inspire the Future to Move the World*. Mexico City: National Bioethics Commission of Mexico, 2015.

[46] Sheila Jasanoff has shown how political cultures and other factors have shaped public policy on reproductive choices differently in the US, the UK and Germany. Sheila Jasanoff, *Designs on Nature: Science and Democracy in Europe and the United States*. Princeton: Princeton University Press, 2005, at 167-170.

[47] See for instance: John M Elliott, Calvin Ho and Sylvia Lim, *Bioethics in Singapore: the Ethical Microcosm*. Singapore: WorldScientific, 2010; Stefan Sperling, *Reasons of Conscience: The Bioethics Debate in Germany*. Chicago: University of Chicago Press, 2013; Duncan Wilson, *The Making of British Bioethics*. Manchester: Manchester University Press, 2014.

1.3 Juridification in ELSIfication

Lars Blichner and Anders Molander explain that juridification is related to the concepts of judicialisation and legalisation. As a descriptive term, juridification has been variedly defined as the proliferation of law or an increase in formal or positive written law, growing monopolisation by legal professionals, expansion of judicial power and the spread of rule-guided action or the expectation of lawful conduct.[48] By their analysis, juridification is a process that takes place within a legal order or a legal order in the making, and has at least five dimensions:[49]

(1) **Constitutive**: A process where norms constitutive of a political order are established or changed to the effect of adding to the competencies of the legal system;

(2) **Legal Expansion and Differentiation**: A process through which law comes to regulate an increasing number of different activities;

(3) **Conflicts Resolution**: A process whereby conflicts are increasingly being solved by or with reference to law;

(4) **Increased Judicial Power**: A process by which the legal system and the legal profession get more power; and

(5) **Legal Framing**: A process by which people increasingly tend to think of themselves and others as legal subjects.

From the standpoint of welfare law, a broadly similar description of juridification has been proffered:[50]

---

[48] Lars Chr Blichner and Anders Molander, Mapping Juridification, *European Law Journal* (2008) 14, 1: 36-54, at 36.

[49] *Ibid*, at 38-39.

[50] Henriette Sinding Aasen, Siri Gloppen, Anne-Mette Magnussen and Even Nilssen, Introduction. In Henriette Sinding Aasen, Siri Gloppen, Anne-Mette Magnussen and Even Nilssen, *Juridification and social citizenship in the welfare state*. Cheltenham: Edward Elgar, 2014, pp 1-20, at 2.

Across the different perspectives, however, there is agreement that juridification broadly refers to processes involving shifts towards constitutive regulations, increased judicial power, more autonomous judicial institutions, more detailed legal regulations, regulations of new areas, and conflicts and problems increasingly being framed in legal and rights-oriented terms ... Juridification includes, but goes beyond, what is commonly referred to as judicialisation – the increasing social and political role of courts – and also brings attention to the changing role and power of elected politicians, bureaucrats and professionals.

In bioethics, juridification has similarly been observed to be operative in the ELSI initiatives attached to major science programs in Canada. José Julián López and Janet Lunau illustrate two specific modes of legal reasoning – analogy and reflective equilibrium – that have been applied in the works of two of the most prominent ELSI legal scholars.[51] Analogical reasoning is the method used to determine an outcome of a new situation by reference to relevant precedents (typically relating to similar situations). Reductionism is arguably the greatest weakness, as well as strength, of this approach as the ability to gloss over novelty and differences enables the generation of closure (or finality).[52] In contrast, reflective equilibrium (in a broadly Rawlsian sense) seeks to generate coherence in moral theorising by simultaneously pitting general theories, principles and considered judgments against each other. Unlike moral theory however, there are fixed parameters in legal reasoning, primarily because legal inquiry is not an open-ended process. Instead, "law is a social technology of dispute resolution, [where] the *telos* of legal reasoning as a knowledge producing practice is to invoke the authoritative sources internal to its practice that will facilitate a resolution".[53] When ELSI questions become juridified through their subsumption to modes of legal

---

[51] José Julián López and Janet Lunau, ELSIfication in Canada: Legal Modes of Reasoning, *Science as Culture* (March 2012) 21, 1: 77-99.
[52] *Ibid*, at 89.
[53] *Ibid*, at 94.

reasoning, the 'expressive capacity' and 'cultural power' of the law is drawn upon to produce closure. This in turn has been found to "resonate with the ELSI field's desire for the practical advanced assessment of technological development".[54]

The normative content of juridification is often unclear as the processes that are typified by Blichner and Molander are not distinct of one another and their mutual interaction could lead to different outcomes, depending on situational and temporal conditions. Owing to the tensions that arise among the different dimensions, as well as the inner tensions within each dimension, attempts at identifying an idealised definition or notion of juridification have met with little success. While juridification could be a precondition for constitutional democracy, the fear is that it could lead to total legal domination if taken to an extreme. In other words, legal certitude may be secured at the expense of (through displacement or subsumption) other conceptions of self and others.[55] For instance, Leila Kawar cautions that juridification can shift the language of governance and thereby contribute to the power of state institutions, but its impact on the substantive rights of subordinated groups may ultimately be limited.[56] In relation to children's rights, concerns have been expressed over the potential risks that juridification might result in dichotomised social relations, especially in educational relationships. In addition, a legal rule could be too limiting through possible exclusion of other factors (e.g. age, ethnicity, economic and religious background) that influence the construction of children's rights.[57] This 'crowding out' by law of other social and political norms and considerations presents the growth of law as uncontrolled and

---

[54] *Ibid.*

[55] *Ibid*, at 53-54.

[56] Leila Kawar, Commanding Legality: The Juridification of Immigration Policy Making in France, *Journal of Law and Courts* (Spring 2014), 2, 1: 93-116.

[57] Didier Reynaert, Maria Bouverne-De Bie and Stijn Vandevelde, Between 'believers' and 'opponents': Critical discussions on children's rights, *International Journal of Children's Rights* (2012) 20: 155-168, at 161-162.

harmful, particularly where juridification fails to meet its intended goal of regulation.[58] There is a further concern that directive-styled (i.e. command-and-control) and comprehensive regulation could divert targets of regulation (such as researchers and doctors) from norm compliance to law compliance, thereby undermining their desire to concern themselves with the normative spirit of the law. In other words, juridification could result in the displacement of professional or communal norms by legal ones, with detrimental effect on professional or communal practices. Such a development could further encourage the pursuit of self-interest and disincentivise trustworthiness and ethical reflexivity.[59] To varying extents, these concerns have already been observed in the IRB review process,[60] but Laura Stark observes that personal and local sensibilities do affect how IRB members decide even if decision-making appears to be systematic due to the constraints of its social configuration.[61]

For these reason, Teubner deploys 'juridification' negatively to denote a phenomenon where legal formalism crowds out other forms of rationalities and so reduce a social phenomenon to a legal one (hence the depiction of juridification as legal pollution).[62] Implicitly,

---

58 Gunther Teubner, Juridification – Concepts, Aspects, Limits, Solutions. In Gunther Teubner (ed.), *Juridification of Social Spheres: A Comparative Analysis in the Areas of Labor, Corporate Antitrust and Social Welfare Law.* Berlin: Walter de Gruyter & Co, 1987, pp 3-48, at 3.

59 Robert Gatter, Human Subjects Research and Conflicts of Interest – Walking the Talk of Trust in Human Subjects Research: The Challenge of Regulating Financial Conflicts of Interest, (2003) *Emory Law Journal* 52: 327-401, at 388-389.

60 Marie-Andrée Jacob and Annelise Riles, The New Bureaucracies of Virtue, *Political and Legal Anthropology Review* (2007) 30, 2: 181-191; and Marie-Andrée Jacob, Form-made Persons: Consent forms as Consent's Blind-Spot, *Political and Legal Anthropology Review* (2007) 30, 2: 248-268.

61 Laura Stark, *Behind Closed Doors: IRBs and the Making of Ethical Research.* Chicago and London: University of Chicago Press, 2012, at 166.

62 Gunther Teubner, Juridification – Concepts, Aspects, Limits, Solutions. In Gunther Teubner (ed.), *Juridification of Social Spheres: A Comparative Analysis in the Areas of Labor, Corporate Antitrust and Social Welfare Law.* Berlin: Walter de Gruyter & Co, 1987, pp 3-48, at 38.

Teubner seems to assume that the 'juridical' component can always and readily be isolated so that the danger of juridification is also a question of 'relative dominance' between formal legal rationality and other competing rationalities.[63] Others have adopted a more moderate view of the normative implications of juridification. Habermas assessed its outcome in the context of the welfare state to be ambivalent. While the welfare state seeks to empower individuals through guarantees of certain individual entitlements under certain specified general legal conditions, the abstraction and administrative formal rationalisation entailed have the effect of reducing the freedoms guaranteed.[64] Gordon Silverstein makes a similar observation in evaluating juridification as legal framing, or the degree to which a debate and the product of that debate in a political process come to be dominated, structured, framed and constrained by a certain part (i.e. law) of that process. He attributes this phenomenon in one part to the increasing role of, and reliance upon, judicial decision-making, legal reasoning, and legal language, and in another part to the legalisation and formalisation of political discourse and of the political process itself.[65] Evaluating developments in the US over the past 50 years, he observes that law and politics have become more intertwined. However, juridification is not an all-or-nothing proposition, but more a question of degree. The juridification of policy can be advantageous if it is the only viable means to achieve certain goals (e.g. overcoming

---

63 *Ibid,* at 40.
64 Jürgen Habermas, *The Theory of Communicative Action* (in two volumes). Boston: Beacon Press, 1987, at 361-363 (Volume 2). As Habermas explains, a juridically structured social welfare necessitates individualisation (through social legislation), which in turn contributes to the erosion of the social fabric. To access their entitlements, these individuals are forced to conform the complexity of their life-situation to the administrative logic of social security. The monetary relief that is obtained might not ultimately address their particular set of interests, needs and desires, which cannot be reduced to monetary terms.
65 Gordon Silverstein, Law's Allure in American Politics and Policy: What It Is, What It is Not, and What it might yet to be, *Law & Social Inquiry* (Fall 2010) 35, 4: 1077-1097, at 1080-1081.

struggles over abortion), but less so if it prevents the production of creative solutions through institutional interaction.[66] Whether
juridification is beneficial would depend on understanding how
institutions interact and constrain each other.[67]

Daniel Loick offers a further perspective on juridification from the
standpoint of the agents themselves. Loick explains that although
Habermas has provided the first sociologically informed account of
the expansion of law in terms of juridification as the colonisation of
the lifeworld, Habermas fails to appreciate the relations of power
within the lifeworld, and also the political struggles that are entailed
in recognition and rights.[68] For this reason, he initially conceives of
the process of juridification as a dilemma: improving the situation of
the disadvantaged by conferring on them particular rights, but
simultaneously reducing their freedom due to erosion of the social
fabric. In the realms of family law and school law, emancipation from
dependence relations in the family or the school is obtained at the cost
of a new dependence on the state and its coercive (and typically non-
reciprocal) powers. To overcome this dilemma, Loick argues that one
must, on the one hand, resist the tendency to underestimate the
reality of subordinative and violent relations in the lifeworld (i.e.
whether in a family or school environment) and, on the other hand,
resist the tendency to de-politicise the struggles for emancipation
in juridification.[69] For Loick, the ambivalent effects of juridification

---

[66] *Ibid*, at 1082.

[67] *Ibid*, at 1093-1094.

[68] Daniel Loick, Juridification and politics: From the dilemma of juridification to
the paradoxes of rights, *Philosophy and Social Criticism* (2014) 40, 8: 757-778, at
759-764.

[69] Loick explains: "To want to overcome exploitation and violence and *at the same
time* to disavow the imperatives of entrenched law and its juridical techniques of
domestication compels agents to extend their political attention in paradoxical
ways: such a politics must always also constitute struggles *for* rights as well as
articulate reservations *against* them. This implies, *on the one hand*: those
particular rights that empower the equality and inclusion of those who so far have
been excluded or subordinated by them or through them, which refers in this

should not be understood as dilemmas, but as paradoxes that arise from the fact that the agents "situated in the lifeworld must simultaneously demand as well as refuse rights".[70]

The capability of the law to transform messy and complex phenomena into de-politicised and calculable cases that are amenable to governance is well recognised.[71] Juridification in this sense tends to have a negative connotation in its reference to the 'colonisation' of social relationships in legal terms.[72] When actions become guided solely by the logic of a legal rule or general legal claim, it creates a false sense of finality in the purported existence of general social consensus and consistency with the requirements of justice.[73] Returning to the 'bioethics-as-public-policy' framework, this study has not found the absolutisation of law. Much to the contrary, the rigidification of social relations that is entailed in juridification is often avoided, save for normative requirements that are considered to be of utmost importance. In theory, the ELSI label suggests that the ethical, legal and social components could be neatly segregated and evaluated. The account presented in this study suggests that, not only are ethical and legal rationalities *not* neatly demarcated, they form an infungible composite with the ethical, the scientific, the medical and the social, the last of which being a sort of incomplete remainder that accentuates the artificiality of the various forms of epistemic fractioning.

---

context primarily to women and children, ought to be multiplied and claimed ... *On the other hand*, to the paradoxes of right correspond a de-privileging of the state as a political center of gravity and its relocation to economic, civil, social and sub-institutional arenas; this entails the creation of conditions for being able to forgo the invocation of rights, the establishment of ... social unities of individuals, the construction of new social relations and experimentation with new life-forms ..." *Ibid*, at 773-774 (emphasis in original).

70   *Ibid*, at 770.

71   Pierre Bourdieu, The force of law: towards sociology of the juridical field, *Hastings Law Journal* (1987) 38, 4: 814-853 at 830.

72   Alan Hunt, Foucault expulsion of law – toward a retrieval, *Law and Social Inquiry* (1992) 17, 1: 1-38.

73   Tom Cockburn, Children and the feminist ethic of care, *Childhood – a Global Journal of Child Research* (2005) 12, 1: 71-89.

For analytical and justificatory purposes, different technical, ethical, legal or social questions may be asked. In practice, the different forms and degrees of abstraction are commingled in order to achieve particular policy goals. My deployment of the term 'juridification' simply suggests the application of legal norms, rationalities, language, techniques and practices in sustaining a particular understanding or knowledge claim. It also serves to denote the contributions of law to the construction of artefacts like human eggs, embryos, chimeras and hybrids. Here, juridification neither precludes *all* other forms of rationality (save for non-public reasons that usurp public purposes), nor provides permanent closure. Much to the contrary, and consistent with the STS notion of co-production, legal rationality of one sort or another has been hybridised with other forms of rationalities, such as ethical and medico-scientific ones, to sustain a bioethical claim and to maintain epistemic openness. At the same time, I am not proposing that juridification necessarily leads to an exclusively legal norm. François Ewald proposes this in drawing a distinction between the juridical (i.e. the institution of law as the expression of sovereign power) and the law (as formulation of norms).[74] Such a viewpoint does not sufficiently account for the distinct characteristics of legal institutions and rationalities. To be sure, I am not thereby saying that the law is so distinct as to become an autopoietic entity. Rather, my argument is that the extremes of reductionism in the representation of law should be avoided.[75]

---

[74] François Ewald, Norms, Discipline, and the Law, *Representations* (1990) 30:138-161, at 138-139. Ben Golder and Peter Fitzpatrick provide convincing arguments on why such an approach is itself limiting and inconsistent with Foucault's analytical agenda. See Ben Golder and Peter Fitzpatrick, *Foucault's Law*. London and New York: Routledge, 2009, at pp 102-107.

[75] Conceptually, there is value in reinstating juridification as a heuristic to understand the role of law and how it operates within a complex socio-political environment, particularly since Habermas appears to have moved away from his narrow conception of juridification as colonisation of the lifeworld in his more recent works. See Jürgen Habermas (tr. William Regh), Between Facts and Norms: Contributions to a Discourse Theory of Law and Democracy. Cambridge MA: MIT

1.4 Bioethics as Governance

In *Discipline and Punish*, Michel Foucault characterises law as the embodiment of sovereign power, or essentially as orders backed by threats. With the rise of disciplinary power, Foucault considers that the sovereign and its power (i.e. law) must necessarily weaken. As society increases in complexity, the old order of law would ultimately be expulsed by the new order of disciplinary powers,[76] and the latter will ultimately prevail over the old right of sovereignty.[77] This limited notion of law has been most thoroughly critiqued by Alan Hunt and Gary Wickham. They observe that, like John Austin before him, Foucault has inflexibly linked law to the sovereign. Law is thereby reduced to criminal law, with the omission of other aspects of law that relate to broader social phenomena and the distribution of social authority.[78] They argue that law has always been involved in, if not preoccupied with, the task of either exercising control over or exempting from control the different forms of disciplinary regulation. Contrary to Foucault's claim that disciplinary power is of relatively recent origin, Hunt and Wickham point out that ethical and processual (or ritualistic) discipline and law were intrinsic to the rationale of state. In addition, Foucault's dialectic approach of setting law against discipline (or 'counter-law') fails to recognise that both forces are concerned with governmentality. They explain that governmentality

---

Press, 1998. See also Mathieu Deflem, The Legal Theory of Jürgen Habermas. In Reza Banakar and Max Travers (eds.), *Law and Social Theory*. Oxford: Hart Publishing, 2013, pp 75-90.

76 Michel Foucault (tr. Alan Sheridan), *Discipline and Punish: The Birth of the Prison*. New York: Vintage, 1995, at Parts I and II.

77 Michel Foucault (tr. David Macey), *'Society Must Be Defended': Lectures at the Collège de France, 1975-76*. London: Allen Lane, 2003, at 39-40.

78 Alan Hunt and Gary Wickham, *Foucault and Law: Towards a Sociology of Law as Governance*. Pluto Press: Finland, 1994, at 60. The authors recognise that law is not Foucault's primary object of concern, although his ultimate interest on the development of a 'punitive rationality' and its implications on freedom have a profound relationship with the question of law.

is the dramatic expansion in the scope of government, featuring an increase in the number and size of the governmental calculation mechanisms, as well as modern bureaucracies. This expansion occurred at about the same time as a number of other themes, including the emergence of the reason of state, the emergence of the problem of population, the birth of modern political economy, the move towards liberal securitisation, and the emergence of the human sciences as new mechanisms of calculation. In particular, it is the reason of state that requires the government to decipher the mystery of the state and calculate the correct principles for its ordering.[79]

Foucault's negative framing of (positive sanction-based) law appears more ambivalent in his later works.[80] In differentiating biopower as applicable to populations in contrast to disciplinary power that individualises bodies, he seems to recognise that it would be too simplistic to regard government as concerned only with control or domination.[81] The state must necessarily draw on both its sovereign power, as well as disciplinary (and bio-)powers in order to maximise the capabilities and wellbeing of its population. While alluding to the interaction between old and new forms of power, he continues to point to juridical regression, although accepting the increasing importance of law as norm.[82] However, Foucault appears to have provided his most positive affirmation of state law in his discussion of ·

---

[79] *Ibid,* at 76.

[80] The negative framing of law (as opposed to the more 'productive' discipline) is perhaps most evident in his discussion on Power/Knowledge. See Michel Foucault (tr. Colin Gordon *et al.*), *Power/Knowledge: Selected Interviews and Other Writings 1972-1977.* Brighton: Harvester Press, 1980, at 119, 122 and 139.

[81] Even then, Foucault continues to regard discipline and law to be incompatible or competing: Michel Foucault (tr. Robert Hurley), *The Will to Knowledge: The History of Sexuality, Vol. 1.* Harmondsworth: Penguin, 1979, at 97; 137-139. See also Michel Foucault (tr. David Macey), *'Society Must Be Defended': Lectures at the Collège de France, 1975-76.* London: Allen Lane, 2003, at 38-39.

[82] Michel Foucault (tr. Robert Hurley), *The Will to Knowledge: The History of Sexuality, Vol. 1.* Harmondsworth: Penguin, 1979, at 144.

governmentality as a new power-complex of the modern state. This notion relates to an: [83]

> ... ensemble formed by institutions, procedures, analyses and reflections, calculations, and tactics that allow the exercise of this very specific, albeit very complex, power that has the population as its target, political economy as its major form of knowledge, and apparatuses of security as its essential technical instruments.

Far from expulsion, sovereign law remains an integral (albeit hybridised) part of a triangulation of law, disciplines and administration, as Rose, Valverde and others have read Foucault.[84] But what about Foucault's worry that biopower will be wielded by the state as justification for the most draconian of interventions to subdue populations unto its will?[85]

Foucault did not have the opportunity to consider how bioethics as governance relates to biopower. As Jonathan Montgomery explains, bioethics as a governance practice comprises distinctive institutions and structures to mediate disagreements over many bioethical issues in a morally pluralistic society, to facilitate sufficient consensus to enable public policy choices to be made, to maintain public confidence

---

[83] Michel Foucault, Ethics: Subjectivity and Truth. In Paul Rabinow (ed.), *Essential Works of Michel Foucault, 1954-1984.* The New Press: New Press: 1997, at 20. See also: Michel Foucault, Governmentality. In Graham Burchell, Colin Gordon and Peter Miller (eds.), *The Foucault Effect: Studies in Governmentality.* Hertfordshire: Harvester Wheatsheaf, 1991, pp 87-104. Foucault explains (at 102): "We need to see things not in terms of the replacement of a society of sovereign by a disciplinary society and the subsequent replacement of a disciplinary society by a society of government; in reality one has a triangle, sovereignty-discipline-government ...".

[84] Nikolas Rose and Mariana Valverde, Governed by Law? (1998) *Social and Legal Studies* 7: 541-551; Anthony Beck, Foucault and Law: The Collapse of Law's Empire (1996) *Oxford Journal of Legal Studies* 16: 489-502; Duncan Ivison, The Technical and the Political: Discourses of Race, Reasons of State *Social and Legal Studies* (1998) 7: 589-594.

[85] Michel Foucault, *History of Sexuality* (Volume 1). New York: Vintage Books, 1990, at 137.

and avoid social conflict.[86] The institutionalisation of bioethics into specific forms such as committees, regulatory bodies and commissions in many countries is a historical contingency that arose in response to research scandals and the resulting perception of a need to restrain irresponsible science.[87] As we have earlier considered, bioethics is itself committed to sustaining pluralism through public debate and democratic decision-making owing to the socio-political conditions through which it emerged.[88] To varying degrees, it has in different places and at different times assumed features of 'public reason', and in this role, both enabled and facilitated the examination, justification and use of scientific knowledge.[89]

By avoiding an excessively narrow understanding of law only as 'orders backed by threat', this study shows that the law in its various constituents and forms has been an intrinsic part of bioethics as applied in public policy and in the governance of human biomedical research. As we shall see, the work of the BAC must be understood in terms of its ongoing interactions with other governmental agencies and with the disciplines of ethics, medicine and the sciences, among others. The development of a rationality of state encompasses not only 'punitive rationality,' which Foucault equates to formal law, but also disciplinary power, encapsulated in rituals, processes, techniques and norms that make up and legitimise this notion of 'law' and more. As subsequent chapters will show, the ultimate backing that institutions of law provide to the construction of eggs, embryos, hybrids and chimeras has been critical in securing public trust and legitimacy. This hybridisation of law and disciplines is also important in illustrating the relationship between law and biomedical sciences. Consistent with the notion of co-production, both law and discipline

---

86 Jonathan Montgomery, Bioethics as a Governance Practice, *Health Care Analysis* (2016) 24, 1: 3-23, at 5.
87 *Ibid*, at 13-16.
88 *Ibid*, at 17-18.
89 *Ibid*, at 18-20.

powers co-construct and reinforce dominant social understandings of security, progress and collective good.[90] In deliberating over the varied applications of human pluripotent stem cell research, a holistic understanding of scientific development would not be possible without simultaneously engaging with legal facticity in the distinctions between subject and object, permissible and non-permissible, human and non-human, property and non-property, and so forth. From this standpoint, the law is arguably no more distinct as a cultural institution than medical science(s).[91]

Hunt and Wickham rightly observe that law is increasingly concerned with 'normative formation', so that the phenomenon of normalisation is not the exclusive domain of disciplinary powers. A more adequate account needs to stress a persistent increase in the range, scope and detail of legal intervention that produces a general movement towards an expanding legalisation and juridification (read 'hybridisation') of social life.[92] In a more recent contribution, Nikolas Rose *et al.* similarly argue that governance *is* intellectual innovation rather than some blueprint of dominance that "falls out of the clear blue sky",[93] and that it is questionable that one should find a single form of governance (or government) that is at once coherent, consistent and absolute:

> The assemblage nature of government always suggests that rationalization – the process of rendering the various elements internally consistent – is never a finished process. Rationalities are

---

90 Sheila Jasanoff, Making Order: Law and Science in Action. In Edward J Hackett, Olga Amsterdamska, Michael E Lynch, Judy Wajcman, Wiebe E Bijker, *Handbook of Science and Technology Studies*. Cambridge MA: MIT Press, 2007 (3rd Edition), pp 761-789, at 772.

91 See generally: Mark Kelman, *A Guide to Critical Legal Studies*. Cambridge MA: Harvard University Press, 1987.

92 Alan Hunt and Gary Wickham, *Foucault and Law: Towards a Sociology of Law as Governance.* Pluto Press: Finland, 1994, at 66.

93 Nikolas Rose, Pat O'Malley and Mariana Valverde, Governmentality, *Annual Review of Law and Social Science* (2006) 2:83-104, at 92.

constantly undergoing modification in the fact of some newly identified problem or solution, while retaining certain styles of thought and technological preferences.[94]

Quite sensibly, Rose *et al.* argue that one should eschew static abstraction, and focus instead on analysing the 'technologies' that govern habits, morality and ethics.[95]

In focusing on the artefacts of human pluripotent stem cell technology, there is in practice no clear demarcation among 'governed', 'self-governed' and 'governor', although these are helpful as a starting point and general heuristic references. To my mind, the governed/self-governed/governor formulation runs along the same conceptual strand as Marilyn Strathern's audit/policy/ethics triad. In this regard, she considers that social and cultural worlds are brought closer together with the language of ethics, and both audit and ethics are structuring social expectations in such a way as to create new principles of organisation.[96] Drawing from Annelise Riles, Strathern observes that the way in which ethics, audit and policy describe themselves point to their implication in one another, so if audit/policy/ethics is really a triad of emergent practices or a set of related trajectories, then audit (i.e. accountability in a widely acceptable and mobile cultural form) is just one among many changing features of social life. Applying Strathern's rationale to Hunt and Wickham, the governed/self-governed/governor formulation will ultimately relate back to the justifications and reasons for governance.

Marilyn Strathern indicates that the 'policy' of interest to anthropological enquiry is an arena where governments re-invent society and promote cultural change. For instance, the New Right discourses

---

94 *Ibid*, at 98.
95 *Ibid*, at 97.
96 Marilyn Strathern, Accountability ... and ethnography. In Marilyn Strathern (ed.), *Audit Cultures: Anthropological studies in accountability, ethics and the academy*. London: Routledge, 2000, pp 279-304, at 281.

of the 1980s embedded certain conceptualisations of the 'individual' (person) in a nexus including 'freedom,' 'market', 'enterprise' and 'family.'[97] It incorporates a particular vision of the way in which people relate to the state. It was a relationship that could be mediated by, or translated into, ideals of how people would relate, as individuals and family members, to the 'market', and new 'customers' were invented.[98] Government defined the state's role as guardian or guarantor of value so that 'performance', which commonly took the form of good practice and good financial management, was subject to 'selectivity' based on 'measures' used as a bureaucratic yardstick. Auditing becomes an example to add to all the myriad ways in which people govern themselves and the social state gives way to the enabling state.[99] In promoting value for money and economic efficiency, persons and organisations are being assisted to provide public assurance of their viability. When, as in higher education, 'individuals' become conscious of themselves as 'performers', seemingly 'in control' of their performance, the bureaucratic reflexivity involved is part of their relationship to the enabling state.[100]

It is crucial to recognise law as a purposeful enterprise in order to understand juridification in bioethics (as governance practice) more holistically. Perhaps the context of bioethics makes this point all the more obvious, as the justification for governance – particularly where the attribution and distribution of agency and duty are concerned – raises a more fundamental issue about the relationship between legal

---

[97] *Ibid*, at 288.

[98] Strathern notes (*Ibid*, at 299: see footnote 16 in text) the critique of Heelas and Morris's *The Values of the Enterprise Culture: the Moral Debates* (1992): the traditional enterprise virtues of responsibility and discipline had been eclipsed by the runaway success of promoting consumerism and the ethic of wealth creation. These are in turn made visible by separate organs dedicated to accountability and quality control.

[99] Strathern refers to Nikolas Rose's *Powers of Freedom: Reframing Political Thought*. Cambridge: Cambridge University Press, 1999: *Ibid*, at 289.

[100] *Ibid*, at 290.

norms and moral ones. To regard law as nothing more than a 'one-way projection of power' is consequently a failure to not only recognise that the law has a meaningful content, but also to omit the opportunity to situate legal values normatively. Writing in the aftermath of the Second World War, Lon Fuller shows us that the law is not purely functional, but has substantive moral content, in terms of both its effects ('external morality') and its intrinsic qualities ('internal morality'). As a necessarily progressive enterprise, law is also aspirational in striving towards the fundamental purposes for which it subsists. One such purpose, as Fuller identifies, is the facilitation of social life through communication, coordination and mutual understanding.[101] This purpose engenders the internal morality of law, and is embodied in principles like respect for persons and certain virtues that Fuller identifies as essential for meaningful engagement in the public sphere.

Ronald Dworkin considers that most, if not all, of the virtues encompassed in Fuller's internal morality of law may be summed up in the quality of integrity of law, or public morality (which is not to be confused with popular morality). In the socio-political context of Anglo-American legal systems, integrity relates to the internal consistency of the system of rules and principles in past decisions of the courts and other political institutions. These rules and principles form the public morality of a community of people, and from which the rights and responsibilities of its members are derived. These rights and responsibilities constitute the phenomenon of law, not only in the understanding among citizens but also in the behaviour of

---

[101] Lon Fuller, *The morality of law*. New Haven: Yale University Press, 1969, at 185-186. Adopting a similarly purposive approach to thinking about technological futures through law, Graeme Laurie *et al.* observes that "law has a positive social shaping role aimed at encouraging just outcome." See: Graeme Laurie, Shawn H E Harmon and Fabiana Arzuaga, Foresighting Futures: Law, New Technologies, and the Challenges of Regulating for Uncertainty, *Law, Innovation and Technology* (2012) 4, 1: 1-33, at 12.

legislators and judges in particular. Crucially, the quality of integrity requires fidelity to public morality in all activities relating to the creation, administration and adjudication of law. Given that past decisions need not necessarily reflect popular morality, public morality with which the law is aligned may differ accordingly.[102]

A more principled construction of public morality is implicit in Jürgen Habermas's principle of democracy. He argues that this principle establishes not only a procedure for legitimate decision-making, but also steers the production of the legal medium itself. Whereas morality encompasses internally constituted argumentations that are both necessary and sufficient, the democratic principle is chiefly concerned with creating a system of rights and a language that enables a community of people to understand themselves as a voluntary association of free and equal consociates under law. In other words, legal norms (as public morality) have an artificial character in constructing actors within an abstract community and regulating the external relations among them. Unlike Kant's critical perception of legal abstraction in legality or juridical form however, Habermas does not consider legality as limitations of morality. He instead suggests that there is a complementary relationship between law and morality. From a sociological standpoint in particular, the constitution of legal form is necessary to offset the weaknesses of morality in postmodernity. With modernisation and the collapse of traditional ethical life, morality that is detached from habit and customary law becomes inoperative and ineffective. In contrast, law is simultaneously a system of knowledge and a system of action. Because values-orientations are interwoven with a system of actions, law is immediately effective. Legal subject is thereby unburdened by cognitive, motivational and organisational demands in ways that the person as a moral subject will be.[103] If Fuller, Dworkin and Habermas

---

102 Ronald M Dworkin, *Law's Empire*. Oxford: Hart Publishing, 1998, at 97.
103 Jürgen Habermas (tr. William Rehg), *Between Facts and Norms: Contributions to a Discourse Theory of Law and Democracy*. Cambridge MA: MIT Press, 1998, at 115.

are correct in their purposive reading of law, then juridification in bioethics as governance practice must *pro tanto* be construed in terms of the extent that the law has articulated and supported fundamental and essential public values that are necessary to support meaningful social life.

1.5 Overview of Juridification in Bioethics

In thinking what is 'legal' about bioethics, I have applied Actor-Network-Theory (ANT) in an attempt to map out a particular network of agents, things and locations by legal norms, rationalities, techniques and practices across spatial, material, social and ideological dimensions. I hope to provide a more nuanced account of bioethics as governance practice by revealing how law as a knowledge system has interacted and (as I will show) hybridised with other knowledge systems.[104] In the Annex on Methodology and ANT, I have set out the reasons why ANT is effective as a mode of inquiry that renders visible connections and interactions that are not obviously so. I want to emphasise here the importance of rendering visible the 'nuances' of governance practices within a 'bioethics-as-public-policy' framework. As I have explained, the dualism that is implicit in the early accounts of law (and juridification) by Habermas (i.e. legal sphere vs. non-legal sphere) and Foucault (i.e. sovereign power vs. disciplinary powers) lack explanatory power and analytical robustness. In framing and pitting law as sovereign power against non-sovereign power for instance, it becomes impossible to understand how the different knowledge systems and/as modalities of power interact within bioethics and the way that they shape (and co-produce) each other. Latour's criticism of Durkheim's dualism of 'self-contained individuals'

---

[104] Sheila Jasanoff, Making Order: Law and Science in Action. In Edward J Hackett, Olga Amsterdamska, Michael E Lynch, Judy Wajcman, Wiebe E Bijker, *Handbook of Science and Technology Studies*. Cambridge MA: MIT Press, 2007 (3rd Edition), pp 761-789, at 779.

fighting for a place in a 'self-contained society' as an ultimately sterile analysis could also be applied to this aspect of Foucault's analytic.[105] As Latour describes the problem, "we have lost the precise conduits through which what we call 'the whole' actually circulates".[106] In applying ANT, I also hope to better understanding how different modalities of power interact to constitute bioethics as a spatial dimension within which co-production occurs. For instance, Bruno Latour shows the link between politics and expertise in his account of a fundamental transformation brought about by the discovery of microbes by Louis Pasteur, and the alliance between his followers (referred to as Pasteurians) with the hygienists.[107] It was in the 'limited space' of the laboratory that abstraction and ascription were possible. Latour's analysis points to the significance of the relationship between physical and ideological spaces, which is often overlooked. An informant once commented that regulatory development in Singapore is mirrored in the 'phased' construction of the Biopolis, the physical location where much of life sciences research is conducted.[108]

ANT enables us to think about juridification not only as the ways that the law has contributed to bioethics as governance practices, but also as dynamic 'spaces' within which particular interactions are sustained. The conduits that we find are continuously made and re-made within spatial-temporal intervals, as significant degrees of learning and responsiveness are very much part of policy work. These 'spaces' are also another way of recognising the inevitability of fractals, as Marilyn Strathern observes, because ethnographic

---

[105] Bruno Latour, Networks, Societies, Spheres: Reflections of an Actor-Network Theorist, *International Journal of Communication* (2011) 5: 796-810, at 803.

[106] *Ibid*, at 805.

[107] Bruno Latour and John Law, *The Pasteurization of France*. Cambridge MA: Harvard University Press, 1988.

[108] Interview with CR2, 10 September 2008. See also Axel Gelfert, Before Biopolis: Representations of the Biotechnology Discourse in Singapore, *East Asian Science, Technology and Society: and International Journal* (2013) 7, 1: 103-123, at 106.

representations are always partial.[109] In other words, the 'spaces' within which juridification subsists are explicit recognition of epistemic limits, while simultaneously illustrating a particular power-complex at work. ANT thereby also enables a re-casting of juridification to mean more than the collections of legal processes identified by Blichner and Molander. One modality of power responses to and co-produces the other, and they collectively co-construct and sustain epistemic claims and the various artefacts we are concerned with in this study. Given the nature of co-production, my study detracts from those who present juridification narrowly. An inquiry into the role of law in bioethics not only explicates the 'spaces' within which change is possible, but also as an emergent composite of ways in which knowledge is presented, tested, verified and used in the public sphere.

The chapter that follows considers how juridification has enabled progress through bioethics in public policy and biomedical research governance. Bioethics was the discursive space within which a politically justifiable compromise was attained, at first in bioethical discussions in the US and the UK, and then in a bioethical form that extended across the world in terms of, for example, the 14 day limit. This development paved the way for the use of early human embryos in *in vitro* studies, and subsequently for the use of early animal embryos with human material, as well as in *in vivo* studies involving sentient animals. By considering the interactive dynamics between the governance regime and technological progression from *in vitro* fertilisation (IVF) onwards, the discussion adds to current under-standing of society as not simply 'reacting' to the impact of new scientific developments, or of law as not necessarily lagging behind technological advancements. It shows how human embryo and pluripotent stem cell research are deeply connected through bioethics and its constituent knowledge systems (including law) with the

---

109 Marilyn Strathern, *Partial Connections*. Savage ML: Rowman & Littlefield Publishers, at xxiv and 53.

prospect of improved medical and economic possibilities for the future. In other words, therapeutic promise that is offered by human embryo research and Somatic Cell Nuclear Transfer (SCNT) – so central to the construction of the common good – is itself an outcome of bioethical discourse. To take a closer look at juridification in this context, legal inscription of some form was necessary to overcome moral ambiguity in the status of a human embryo. In this respect, bioethical and regulatory innovation in the UK has been instructive for countries like Singapore, where bioethics was drawn on by policymakers to devise a normatively moderate space that made the establishment of a regulatory infrastructure possible. This infra-structure in turn enables and supports human pluripotent stem cell research by giving inter-subjective meaning to the research. Perhaps the most innovative aspect of this innovation in governance practice is the deployment of law in policy sense-making. Legal inscription was not applied with the intent of foreclosing future discussion on the status of the embryo, but has been clearly expressed to be subject to review. For instance, it has been queried if the requirement of dual level of review in a number of jurisdictions for human embryonic stem cell (hESC) research (discussed in Chapters 2 and 4) is still justifiable, or if standard review would suffice.[110] A recent scientific development may well provide the occasion for the 14 day limit to be revisited.[111]

This innovation in governance further enabled development in research involving human-animal combinations (HACs) at various stages of growth. In contrast to the relatively more remote question of 'When life begins?', human-animal chimeras and hybrids present equally fundamental questions like 'What makes us human?', and

---

[110] Timothy Caulfield *et al.*, Research ethics and stem cells: Is it time to re-think current approaches to oversight? *EMBO reports* (2015) 16, 1: 2-6.

[111] Scientists at the University of Cambridge have devised a new technique that allows embryos to develop in vitro up to 13 days after fertilisation. Understanding embryonic growth beyond the 14-day limit could open up new avenues of research that could help improve the chances of success of IVF. See: Insoo Hyun, Amy Wilkerson and Josephine Johnston, Embryology Policy: Revisit the 14-day rule, *Nature* (2016) 533, 7602: 169-171.

'What is the moral status of chimeric and hybrid animals?' Here again, legal inscription has been an important form of boundary work in countries like the UK and Singapore. In this chapter, I argue that these phenomena are indicative of progress in bioethics, as well as in public policy. A secondary objective of this chapter is to provide a succinct overview of the regulatory landscape in the US, UK and Singapore, with reference to international norms set out by the International Society for Stem Cell Research (ISSCR). It should hopefully be clear that the governance of biomedical research emerged to be a hybrid of ethical and scientific norms and practices that are sustained by a regulatory framework that is built upon public values that have been identified in part through public engagement. Finally, this chapter concludes by proposing that pragmatism underscores juridification in bioethics, not in a demeaning way, but rather as a means of working towards the ideals of the common good and of political liberalism.

Chapter 3 examines juridification as legal reasoning (more precisely, as syllogistic reason and analogy), and comparative law as legal technique and practice, applied in creating normative positionality through the practice of comparison within a 'bioethics-as-public-policy' framework. Comparison cuts across the knowledge systems of law and disciplinary powers, and is done for the purposes of interpretive sense-making and drawing relationalities. Within a policy setting, it is performed as technocratic practice and self-knowledge. It should be no surprise to find that the logic of comparison and comparative law has for a time been brought into the service of state, although not necessarily directed at the exercise of coercive power.[112] Situating the practice of comparison epistemically is challenging because bioethics is not represented by a single goal, intellectual tradition, methodology or epistemological orientation.[113] It does appear to be ubiquitous and is almost taken-for-granted,

---

112 Annelise Riles, *Rethinking the Masters of Comparative Law.* Oxford & Portland: Hart Publishing, 2001, at 6.
113 Renée C Fox and Judith P Swazey, *Observing Bioethics.* New York: Oxford University Press, 2008, at 9.

and to that extent, somewhat lacking in reflexivity. Consequently, comparison of regulatory provisions or policies has generally been assumed to have a legal character. It operates largely on the implicit assumption that since law or legal discourse is a constituent of, or contributor to, the epistemology of bioethics, it should follow that bioethics could be equivalent to law. As the analysis in this chapter will show, quite the opposite occurs in that de-juridification has been the first step to comparison in this 'bioethics-as-public-policy' framework. From a jurisprudential standpoint, such a reversion to a meta-law position lends support to the argument of Hans Kelsen that the normative basis of law may not be different from those of other important social institutions.

Interestingly, given that a bioethical inquiry could already have a particular ethical framing or lineage, it is necessary to consider if the comparison is merely justificatory rather than investigative and/or constructive. In other words, a question to consider is whether the comparison is 'real' in its suggestion of similarities and/or differences. I argue that comparison could be both investigative and constructive, thus blurring the distinction between technique and epistemology. In the study reported in this book, comparative projects have generated many comparative tables, some of which have been set out in this chapter. My intent is not to communicate information, since the policy or regulatory positions of a number of countries have changed since the time that these comparative tables were constructed (although I have attempted to provide pertinent updates in the accompanying footnotes, where applicable). Instead, these comparative tables are intended to illustrate how comparison enables association and establishes solidarity of one jurisdiction with other 'like-minded' jurisdictions. Standards (or 'best practices' in some situations) and expectations are invariably implicit in these tables. Re-juridification occurs, through a 'scripting' process, when these standards and expectations are consolidated and systematised for one reason or another.

We examine (re-)juridification in the ossification of relationalities in terms of the scripting process within a 'bioethics-as-public-policy' in Chapter 4. This study makes a number of findings. First, the 'script' or constituted knowledges are profoundly influenced by the scripting process, and are to that extent relatively open-ended.[114] Scripting occurred across different 'scripts' and on a global scale. It is argued that the character of the 'script' is broadly defined by particular 'focal points' that serve as linkages. In theory, this provides a relatively novel account of 'legal globalisation' that occurs in a policy environment. Second, documents have been found to play a crucial role in the forming of relationalities through linkages. They functioned in essence as 'script-carriers'. Taking these two findings together, this research demonstrates the importance of close reading of text and multi-sited analysis as methodologies. Third, the script possesses a limited anthropological content, which is both relational and normative.

This chapter also provides a relatively elaborate analysis of the ossification of relationalities through the instrumentality of documents scripted by the US National Academy of Sciences, the International Society for Stem Cell Research, the California Institute for Regenerative Medicine, the UK Academy of Medical Sciences (AMS), the Danish Council of Ethics, and to a more limited extent, the German Ethics Council and the European Union. It is further considered how all of these documents, as well as the scripting process engendered, have impacted or otherwise relate to those of the BAC in Singapore. While none of these developments have been actively coordinated among these various countries and organisations, a degree of epistemic consolidation is apparent, particularly in terms of the juridical boundaries. For instance, there is general

---

[114] My use of the term 'script' is inspired by Latour's ANT, where networks confer qualities and instil motivations to actors through establishing roles as scripts. The process of scripting relates more generally to 'translation' in ANT although I hesitate to use this term as the outcome need not necessarily result in inscriptions or immutable mobiles.

consensus that the implantation of a cytoplasmic hybrid embryo in a womb should be prohibited. In this respect, this chapter provides an illustration of how bioethical standards have emerged for the governance of human pluripotent stem cell research. Also interesting is that a relatively similar form of hybridised bioethical approach (all-inclusive of public engagement) appears to have been adopted by the different countries considered. This could be a reason why such a 'scripting' process from the bottom-up has been far more productive in epistemic terms than a broadly similar endeavour that was initiated in the 56th Session of the United Nations General Assembly between 2001 to 2002.[115]

In Chapter 5, we consider the juridification of *generic* nascent life, by studying the ways in which the BAC in Singapore, and the AMS in the UK, constructed human-animal combinations as regulatory objects (and subjects). It is argued that the juridical techniques of categorisation, systematisation, distantiation and objectification have been deployed in the process. In categorisation, the BAC first grouped together the different types of human-animal combinations that can be purposefully created by scientists. Following this, it systematically selected two main types of combinations – animal chimeras and cytoplasmic hybrids – to direct its attention to. Mainly through a documentary process, these biological constructs are then objectified, and distantiation is achieved mainly through the device of public consultation. Application-wise, these objects could be regarded as

---

[115] To be sure, I am not suggesting that we now have a 'script' on human pluripotent stem cell research that all at once flows eloquently and coherently, Rather, the sort of 'script' that we have has been described as 'a patchwork of patchworks': Timothy Caulfield *et al.*, The Stem Cell Research Environment, *Stem Cell Reviews and Reports* (2009) 5, 82-88. However, there are categorical traits or features that are shared across some or many jurisdictions. I have referred to these as 'focal points'. See: Rosario M Isasi and Bartha M Knoppers, Mind the Gap: Policy Approaches to Embryonic Stem Cell and Cloning Research in 50 Countries, *European Journal of Health Law* (2006) 13: 9-26; Rosario M Isasi and Bartha M Knoppers, Beyond the permissibility of embryonic and stem cell research: substantive requirements and procedural safeguards, *Human Reproduction* (2006) 21, 10: 2474-2481.

metaphorical models of 'Seeing-As' that are created to displace their more commonly perceived equivalents in folk knowledge. However, it is further argued that chimeras and hybrids should more accurately be understood as placeholders, or metaphorical models of 'Seeing As-If'. This reference better represents the temporal and 'open texture' qualities of these constructs, particularly since both chimeras and hybrids are neither strictly 'human' nor 'non-human' in legal epistemology. Nevertheless, it is important to recognise that these constructs are not only biological, but also regulatory subjects. The political significance of this is that chimeras and hybrids could then fall under regulatory control, thereby enabling research to proceed on a 'regulated' basis. For the purposes of this study, the regulatory nature of chimeras and hybrids suggests that the techniques deployed have legal character and/or content.

The bioethical construction of HACs as regulatory objects through juridification has the effect of what Étienne Souriau and Bruno Latour term as 'instauration'. Although ontological security has been reinstated or re-established for the *homo sapiens* species even while research involving HACs is permitted to advance within the 'bioethics-as-public-policy' framework, the identity and uniqueness of humankind could no longer be perceived in the same light. The contingency of alterity gives rise to risks, not only from the prospect (however remote) of its occurrence, but also from the uncertainty of risks that could arise from biological artefacts that we do not completely understand or know. While juridification may point to manageable risks, instauration makes uncertainty in risk-taking explicit.

The notion of 'risks' within a 'bioethics-as-public-policy' framework is discussed in Chapter 6. If we consider risks to be an expression of indeterminacy that arises from participatory engagement, the act of instauration invites us to think hard about whether risks can always be quantified and neatly managed away. In bioethical analysis, it is usually asked at the initial stage whether scientific knowledge can help lend greater certainty to a situation by quantifying certain risks. In the context of human oocyte (or egg) donation for human pluripotent stem cell research, the risk of ovarian hyper-stimulation was a quantifiable risk that was set apart and made an explicit subject of the informed consent process. In this sense, a female research participant would be objectified and individualised twice over – once as a matter of scientific objectification and again in the ethico-juridical requirement of informed consent. Risks that could not be quantified in scientific knowledge are regarded as 'uncertain' risks that must be judged, not only as a matter of voluntary choice on the part of a research participant, but also on the basis of public values. In this chapter, we first consider scientific objectification as expressed and practised in the epistemic history of risk assessment, management and communication. We then consider the 'remainder' problem, in terms of how the BAC has sought to address the scientifically disputed elevation in risk of cancer that egg donation could cause, and the risk that certain groups of women could be exploited. Curious enough, the bioethical position arrived at, on the basis of fairness to healthy women who might donate eggs purely for research use, would also exclude these women as they are likely to be succumbed by the burden of judgment. Arguably, public engagement did not (and perhaps could not) redress the fragmentation and individualisation that the risks of egg donation generated.

However, public engagement as an exercise quite independent of the concern with risks has helped to constitute a public sphere for bioethics. Focusing on the 'public' of the BAC's consultation paper on egg donation, it essentially comprised a loose association of institutions and individuals that is akin to a 'network', but also seemingly 'random' organisations and individuals drawn to the subject for a variety of reasons. For this reason, the 'public' of the BAC is broadly depicted as a 'public sphere', wherein the ideals of reciprocity, inclusiveness, pursuit of the common good, and perhaps even a public rationality, are implicit. More importantly, it is necessary to query what is being done in the 'public sphere' and why. Where the BAC's recommendations on egg donation are concerned, engagement in the public sphere served to affirm the non-commercialisation of human bodily materials and body parts as a public value, and to allocate bioethical responsibilities on that basis. While the BAC was not established primarily to engage the public, public engagement has become an important means of filling epistemic 'gaps' in bioethical knowledge and of securing legitimacy. This development presents important questions as to the nature of bioethical bodies like the BAC and the establishment of bioethics as an emergent civic epistemology. These questions are taken up in the final chapter of the book.

While risks objectify and individualise, learning and knowledge generation are also engendered. Chapter 7 focuses on the latter, firstly in terms of how risks have themselves contributed to the shaping of bioethical governance in quite a unique way. Most fundamentally, state intervention in the practice of biomedical science is indirect, and primarily through the intermediation of bioethical bodies like the BAC. At least in the case of Singapore, such an arrangement has arguably constituted the BAC as a pseudo-juridical entity in five respects:

(1) It has real links to state and juridical institutions;

(2) It deploys legal norms, rationalities, techniques and language in a relatively pervasive manner;

(3) It has juridical form;

(4) It creates legally informed sociality; and

(5) It promotes integration through intermediation.

This study also finds that a combination of legal and non-legal rationalities could be viewed as technologies of risk and precaution, which in turn create a rationale for governance. In this respect, it is important to recognise that the law is itself cognitively and normatively open, in a way that Mariana Valverde and others have described the legal conception of risks as a 'common fund of knowledges'. This recognition is necessary to appreciate how juridification operates in the constitution and implementation of bioethics as anticipatory knowledge and governance.

If one agrees that bioethical bodies are, to varying degrees, pseudo-juridical bodies, I have for this and other reasons argued that the form of reasoning that finds application by these bodies bears remarkable semblances to the Rawlsian conception of public reason. While the merits of a more discourse-based notion of public reason have been highlighted by a number of scholars including Onora O'Neill, this study does not provide convincing evidence for one conception or the other. It only explains and illustrates why public reason is especially appropriate for bioethical decisions, particularly when political compromises are entailed. Finally, this study presents bioethics as comprising social and institutional practices by which its public spheres, variously construed, construct, review, validate and deliberate over politically relevant knowledge. By the formulation presented by Sheila Jasanoff and Clark Miller, bioethics is arguably a civic epistemology. This feature is an important way in thinking about how bioethics as governance practice is not (and should not) be purely regulatory or legal, but has a more hybrid quality. It is also emergent, in a sense that it does not have, and perhaps never will achieve, complete internal coherence of political philosophy. This is, in my view, a merit that is worth sustaining.

2

Regulating Human Pluripotent Stem Cell Research

Bioethics has had an important role in guiding deliberations over debates on artificial reproductive technologies like *in vitro* fertilisation (IVF), and has successfully framed human embryo research as indispensable to medical progress, particularly in the therapeutic promise of regenerative medicine. There is no single, universally agreed definition of regenerative medicine, and it broadly refers to novel biotechnologies that are directed at restoring, maintaining or enhancing tissue, cell or organ function by stimulating or augmenting the body's inherent capacity to self-repair. The long term goal is to harness the regenerative potential of both hESC and iPSC to restore functionality in the body. Currently, clinically applied cell therapies are limited to a patient's own 'adult' stem cell lines, or 'autologous' cells.[116] However, the moral status of a human embryo

---

[116] Andrew Webster, Introduction: The Boundaries and Mobilities of Regenerative Medicine. In Andrew Webster (ed.), *The Global Dynamics of Regenerative Medicine: A Social Science Critique*. Basingstoke and New York: Palgrave Macmillan, 2013, pp 1-17, at 3-4. Reviewing corporate and patent data, efforts to commercialise stem cell treatments have been found to concentrate on three therapeutic areas: cardiovascular, gastrointestinal and the central nervous system. See: Graham Lewis, Regenerative Medicine at a Global Level: Current Patterns and Global Trends. In Andrew Webster (ed.), *The Global Dynamics of Regenerative Medicine: A Social Science Critique*. Basingstoke and New York: Palgrave Macmillan, 2013, pp 18-57.

has not been successfully resolved. This hurdle was surmounted in a number of jurisdictions through an explicit inscription of the therapeutic promise into law or regulation, where this hope has become a central justification for human embryo and pluripotent stem cell research.[117] A corresponding legal framework has been developed in these jurisdictions, and it continues to sustain the hope of realising the promise of medical progress. An illustration of this was when, in August 2009, two pro-life researchers sued the US government for violating a 1995 law that prohibits federal funding of research in which a human embryo is destroyed.[118] This lawsuit was initiated when the National Institutes of Health (NIH) published its revised guidelines after US President Barack Obama lifted an earlier presidential order (formalised by then US President George Bush) that restricted US government funding to research involving a small number of existing hESC lines.[119] The complainants argued that if a funded project involves the use of an embryonic stem cell, then an embryo necessarily has been destroyed. In addition, they theorised that more embryos would be 'subjected to risk' as increased US government funding of hESC research will incentivise the destruction of more embryos to increase the supply of hESC lines. The complainants were initially successful in obtaining a preliminary injunction to suspend federal funding of hESC research, but this was

---

[117] Beatrix Rubin has discussed inscription of the therapeutic promise in law in Germany, Britain and the US. See: Beatrix P Rubin, Therapeutic Promise in the Discourse of Human Embryonic Stem Cell Research, *Science as Culture* (2008) 17, 1: 13-27, at 21-22.

[118] The Dickey-Wicker Amendment prohibits NIH from funding "(1) the creation of a human embryo or embryos for research purposes; or (2) research in which a human embryo or embryos are destroyed, discarded, or knowingly subjected to risk of injury or death greater than that allowed for research on foetuses in utero under 45 C.F.R. 46.204(b) and 42 U.S.C. § 289g(b)." See *Consolidated Appropriations Act*, 2012, Pub. L. No. 112-174, § 508.

[119] National Institutes of Health, *Guidelines for Human Stem Cell Research*, 74 Fed. Reg. 32, 170 (July 7, 2009).

overturned by the US Court of Appeals for the District of Columbia.[120] In essence, the Court of Appeals held that it did not have the legal authority to interfere with the NIH's decision to increase the number of existing hESC lines that could be used in US government funded research as the NIH was acting within a reasonable interpretation of the legislative provision. At the legal front at least, this attempt to cease US government funding of hESC research was ended when the US Supreme Court declined to hear a final appeal by the complainants.

This chapter considers the contributions of law (and regulation) in enabling progress in bioethics, initially in the use of early human embryos in *in vitro* studies, and subsequently in the use of early animal embryos with human material, as well as in *in vivo* studies involving sentient animals. By considering the technological pro-gression from IVF onwards, the discussion adds to current under-standing of society as not simply 'reacting' to the impact of new scientific developments,[121] or of law as not necessarily lagging behind technological advancements. It shows how human embryo and pluripotent stem cell research are deeply connected through bioethics and law with the prospect of improved medical and economic possibilities for the future. We begin, in the section that follows, by briefly considering the therapeutic promise that is offered by human embryo research and SCNT. The current state of scientific knowledge and practice is essentially limited and structured by a middle ground perspective on the moral status of a human embryo. As we have considered, the use-derivation distinction that is applied by the NIH is an example of one such perspective. Lacking in internal consistency, the weakened epistemic quality of this and similar perspectives precludes it from singularly grounding public policy on hESC and related research. Legal inscription of some form is necessary, and

---

[120] *James L Sherley and Theresa Deisher v Kathleen Sebelius, in her capacity as Secretary of the Department of Health and Human Services, et al.,* 644 F. 3d 388 (D.C. Cir. 2011).

[121] Ingrid Geesink, Barbara Prainsack and Sarah Franklin, Stem Cell Stories 1998-2008, *Science as Culture* (2008) 17, 1: 1-11, at 5.

in this respect, bioethical and regulatory innovation in the UK are considered. The UK experience has been instructive for countries like Singapore, where bioethics was drawn on by policymakers to devise a normatively moderate space that enabled the establishment of a regulatory infrastructure, which in turn enables and supports human pluripotent stem cell research. A further development engendered in SCNT and iPSC is also considered. This pertains to human-animal combinations at various stages of growth. In contrast to the relatively more remote question of 'When life begins?', human-animal chimeras and hybrids present fundamental questions like 'What makes us human?', and 'What is the moral status of chimeric and hybrid animals?' Here again, legal inscription has been an important form of boundary work being done in countries like the UK and Singapore. It is suggested that these phenomena are indicative of progress not only of law, but also in bioethics. A secondary objective of this chapter is to provide a succinct overview of the regulatory landscape in the US, UK and Singapore, with reference to international norms set out by the ISSCR. Finally, this chapter concludes by proposing that pragmatism underscores juridification in bioethics, not in a demeaning way, but rather as a means of working towards the ideals of the common good and of political liberalism.

2.1 The Embryo Rendered Visible

The creation of embryos outside of the body of a woman became possible through IVF. Generally, eggs are surgically removed from a woman and fertilised in a petri-dish and then re-introduced into the womb. It is common practice for more than four eggs to be fertilised so that several embryos will be introduced in order to achieve a higher rate of reproductive success.[122] Very often, spare (or supernumerary)

---

[122] Scientific information in this Part is derived primarily from the *Report on the Ethical, Legal and Social Issues in Human Stem Cell Research, Reproductive and Therapeutic Cloning* (June 2002) of the Bioethics Advisory Committee and *Stem Cells: A Primer* issued by the US National Institutes of Health (May 2000).

embryos result from IVF since not all embryos will be implanted into the womb. These embryos are either stored for future use by the donees or, with the consent of the donees, donated to another infertile couple or given to research.

The availability of donated embryos made it possible for hESC research to be conducted. At the point of fertilisation where a sperm cell fuses with an egg cell, an embryo is formed. The embryo begins to develop at this point through a series of cell division so as to, in effect, become a composite (from single to double and then quadruple celled and so on) of functionally identical and unspecialised cells. These unspecialised embryonic cells are embryonic stem cells, which researchers have developed an interest in. Embryonic stem cells are a group of cells unique for their ability to divide for indefinite periods in culture and essential for their ability to differentiate into specialised cells such as muscle, blood and bone cells. The latter feature has been termed pluripotentiality. However, embryonic stem cells are only one of three known types of stem cells with these unique features. The other two types of stem cells are embryonic germ cells that are derived from foetuses and adult stem cells that are derived from tissue such as bone marrow and umbilical cord blood. Embryonic germ cells and adult stem cell also proliferate and serve to continually renew tissue throughout an individual's life, but the general view is that as these two types of stem cells are developed in an environment where cells are already relatively well differentiated or specialised. Consequently, they are less pluripotent relative to embryonic stem cells.

As we have considered, researchers hope to harness the vast therapeutic benefits that the knowledge of pluripotent stem cells can confer as 'cell replacement therapy'. Cell replacement therapy is in essence the only viable form of treatment for medical conditions such as Parkinson's disease. By this intervention, pluripotent stem cells could be introduced into a degenerating brain so as to counter or retard the degeneration process by themselves becoming brain cells to replace the degenerated cells. The manner in which such embryonic stem cells are procured involves a more elaborate process known as therapeutic cloning.

In therapeutic cloning or SCNT, an egg cell is enucleated and replaced with the nucleus of a specialised cell extricated from the relevant donor. The re-constituted egg cell is then induced to initiate cell division as though it has been fertilised by a sperm cell. The embryonic stem cells that arise from cell division are extracted from the embryo and implanted back into the donor so that they may specialise into the required cells in order to replace the damaged target cells. The principal advantage that therapeutic cloning has over organ transplant is that embryonic stem cells are unlikely to be rejected by the host system since they are essentially genetically identical to the host cells. In addition, therapeutic cloning will have a much broader scope of application since certain tissues (such as the brain) may not be replaced in its entirety by present technological knowledge.

At the same time, researchers are gaining knowledge on how specialisation in cells may be reversed. Every cell in a human person contains the full genetic description of that person. On this basis, a specialised cell (such as a heart cell) may be reconfigured into another cell (such as a lung cell) if it is able to regain its pluripotency that it first possessed at the embryonic stage. As we shall see, hECS research has contributed to the ability to reprogramme differentiated (somatic) cells back to their pluripotent state, although it is still premature to say if it can be safely and effectively applied for therapeutic purposes.

Embryonic stem cell research and therapeutic cloning have attracted much controversy, which at its core, relates to the moral status of a human embryo. A related concern is that of human repro-ductive cloning. Therapeutic cloning is technologically the same as that which may be used for human cloning. Hence, the concern is that by allowing therapeutic cloning, human civilisation is led down the slippery slope towards also allowing human reproductive cloning.

2.2 Unsettled Moral Status of an Embryo

The moral status of a human embryo remains obscure as questions associated with it (like 'When does life begin?' or 'Is there a right to reproduce?') are unlikely to be free of moral objections from all quarters. Some people are fundamentally opposed to all forms of embryo research as they believe that a human embryo is morally equivalent to a human being and should be treated in the same manner as an adult person.[123] In particular, proponents of this view argue that ensoulment begins at conception so that upon fertilisation, the embryo acquires distinct personality.[124] Famously, the official view of the Roman Catholic Church is that the human being is to be respected and treated as a person from the moment of conception.[125] And even if embryos are not yet persons, they should be regarded as morally distinct for possessing the potential to become human beings.

Others do not find such a position to be justifiable. Certain properties (such as sentience and consciousness) are morally significant to the ways that an organism should be treated. Furthermore, the sort of moral status that an organism has does not depend on the potential of developing these properties, but on properties that the organism has now or has had in the past.[126] Under this view, an embryo has no sentience, cannot feel pain and has never been a human person. Given these, it cannot be said to have any moral interests – a concept that may perhaps be best understood as something an entity assumes in

---

123 Tadeusz Pacholczyk, The Wisdom of the Church is in her Silence, Too, *National Catholic Register*, 10 August 2003).

124 *Ibid.*

125 Congregation for the Doctrine of the Faith, *Dignitas Personae: On Certain Bioethical Questions*. Vatican City: Congregation for the Doctrine of the Faith, 2008. One of the fundamental ethical principles affirmed in the document is (at paragraph 4 of the First Part): "The human being is to be respected and treated as a person from the moment of conception; and therefore from the same moment his or her rights as a person must be recognised, among which in the first place is the inviolable right of every innocent being to life."

126 Frances M Kamm, *Bioethical Prescriptions: To Create, End, Choose, and Improve Lives*. Oxford and New York: Oxford University Press, 2013, at 153-154.

conjunction with the development of certain mental or physical attributes. The notion of ensoulment at conception, while containing some elements of moral thinking, does not automatically give rise to moral considerations by virtue only of the religious nexus. If an embryo has intrinsic worth, then all embryos whether super- numerary or otherwise created should be treated in the same manner for moral consistency. However, the 'embryo rescue cases' aptly illustrate that such a view is not only contrary to common sense, but could result in even greater wrongs in real-life.[127] As Robert Lee and Derek Morgan (citing Jonathan Glover) explain in the following passage:[128]

> [N]o one denies that [the pre-embryo] is alive, and that it is surely a member of our species rather than any other ... but ... It is widely assumed that qualifying as a human being is sufficient to guarantee the possession of a right to life. But this assumption is questionable, and perhaps derives much of its plausibility from our thinking of 'human beings' in terms of our friends and neighbours. An embryo is not the kind of human being you can share a joke with or have as a friend.

In addition, an embryo that is produced through nuclear transfer (or SCNT) does not involve fertilisation although an embryo does arise from the process. Proponents of this view also reject the argument that an embryo is a potential human being – since this proposition assumes that the embryo possesses the physical integrity, as well as the appropriate environmental conditions, to go to term. Even in natural procreation, one or both of these conditions are

---

[127] Katrien Devolder provides a generic explanation of such cases, where a fire fighter has to decide between rescuing a freezer that contains 1,000 supernumerary embryos or an employee from a burning warehouse, but not both. If embryos are regarded as having full moral status, the logical choice will be inconsistent with commonly held intuitions. See Katrien Devolder, *The Ethics of Embryonic Stem Cell Research*. Oxford: Oxford University Press, 2015, at 18.

[128] Robert Lee and Derek Morgan, *Human Fertilisation & Embryology: regulating the reproductive revolution*. London: Blackstone Press, 2001, at 64.

observed to be absent in approximately four out of five cases. It remains unsettled whether any sensible distinction may be drawn between 'destruction' of an embryo in human embryonic stem cell research and spontaneous 'abortions' that occur in natural conception.

It is not difficult to understand why the view that human embryos have full moral status is difficult to defend. Where public policies and the policies of professional research bodies are concerned, there appears to be a level of consensus that embryos have what Katrien Devolder terms as an 'intermediate moral status', or "a moral status somewhere in between that of a person and that of an ordinary body cell".[129] Human embryos are considered to have some intrinsic value either because they are human, or because they could attain fully moral status over time if one or more thresholds are met. Consequently, policy measures include those that allow the use of donated supernumerary embryos for research but disallow the creation of an embryo purely for research (the 'discarded-created distinction'), and those that permit the use of embryos for research but not the derivation of hESCs (the 'use-derivation distinction').[130] Even within this intermediate moral status, Devolder sets out three different degrees of intrinsic value that could be ascribed to human embryos: very high, lower, and low. Her explanation of the implications is as follows:[131]

> Those who accord a very high intermediate moral status to the embryo are more likely to support the moral distinction between iPSC and embryonic stem cell research, those who accord a somewhat lower moral status may rather choose the use-derivation distinction, and those who accord a low intermediate moral status to the embryo might opt for the discarded-created distinction.

---

[129] See Katrien Devolder, *The Ethics of Embryonic Stem Cell Research*. Oxford: Oxford University Press, 2015, at 18.

[130] *Ibid*, at 23.

[131] *Ibid*, at 138.

To be sure, the moral lines that Devolder has drawn to illustrate the different middle-ground positions are derived through her conceptual analytic of 'causal distance',[132] rather than through policy analysis. Public policy encompasses a much wider forum and a broader set of considerations. For instance, it necessarily includes those who do not consider human embryos to have any intrinsic value. And for those who hold this view, it would not be morally acceptable to disregard the health and interests of actually existing people, to further a particular ideological cause. Furthermore, embryos that are used in research were not created out of gross disrespect for human life as they would be created for reproductive purposes or if supported by very strong scientific justifications. In neither case is there any intent to kill. One may press this point in questioning if it is morally superior to conduct embryonic research for the purposes of advancing therapies for devastating diseases than it is to invite loss of early life just to have a child. There are no ready answers to these questions, and the moral status of a human embryo continues to be a challenging epistemic project. At a more practical level, many jurisdictions have pressed on through a regulatory approach. The approach that has been adopted in the UK is considered because it has been in many ways pioneering, and has had significant impact on other jurisdictions, including Singapore.

2.3 Regulatory Approach in the UK

The United Kingdom is one of a few countries that has moved beyond the impasse of normative indeterminacy in relation to human embryological research. In particular, it has established a comprehensive legal regime that is administered by a dedicated regulatory body – the Human Fertilisation and Embryology Authority

---

132 *Ibid*, at 137-138; 152. The term 'causal distance' may also be referred to as 'indirectness', as both terms relate to the proximity of one's connection to the ultimate wrongdoing; this being the destruction of a human embryo from full or intermediate moral status point of view.

(HFEA) – to govern the use of human sperm, oocytes (or eggs) and embryos, as well as derivatives thereof, in research and fertility treatments. The regime itself was a response to the birth of Louise Brown on 25 July 1978, the first test-tube baby conceived through IVF, which was at that time a highly experimental procedure pioneered by Robert Edwards and Patrick Steptoe. To allay public concerns over the welfare of children born through IVF and possible abuses of the technology, a Voluntary Licensing Authority was initially set-up to oversee the use of IVF techniques. As it was unclear to the British government if IVF should be permitted at all, and if so, how it should be regulated, an expert committee chaired by philosopher Mary Warnock (later Baroness Warnock) was appointed to develop principles for the regulation of IVF and embryology. This initiative was also the first formal inquiry into the various challenges presented by developments in medicine and science related to human fertilisation and embryology in the UK.

The Committee of Inquiry into Human Fertilisation and Embryology published its report (generally known as the 'Warnock Report') in July 1984, [133] which formed the basis for the *Human Fertilisation and Embryology Act* (HFE Act). Among the recommend-dations made by the Committee of Inquiry is the establishment of a statutory licensing authority both to regulate fertility services determined as a matter of policy to be subject to regulatory control and to license research involving the use of embryos in circumstances where this is justified by the objectives of the research. This was necessary to allay public anxiety by keeping a number of specific technologically-assisted reproductive techniques and procedures, as well as other experimental techniques, under constant review

---

[133] Mary Warnock (Chairperson), *Report of the Committee of Inquiry into Human Fertilisation and Embryology*. London: H.M.S.O., Cmd. 9314, 1984. The Warnock Report addressed, in the main, the ethical, legal and social issues associated with the utilisation of technologically assisted reproductive techniques for the alleviation of infertility.

through the agency of the statutory authority. In addition, the statutory authority will also consider if further restrictions are required. The recommendation to establish the statutory authority was taken up by the British government[134] and the HFE Act was passed in 1990. Parliament further empowered the HFEA created under the legislation to license research – a matter which was left open in the White Paper. Broadly speaking, the HFEA is said to have developed five ethical principles from the legislation, its deliberation over real cases and through widespread public consultation:

(1) The assurance of human dignity, worth and autonomy;

(2) The welfare of the potential child;

(3) Safety is given great weight;

(4) Respect for the status of the embryo; and

(5) The saving of life as an acceptable use to which new advances in embryology may be put.[135]

It is now clear that IVF has started a long chain of technological developments that include intracytoplasmic sperm injection, pre-implantation genetic diagnosis and human leukocyte antigen (HLA) typing. Embryo research raised concerns over human cloning, which prompted the British government to enact the Human Reproductive Cloning Act to prohibit reproductive cloning. However, embryo

---

[134] The government followed up on the recommendations presented in the Warnock Report with the White Paper (Human Fertilisation and Embryology: A Framework for Legislation (Cm 259)). The White Paper provided for the establishment of a statutory licensing authority to regulate "infertility services" but left open the issue of embryonic research which Parliament could have either prohibited or permitted by way of licensing. In contextualising the provisions, the White Paper indicated that about 7,000 babies a year are born in the UK with an obvious single gene inherited defect. In addition, it was indicated that IVF could alleviate male infertility, which was the sole cause in about 30% of cases of infertility.

[135] Ruth Deech and Anna Smajdor, *From IVF to Immortality: Controversy in the Era of Reproductive Technology*. Oxford: Oxford University Press, 2007, at 5.

research (including therapeutic cloning) is allowed on a regulated basis. Essentially, any research involving a human embryo must be for a "principal purpose" considered "necessary and desirable" under the legislation.[136] In keeping with the recommendations of the Warnock Report, research can only be performed on an embryo for a maximum of 14 days or until the primitive streak appears. As Baroness Warnock subsequently explains, there are good scientific reasons for distinguishing between an embryo before 14 days and an embryo after that stage. While not a perfect indicator, it cannot be said to be any more arbitrary than the question of 'When does life begin?' Her explanation is instructive:[137]

> Sperm and eggs, though human and alive, do not count as 'human life' in the sense required; it is only when they have come together that a human individual is created who has the potential to become a human person. This belief, though now often couched in terms of the individual's DNA, already incorporated in the cells making up the embryo, in fact owes a good deal to Aristotle, who not only had no notion of DNA, but did not even know of the existence of human eggs, speculating that an embryo was formed by male sperm somehow thickening female blood within the uterus. He held that a human being begins to exist when the specifically human form of life enters the embryo at a fixed date, earlier for males than females. There were three kinds of life or soul; the vegetative, shared by all living

---

136 The principal purposes have been set out as: (a) increasing knowledge about serious disease or other serious medical conditions, (b) developing treatments for serious disease or other serious medical conditions, (c) increasing knowledge about the causes of any congenital disease or congenital medical condition that does not fall within paragraph (a), (d) promoting advances in the treatment of infertility, (e) increasing knowledge about the causes of miscarriage; (f) developing more effective techniques of contraception, (g) developing methods for detecting the presence of gene, chromosome or mitochondrion abnormalities in embryos before implantation, or (h) increasing knowledge about the development of embryos. See Human Fertilisation and Embryology Act 2008, Schedule 2, paragraph 3.

137 Mary Warnock, *Making Babies: Is there a right to have children?* Oxford: Oxford University Press, 2002, at 33-34.

things, including plants; the sensitive, shared by all animals, including man; and the rational peculiar to man. When Aristotle's speculations were discovered and taken over, first by Thomas Aquinas and later as the official doctrine of the Church, there was much discussion of the exact timing of this entry of the human life, or soul, into the body. Of course by now the concept of 'the soul' had entirely changed since the days of Aristotle, the soul being now a thoroughly Christianized entity, immortal, and in a special sense in the hands of God, and of infinite value. It was gradually agreed that one could not be sure of the exact time at which ensoulment took place, and therefore, to be safe, it must be assumed that it was at the moment of conception, or fertilisation.

There is nothing sacrosanct in the 14 day rule, or indeed anything else in the Warnock Report. Its concern was essentially pragmatic, and its recommendations were acknowledged to require periodic review. In January 2004, a review of the HFE Act of 1990 was announced by the government, in view of technological developments and changing social values. Along with the Human Reproductive Cloning Act, this 1990 legislation has been replaced by the HFE Act of 2008. For the purposes of this book, two key provisions of the 2008 legislation are to be noted: first, it ensures that regulation applies to all human embryos handled outside the body and regardless of the process used in their creation; and second, it ensures 'human-admixed' embryos created from a combination of human and animal genetic material for research are regulated. The regulation of 'human-admixed' embryo will be further discussed below.

2.4 Drawing on Bioethics as a Deliberative Space

Singapore's interest in SCNT came about a decade later, when various policy initiatives were introduced to expand the country's biomedical research capability. In 2001, the BAC announced that it would deliberate on ethical, legal and social issues that arise from human cloning and embryonic stem cell research. Similar to the US and the

UK, the moral status of an embryo is central to the controversy. Partly for this reason, the Warnock Report served as an important reference source.

The moral status of an embryo is, under a broad assessment, normatively indeterminate in the absence of a determinate knowledge or institutional structure that provides a 'right' answer to the normative question of when life begins.[138] In this respect, a normative standard should not be regarded as a single system of normative inquiry, but of a composite of systems that one would often find when confronted with certain issues set within a particular societal context. The normative status of an embryo is perhaps not entirely indeterminate. When interpreted against a Christian moral theological system of normative inquiry at least, one would discover a normative prescription that requires compliance independently of any process of rationalisation.[139] Pre-existing institutions or systems of normative inquiry follow from a broader appreciation of the notion that human societies are not structured in normatively neutral ways. They are embedded historically in the common heritage and experience of some of their members in a designate time and place, and it is this cultural context that (at least from a policy standpoint) prescribes normative standards.[140]

At the time the BAC was deliberating on the subject of cloning and stem cell research, a majority of institutions in Singapore have not formulated a viewpoint for the simple reason that there was no need, up to that point, to engage the ethical issues that the subject

---

[138] Determinacy is described as having the effect of marking a belief in existence: Benjamin Gregg, *Coping in Politics with Indeterminate Norms: A Theory of Enlightened Localism*. New York: State University of New York Press, 2003, at 77.

[139] *Ibid*, see Chapter 4 generally. Gregg contrasted the normative indeterminacy of this kind of knowledge with those that are of epistemic determinacy or knowledge which is definite and normative determinable and is a matter of action.

[140] *Ibid*, at 3.

presented. [141] Nevertheless, there was general awareness of the ethical issues through various sources including reports carried over the media and in expert resources including professional journals and meetings. The common perception was that the debate over human stem cell research and cloning was primarily religious in character so that outside of a religious context, it was difficult to engage the discussion. It was within this situational setting that the BAC considered it necessary to develop a more representative and less constrained system of inquiry. This was essentially done by establishing a separate deliberative space for the purpose of allowing citizens to contribute to policy development based on broader political and social values, and in the public interest.

Arguably, the approach that was adopted by the BAC could be characterised as 'post-empiricist' in its use of interpretive (hermeneutic) and discursive (deconstructivist) techniques to demonstrate that subjective presuppositions and assumptions play a significant role in directing our perceptual processes and in pre-shaping perception on what is generally taken to be strictly empirical factors. [142] More specifically, communicative and argumentation processes have been deployed. Its rules of discourse are akin to the rules of evidence in legal proceedings and normative discourse in political philosophy, with emphasis on integrating normative and empirical modes of discourse in order to secure legitimacy with the public, the biomedical scientific community and with the government.

When faced with norms that are indeterminate, the BAC sought to transcend tension between more limited conditions of a local standpoint and the less limited conditions of a perspective beyond.[143]

---

[141] Bioethics Advisory Committee, *Ethical, Legal and Social Issues in Human Stem Cell Research, Reproductive and Therapeutic Cloning.* Singapore: Bioethics Advisory Committee, 2002, at pp 12-13.

[142] Frank Fischer, *Reframing Public Policy: Discursive Politics and Deliberative Practices.* New York: Oxford University Press, 2003, at 14.

[143] Benjamin Gregg, *Coping in Politics with Indeterminate Norms: A Theory of Enlightened Localism.* New York: State University of New York Press, 2003, at 161.

This system of policy inquiry starts with the society's cultures, understandings and practices but with the goal of transcending them. It passes over present tensions by resisting recourse to universal criteria. Metaphorically, this is akin to a decision to build a bridge. While knowledge of all physical laws that are required to build this bridge cannot be described as complete or conclusive, existing knowledge is sufficient to construct a workable structure without the need to first attain complete understanding of physical laws. In other words, the ideological underpinning of the BAC's approach approximates closely to that of pragmatism, which may be clear from the BAC's indication in its SC Report that it was neither to engage in the pursuit of, nor was it within its capacity to inquire into, fundamental 'truths' or universal criteria.[144]

Post-empiricist approaches – notably their emphasis on pluralism of normative standards – are not incompatible with pragmatism, in a sense that Richard Posner has argued that democratic theory is pragmatic.[145] This pragmatic character may perhaps be attributed to the SC Report for the following reasons:

(1) The BAC did not formulate social goals as universal truths. Rather, the end goals (or principles) of 'just' and 'sustainable' were formulated in a way that they were achievable by the normative standard proposed by the BAC;[146]

(2) It follows from (1) that the BAC did not view these end goals as infallible truths. It was for this reason that it also

---

144 Bioethics Advisory Committee, *Ethical, Legal and Social Issues in Human Stem Cell Research, Reproductive and Therapeutic Cloning.* Singapore: Bioethics Advisory Committee, 2002, at 21-22, paragraph 4.

145 Richard Posner's work, *Law, Pragmatism and Democracy.* Cambridge MA: Harvard University Press, 2003, at 64.

146 Bioethics Advisory Committee, *Ethical, Legal and Social Issues in Human Stem Cell Research, Reproductive and Therapeutic Cloning.* Singapore: Bioethics Advisory Committee, 2002, at 21-22.

recommended constant review and the establishment of a regulatory body;[147]

(3) The recommendations of the BAC were formulated to allow some degree of normative determinacy to be attained so that public policy on hESC research and SCNT does not become stagnated. In this regard, the BAC was mindful of the consequences, a feature also present in the end goals formulated;[148]

(4) The recommendations of the BAC do not share in the 'post-modern' scepticism. The recommendations possess arguably limited 'universality' that is derived, not from grounding in universal principles, but from generally accepted best practices encapsulated in bioethical principles and other 'soft law' instruments. For this reason, the BAC carefully analysed bioethical approaches and normative standards in other countries, as well as those embodied in international law or international best-practices instruments. The 'universality' of the recommendations is limited by the temporal and socio-cultural context within which they were developed;[149] and

(5) The indication that the recommendations required constant review connotes a methodology that is experimental. In this respect, the BAC serves as an assessor for Parliament of the changing impact that biomedical sciences have on Singaporean society.[150]

The development of a normatively 'moderated' or middle-ground position required policy analysts to stand away from both the scientific interpretation and the moral theological viewpoint, as though an observer, in order to determine what the broader

---

147 *Ibid*, at 35, paragraph 49.
148 *Ibid*.
149 *Ibid*, at pp 14-20 (Chapter 6) and pp J-1-J-4 (Annex J).
150 *Ibid*, at viii (Recommendations 8, 10 and 11); at pp 32-33, paragraph 42; at 1 (paragraphs 1 to 5).

epistemological issues are. The epistemological issues would in turn determine the extent of moderation required of one or both ideologies (scientific interpretation has been generally treated as a conflicting ideology rather than a transformative force for ease of contrast). This process was premised on the view that scientific interpretation arose out of particular socio-historical contexts so that social meanings and value judgments have been built into scientific practices otherwise described as 'value neutral'. [151] Policy analysts also viewed moral theology as descriptive of one reality in a world of multiple realities, so that there was no 'objective' reality in which any moral ideology could anchor itself.

Again, this process reflects the underlying pragmatism. In bringing together conflicting ideologies, there must be sufficient commonality that needs to be achieved through the identification of aspects of differences that falls beyond the reach of rationalisation. To be sure, 'secularism' is not pragmatism and does not in and of itself have an internally coherent doctrine so as to be regarded as an institution or an ideology. Furthermore, 'secularism' suggests an environment that is devoid of religious ideology but does not go further to indicate if the environment then becomes a 'vacuum' or that it is replaced by another non-religious ideology that should then become a 'religious' ideology. (This would be an impossibility if one accepts the premise that all members of a society are culturally integrated and culture is itself a singular ideology or a composite of ideologies.) A better view may be to think of 'secularism' as an attitude or a product from the interaction of two or more ideologies but even this would not automatically qualify itself as an ideology that has sufficient institutional force to direct conduct. It is however beyond the scope of this work to provide an inquiry into the nature and causes of 'secularism' other than to note that the BAC does not preclude religious ideologies but religious assertions to fundamental 'truths'

---

[151] Lucio Russo, *The Forgotten Revolution: How Science was Born in 300 BC and Why it had to be Reborn.* New York: Springer, 2003, at 385-397.

are moderated to the extent that they could be rationalised, and be rendered comparable within the cultural context of the time.

There was no consensus among the main religious groups in Singapore as to when 'personhood' could be said to begin.[152] On this basis, one could perhaps conclude that at least in ethical policy, human life begins from 14 days of embryonic development, or when the 'primitive streak' becomes evident. From a legal standpoint however, it has been argued that the law is much slower in recognising when human life acquires legal significance, since for instance, a pregnant woman has the discretion to terminate her pregnancy up to 24 weeks from conception.[153] Similarly, the common law relating to inheritance and the Penal Code attribute legal 'personhood' at a much later stage of foetal development.[154] Drawing on the Warnock Report and the bioethical literature that has developed around it, bioethics served as a moderation process, as well as a moderated normative space within which the BAC assumed the role of an interpretive mediator. The development of the sciences on the one hand and moral philosophy on the other has become so 'specialised' that each has evolved into an institutional culture so distinct from the other that there is no common 'language' that may be adopted for members of one institutional culture to communicate with members of the other. In this respect, John Polkinghorne[155] provides a good illustration. The study of cause and effect is undertaken in physics (in the field of quantum physics) as well as in theology (in the doctrine of divine causality).[156] However, the institutional culture within which this concept is developed has

---

152 Calvin W L Ho, Benjamin J Capps and Teck Chuan Voo, Stem Cell Science and its Public: The Case of Singapore, *East Asian Science, Technology and Society: An International Journal* 4 (2010): 7-29.

153 *Termination of Pregnancy Act*, Cap 324, 1985 Rev Ed.

154 Terry Kaan, At the Beginning of Life, *Singapore Academy of Law Journal* (2010) 22: 883-918.

155 John Polkinghorne, *Belief in God in an Age of Science*. New Haven and London: Yale University Press, 1998.

156 *Ibid* at pages 27-32.

become so remarkably technical that only experts in each field will appreciate fully the consequences of the study. It is unrealistic, assuming that it is practicable, for members of one institutional culture to become fully acquainted with the language and practices of another institutional culture in order for a meaningful discussion on issues like hESC research to take place. Even less realistic is for any one institution to forsake its own institutional culture and adopt that of the other for the purposes of effecting dialogue. The intent to involve, and so represent, a wider range of interests, arguments and discourses in the analytical process has been clearly manifested throughout the course of deliberation by the BAC. As Fischer notes, this is achieved partly by emphasising the ways in which people's interest are discursively constructed and the manner in which they come to hold specific interests.[157] The ultimate goal may perhaps be stated as developing a normative position that will raise no reasonable ethical complaint.

The moderated norm took the form of a 'proposed standard' that was grounded in two principles – 'just' outcome and 'sustainable' in consequence. The BAC indicates that the 'just' element is not merely consequential. It possesses substantive (albeit utilitarian) content in that there was an obligation on the part of all institutions to respect the common good, particularly in the sharing of the costs and benefits. In 'sustainable', the BAC also recognised the obligation to respect the needs of generations yet unborn. Taken together, the BAC considered that the best way forward was one that allowed the pursuit of social benefit but in a manner that either avoided or ameliorated potential harm. Application of the 'proposed standard' in policy analysis is akin to the crafting of arguments with the goal of allowing policy engagement by illuminating contentious questions, identifying the strengths and limitations of supporting evidence and elucidating

---

[157] Frank Fischer, *Reframing Public Policy: Discursive Politics and Deliberative Practices*. New York: Oxford University Press, 2003, at 15.

the political implications of contending positions.[158] The 'proposed standard' was essentially drawn from the Warnock Report and presented as an 'intermediate' position. While the moral status is conferred upon an embryo to a level, embryonic research may be conducted but in very limited circumstances:[159]

(a) **Within the 14 Day Limit**: Research may be conducted on an embryo before it reached the 14th day from the day the gametes were fused. However, all such research is to be subject to strict regulation and undertaken only if there is very strong scientific merit in, and potential medical benefit to be derived from, such research. The BAC did not agree with the view that an embryo is merely a collection of cells. While the BAC was prepared to recognise the special status of an embryo before it reached the 14 day limit, it did not consider this special status to be equivalent to the status that a living person would have. Accordingly, the BAC considered it ethical to conduct research on such an embryo on a strictly regulated basis and subject to the conditions stipulated; and

(b) **Beyond the 14 Day Limit**: The BAC considered it unethical for research to be conducted on an embryo that has reached the 14 day limit and that such an embryo would be accorded full status as a person. Many countries have similarly adopted the time limit of 14 days from fertilisation as the ethical boundary, beyond which research on the embryo should not be permissible. The common basis for this time limit is the appearance of the primitive streak at about that time. At that stage, the embryo would be regarded as having developed irreversible individuality and, at that point, become morally significant.

---

[158] *Ibid*, at 201-202.
[159] Bioethics Advisory Committee, *Ethical, Legal and Social Issues in Human Stem Cell Research, Reproductive and Therapeutic Cloning*. Singapore: Bioethics Advisory Committee, 2002, at 29-30, paragraphs 33 to 36.

The BAC clearly indicated that the recommendations that it provided were not intended to resolve the inherent normative indeterminacy – this being the moral status of a human embryo. It did however adopt the view that an embryo is morally more significant than another living organism as necessitated by the cultural conditions of the time. This view may be grounded more in an interest in ensuring that due respect is accorded to a minority perspective (that a human embryo has full moral status) in Singapore, even if it is not taken up in public policy. For this reason, the BAC indicates that the 14 day time limit is not a conclusive statement on when an embryo becomes morally significant. Instead, the time limit is set as a matter of practical necessity so that a 'just' and 'sustainable' position can be attained. That is, one that allows research on hESC research to proceed in view of potential therapeutic benefits that can be procured for the good of all. Since the BAC did not attempt to impute a moral viewpoint, it recommended that the refusal of any individual to be involved in human pluripotent stem cell research as a matter of conscientious objection should be respected. Also noteworthy is that a distinction has not been drawn between supernumerary embryos and an embryo created specifically for research. Under a moderated normative position of the 14 day limit, the moral implications that attend to the use of either types of embryo are equivalent. In addition, they are both equally beneficial as sources of hESC lines. But because intrinsic value (albeit moderated) has been ascribed to a human embryo, there must nevertheless be strong scientific merit in, and potential medical benefit from the research. In the case where an embryo is to be produced exclusively for research, it must additionally be shown that no acceptable alternative exists, and specific approval is obtained from the MOH, on a highly selective, case-by-case basis.[160]

---

160 *Ibid*, at vii–viii.

2.5 From Pluripotency to Chimeras

The recommendations in the SC Report on reproductive and therapeutic cloning include proposals for stringent regulation of human embryonic stem cell research in Singapore and the legal prohibition of reproductive cloning. These were taken up by the legislature with the enactment of the *Human Cloning and Other Prohibited Practices Act* in 2004. As with other major scientific jurisdictions (like the UK as we have considered), the legislation imposes a 14 day limit, so that research involving a human embryo is allowed up to that point in development. And as we shall discuss later on in this work, the 14 day limit has found, albeit for different reasons, wide support among different countries. There has also been general consensus that reproductive cloning is to be prohibited, and a United Nations Declaration was made to that effect.[161]

Although the 14 day rule served to calm the ethical turbulence that was stirred up from the late 1980's onwards, there was no apparent 'gold-rush' into hESC research when the controversy begun to settle from the mid-2000's. Rather than being opportunistic, biomedical researchers attempted to find ethically less contentious means of generating embryonic stem cells that did not entail the destruction of a human embryo. These included harvesting cells from very early embryos prior to implantation (non-harmful biopsy), use of 'organismically dead' embryos, and parthenogenesis. The possibility of harvesting stem cells from embryos prior to implantation was demonstrated when a single cell was taken from an 8-cell mouse embryo. Although not free of criticism,[162] embryonic cells have in fact been removed from human embryos for genetic screening in fertility clinics for many years without any adverse effects on the resulting

---

161 United Nations General Assembly, *Declaration on Human Cloning*, A/Res/59/280, 23 March 2005.
162 Alison Abbott, 'Ethical' stem-cell paper under attack, *Nature* (7 September 2006) 443: 12.

children. Such cells could be a potential source of stem cell lines, with the added advantage of being totipotent and immunologically compatible with the embryo from which they were derived. This technique of deriving hESCs avoids the concern of destroying an embryo, but it raises other concerns as the extracted cell could itself become another embryo (i.e. as an identical twin of the embryo from which it was derived).

Ordinarily, an embryo is diploid in that it contains two different sets of chromosomes, one set from each parent. However, an unfertilised egg can sometimes be induced, by electrical, chemical or physical stimulation, to develop into a type of embryo called a parthenote. In such cases the cell duplicates the chromosome compliment, so the resulting genome (a gynogenome) is again diploid, but with two identical sets of chromosomes. It is also possible to obtain androgenomes by the combination of two sperm nuclei in a single donated enucleated egg. This technique is known as parthenogenesis. A parthenote is not thought to be able to develop into a viable embryo,[163] although at least one instance of a naturally occurring partial parthenote human is known. Some scientists believe the technique avoids some ethical difficulties arising in embryonic stem cell research. However, there is uncertainty as to the utility of the cells for therapeutic purposes, even if tissue from parthenotes is expected to trigger less rejection due to lesser variation in the surface proteins of the cells. The Roslin Institute (also responsible for cloning Dolly the sheep) has reportedly created human parthenotes under license from the HFEA, although this initiative has been opposed by pro-life groups in the UK.[164]

---

[163] Tomohiro Kono, Y Obata, Q Wu, K Niwa, Y Ono, Y Yamamoto, E S Park, J S Seo, H Ogawa, Birth of Parthenogenetic mice that can develop to adulthood, *Nature* (22 April 2004) 428, 6985: 860-864, at 864.

[164] Jonathan Amos, 'Virgin conception' first for UK. *BBC News*, 9 September 2005.

Landry and Zucker[165] have suggested that 'organismically dead' embryos from IVF procedures could be a suitable source of embryonic stem cells. Death, in this context, refers to a cessation of division, so that embryo development is arrested, with no realistic prospect of resumption of division, even though the cells of the 'dead' embryo are metabolically alive. Once dead, donation of stem cells would appear to be uncontroversial, by analogy with use of organs from brain-dead patients.[166] This suggestion is not without difficulties. If an embryo is capable of yielding living stem cells, it is unclear in what sense it is dead. Such a stem cell, or an aggregate of such cells from several embryos, could conceivably be used to create a fresh embryo, in which case the object of the exercise would be defeated. In addition, a high rate of cellular abnormalities may disqualify these embryos as a source of stem cells. For this reason, there is a general preference to confine research to surplus embryos.

The search for an alternative source of pluripotent stem cells did not yield any unambiguously positive result until 2006, when two Japanese researchers (and ironically operating in a society where derivation of hESCs was not considered to be especially controversial) reprogrammed mice fibroblast cells to become pluripotent stem cells. A year later, they were able to do the same with human cell culture, essentially by inducing adult (or differentiated) cells to become pluripotent through genetic manipulation of four genes. The pluripotent stem cells that they produced have since been called

---

165 Donald W Landry and Howard A Zucker, Embryonic death and the creation of human embryonic stem cells, *Journal of Clinical Investigations* (2004) 114: 1184-1186.

166 Giuseppe Testa argues that the attempt to define embryo death in order to equate hESC harvesting to organ transplantation is a poignant display of co-production, where the social design of brain death is re-enacted in the scientific quest for molecular markers of embryo death. The mutual adaptation of moral norms and epistemic practices generates biological artefacts as technological solutions to political controversies. See: Giuseppe Testa, Stem Cells through Stem Beliefs: The Co-Production of Biotechnological Pluralism, *Science as Culture* (2008) 17, 4: 435-448.

induced pluripotent stem cells (iPSCs), and were generated without destroying or manipulating human embryos. One of these researchers – Shinya Yamanaka – was awarded the Nobel Prize in Physiology and Medicine for devising this technique. Of significance is that therapeutic cloning (SCNT) has been noted as having influenced Yamanaka's work.[167] More importantly, iPSC did not render hESC obsolete. Subsequent research by Yamanaka and others shows that there are many epigenetic differences between iPSCs and hESCs. A relatively high level of variations and mutations in iPSCs are thought to have arisen from the original somatic cells from which these iPSCs originated. For this reason, professional research bodies like the ÁMS have noted that while the properties of iPSCs are broadly similar to hESCs, the variations in their properties may reflect incomplete reprogramming, as well as some genetic or chromosomal damage. Even less certain is the relevance of these differences to the prospective clinical use of iPSCs. It has rather wisely been proposed that hESCs remain the 'gold standard' to which iPSCs should be compared.[168]

A further alternative source of pluripotent stem cells that received regulatory attention is human-animal cytoplasmic hybrid embryos, which are derived by transferring a somatic cell nucleus from a human into the enucleated oocyte of a non-human animal. Along with chimeras and transgenic animals, ethical interests and concerns have been on the implication of mixing human and animal characteristics. At the level of genes, such concerns may be more perceptual than real, since identical genetic materials are naturally shared across different species, including humans. It is in the combination of genes that a

---

[167] Zane Bartlett, Induced Pluripotent Stem Cell Experiments by Kazutoshi Takahashi and Shinya Yamanaka in 2006 and 2007. *Embryo Project Encyclopedia*. Arizona: Arizona State University, 2015.

[168] Academy of Medical Sciences, *Animals Containing Human Material*. London: Academy of Medical Sciences, 2011, at 39. Quite independently of being alternatives to hESCs, iPSCs are very important for research into genetic diseases as they are derived from specific patients and may be studied in cell culture or after introduction into animals.

uniquely human genome is defined, since only a very small proportion of human genes are not shared with any other species. But where mixing of tissues in chimeras is concerned, there is reasonable concern when the proportion of certain human biological materials, such as neural tissue, become substantial in a nonhuman species. Interestingly, no jurisdiction has established a broad regulatory framework to govern the creation and use of cytoplasmic hybrid embryos and similar nonhuman species with human material in biomedical research until recently.

2.6 Chimeras and Hybrids as Regulatory Concerns

Broadly speaking, the regulatory framework for basic (i.e. non-therapeutic) human pluripotent cell research has at least two key segments; one that relates to *in vitro* studies using early human embryos, and another that relates to *in vivo* studies involving nonhuman (and mainly sentient) animals.[169] Where the former is concerned, we have already considered how the 14 day rule has emerged as a pragmatic compromise. As for the latter, many countries already have a governance system in place (such as an institutional animal research committee) to ensure that animal research welfare principles are observed. But then, the prospect of creating human-animal cytoplasmic hybrid embryos was presented. It also became more apparent that pluripotent human stem cells, whether derived from an embryo or through iPSC, will need to be introduced into nonhuman animals at different stages of growth in order to test the level of pluripotency in the stem cells.[170] With these developments, the regulatory framework needs to be extended to cover early

---

[169] Göran Hermerén, Ethical considerations in chimera research, *Development* (2015) 142: 3-5. See also: Insoo Hyun, From naïve pluripotency to chimeras: a new ethical challenge? *Development* (2015) 142: 6-8.

[170] Jamie A Hackett and Azim M Surani, Regulatory principles of pluripotency: from the ground state up, *Cell Stem Cell* (2014) 15, 416-430.

human and human-nonhuman chimeric or hybrid embryos, as well as animals that contain human materials.

For reasons that will be discussed further in Chapter 5, cytoplasmic hybrids fall within the expanded regulatory purview of the HFE Act 2008, with the addition of a new category of 'human admixed embryos'. In addition to cytoplasmic hybrids, four other types of 'human admixed embryos', or embryos that contain human and animal material in equal proportion or with human material in predominance are: human-animal hybrid embryos, human transgenic embryos, human-animal chimeras and any embryo which contains both human nuclear or mitochondrial DNA and nuclear or mitochondrial DNA of an animal, but where the animal DNA is not predominant.[171] Under the HFE Act, a licence is required to create, keep or use human admixed embryos *in vitro*, for a principal purpose that has been considered earlier in this chapter. In addition, the following activities are specifically prohibited under the HFE Act:[172]

(a) Placing any embryo or gametes, other than permitted embryos or gametes, into a woman;

(b) Placing a human embryo in any nonhuman animal;

(c) Placing a human admixed embryo in an animal; and

(d) Keeping or using a human embryo, or a human admixed embryo, after either the appearance of the primitive streak or 14 days of development.

Beyond cytoplasmic hybrid embryos, a more comprehensive framework that would apply to chimeras, hybrids and transgenic animals has been proposed by the AMS in 2011. At that time, regulatory gaps were already recognised as a research organism could conceivably fall outside of the purview of either the HFEA (and

---

[171] *Human Fertilisation and Embryology Act* 1990 (as amended in 2008), Subsection 4A(6).

[172] *Ibid*, Subsections 3(2), 3(3), 4A(3), and 4A(4).

Department of Health, more generally) or the Home Office, which regulates animal research under the *Animals (Scientific Procedures) Act* 1986.[173] For instance, it could be queried if the Home Office would be the appropriate authority to regulate a cytoplasmic hybrid embryo that has predominantly animal material. The recommendation by the AMS for the Home Office and the HFEA to work together in developing and maintaining "a smooth, functionally integrated operational interface at the boundaries of their areas of responsibility" was taken up and addressed by the British government.[174] An online navigation platform known as the UK Stem Cell Tool Kit has been established as a reference tool for those interested in developing a programme of human stem cell research and manufacturing, including clinical applications.[175] The Tool Kit applies only to the regulation of human stem cells and their use in the laboratory and clinical settings. A separate guidance has also been issued by the Home Office on the use of human material in animals.[176] It advices that an application for project licence may take some time to prepare, especially if it describes a novel or complex programme of work or raises matters of significant public interest. It further advises the applicant to discuss a draft application with a Home Office inspector, as well as with other experienced project licence holders at an early stage in order to expedite the application.[177] Complex applications (such as one that requires clarification as to the meaning of 'predominant' in relation to a human admixed embryo) may be evaluated by the Animals in Science Committee (ASC), with appropriate co-opted experts.[178] The ASC is an independent non-departmental public body that is

---

[173] *The Animals (Scientific Procedures) Act* 1986 (as amended by SI 2012/3039).

[174] Academy of Medical Sciences, *Animals Containing Human Material*. London: Academy of Medical Sciences, 2011, at 113.

[175] See: http://www.sc-toolkit.ac.uk/home.cfm

[176] UK Home Office, *Guidance on the use of Human Material in Animals*. Advice Note 01/16, January 2016.

[177] *Ibid*, at 6.

[178] *Ibid*, at 8.

responsible for providing impartial, balanced and objective advice to the Secretary of State (Home Office) and to local animal welfare and ethical review bodies on issues relating to the use of animals in scientific procedures. It assumes the role of the national body that the AMS has proposed under its rubric for regulatory review whereby all experiments involving animals containing human material (ACHM) are classified into one of three categories:[179]

Category 1: The great majority of ACHM experiments which do not present issues beyond those of the general use of animals in research. The level of regulatory oversight is the same as other animal research (i.e. usual ethics review and/or animal welfare review). For instance, a mouse model may be used to test the development and functioning of hESCs before the study is carried out in humans.

Category 2: A limited number of ACHM experiments that should be permissible subject to additional specialist scrutiny by the ASC, on a case-by-case basis. Authorisation may require such experiments to be carried out on an incremental or graduated basis. Experiments that would fall within this category include those that:

- Substantially modify an animal's brain with the potential of making the brain function more 'human-like', particularly in large animals;

- May lead to the generation or propagation of functional human germ cells in animals;

- Could be expected to significantly alter the appearance or behaviour of animals, affecting those characteristics that are perceived to contribute most to distinguishing the human species from its close evolutionary relatives; or

---

[179] *Ibid*, at 13-15; See also: Academy of Medical Sciences, *Animals Containing Human Material*. London: Academy of Medical Sciences, 2011, at 110-111.

- Involve the addition of human genes or cells to nonhuman primates (NHP).

Category 3: A very small number of experiments which should not be permitted at this time as they either lack compelling scientific justification or raise very strong ethical concerns. Such experiments include those that:

- Allow the development of an embryo, formed by pre-implantation mixing of NHP and human embryonic or pluripotent stem cells, beyond 14 days of development or the signs of primitive streak development (whichever occurs first), unless there is persuasive evidence that the fate of the implanted human cells will not lead to 'sensitive' phenotypic changes in the developing foetus;

- Transplant sufficient human-derived neural cells into a NHP as to make it possible, in the judgment of the ASC, that there could be substantial functional modification of the NHP brain, such as to engender 'human-like' behaviour. Assessing the likely phenotypic effect of such experiments will be informed by prior work on other species (possibly including stem cell transfer between NHPs) or by data on the effects of 'graded' transplantation of human cells into NHPs; or

- Breed animals that have, or may develop, human derived germ cells in their gonads, where this could lead to the production of human embryos or true hybrid embryos within an animal.

Where Category 2 experiments are concerned, review by the ASC will focus on the ethical and safety issues, as well as the potential value of the research.[180] As general requirements, these experiments must ensure that the animals involved are protected from avoidable suffering and their use in scientific procedures must be demonstrated to be necessary. The experiments must also be supported by strong

---

[180] *Ibid*, at 16-17.

scientific justification and legitimate requirements of industry, where applicable. Members are appointed to the ASC based on their skills, expertise and experience (rather than as representatives of any organisation or interest group), which would include animal welfare, veterinary science and neuroscience. Lay members with an interest in ethical issues arising from the use of animals in scientific research have also been appointed to the ASC. When necessary, individuals with particular expertise may be co-opted to assist in evaluating more specialised issues that arise from the proposed experiments. In conducting their review, all members are expected to work in the public interest.

The evaluative framework presented by the AMS was originally proposed by National Academy of Science (NAS) in the US,[181] and was also adapted by the ISSCR in its 2006 and 2008 guidelines for the conduct of pluripotent stem cell research. The relationship among these professional bodies and their normative documents will be discussed in Chapter 4. Here, we only need to note that while the US has no national stem cell oversight commission or centrally authorised committee, the oversight mechanism proposed by the NAS in the form of Embryonic Stem Cell Research Oversight (ESCRO) committees and enhanced IRB review of the procurement of human biological materials used to derive new stem cell lines have been voluntarily adopted and implemented by research institutions. ESCRO committees are intended to complement existing IRB and Institutional Animal Care and Use Committee (IACUC) oversight, as well as to coordinate the review of all stem cell research based on the categorical scheme discussed above.[182] The ISSCR has similarly

---

[181] National Academy of Science. *Final report of the National Academies' human embryonic stem cell research advisory committee* and *2010 amendment to the National Academies' guidelines for human embryonic stem cell research* amended as of May 2010. Washington DC: National Academies Press, 2010. In Section 7, a dedicated and additional review by an ESCRO committee has been recommended.

[182] For a more detailed description of the oversight regime in the US and its relationship with that proposed by the ISSCR, see: Insoo Hyun, *Bioethics and the*

proposed for ethically sensitive stem cell research experiments to undergo a specialised oversight process, termed 'Stem Cell Research Oversight' (SCRO).[183] Essentially, SCRO is carried out by stem-cell specific experts in science and ethics, and comprises the three categories of research much like the ones considered above. Category 1 relates to relatively routine experiments involving existing hESC lines, and typically only streamlined administrative approval is necessary. Category 2 comprises experiments that require special scrutiny, such as those that attempt to derive new hESC lines. Category 3 identifies experiments that are impermissible, such as extending *in vitro* culture of human embryos beyond 14 days. Where human-animal chimera or hybrid experiments are concerned, the system of review is similar to the one proposed by the AMS.[184] But whereas the NAS and the NIH disallow experiments in which human embryonic or pluripotent stem cells are introduced into NHP blastocysts, neither the AMS nor ISSCR has adopted this restriction. More recently, the NIH announced that it will not fund research in

---

Future of Stem Cell Research. Cambridge and New York: Cambridge University Press, 2013, at pp 81-95.

183 International Society for Stem Cell Research, *Guidelines for the conduct of human embryonic stem cell research*, 2006. See Section 10. The 2008 guidelines of the ISSCR are not discussed as they relate to clinical translation, which is beyond the scope of this work.

184 The Ethics and Public Policy Committee of the ISSCR published a report that specifically addressed ethical concerns in research involving human-animal chimeras. It emphasises the importance of animal chimeras as research tools and cautioned against 'stem cell exceptionalism'. While general animal welfare principles will apply in most cases, it did express a general concern of developing human sentience in animals. Recommendations directed at avoiding this outcome include conducting research on non-sentient constructs before research on sentient animals, monitoring and data collection should be based on a sound assessment of the development trajectories that are likely to be affected (taking into account epigenetic effects), and assessing animal welfare on a regular basis. International Society for Stem Cell Research, Ethical Standards for Human-to-Animal Chimera Experiments in Stem Cell Research, *Cell Stem Cell* (2007) 1, 4: 159-163. See also: International Society for Stem Cell Research, Ethics Report on Interspecies Somatic Cell Nuclear Transfer Research, *Cell Stem Cell* (2009) 5, 1: 27-30.

which human pluripotent cells are introduced into non-human vertebrate animal (i.e. not only NHP) pre-gastrulation stage embryos.[185] It also indicates that, in view of the rapid expansion of potential research models employed beyond the small number of prohibited research where human pluripotent cells are introduced into animals,[186] a deliberative process is being undertaken to evaluate the state of the science, the ethical issues and the relevant animal welfare concerns.

Meanwhile, the ISSCR published its revised guidelines for stem cell research and clinical translation in 2016.[187] While SCRO remains the main oversight process for pluripotent stem cell research, the ISSCR has excluded the derivation of iPSC from specialised review. The reason for this is that it does not engender the same sensitivities as the derivation of hESC lines.[188] However, specialised review is still required for the use of human iPSCs to achieve human-animal chimerism of the central nervous system or through admixing human iPSCs with human embryos. There are two other important features to the 2016 guidelines. First, a set of core ethical principles have been identified to guide the review of basic and clinical stem cell research, these being: integrity of the research enterprise, primacy of patient welfare, respect for research subjects, and transparency and social justice.[189] It is premature to say how these ethical principles will be

---

[185] National Institutes of Health, *NIH Research Involving Introduction of Human Pluripotent Cells into Non-Human Vertebrate Animal Pre-Gastrulation Embryos*, NOT-OD-15-158, 23 September 2015.

[186] National Institutes of Health, *Guidelines on Human Stem Cell Research*, 2009. For a comparison of requirements under the NIH guidelines with those of the NAS and the ISSCR, see: Karen H Rothenberg and Michael R Ulrich, NIH Guidelines on Human Embryonic Stem Cell Research in Context: Clarity of Confusion, *World Stem Cell Report 2010*, pp 89-98.

[187] International Society for Stem Cell Research, *Guidelines for stem cell science and clinical translation*, 2016.

[188] George Q Daley, *et al*. Setting Global Standards for Stem Cell Research and Clinical Translation: The 2016 ISSCR Guidelines. *Stem Cell Reports* (2016) 6: 1-11, at 2.

[189] International Society for Stem Cell Research, *Guidelines for stem cell science and clinical translation*, 2016, Section 1.

implemented, but principles like transparency and social justice will have important implications beyond the review process. Second, an additional process of embryo research oversight (EMRO) has been proposed for both hESC research and any human embryo research that does not explicitly pertain to stem cells or stem cell lines.[190] The latter includes single cell analyses, genome modification and embryo chimerism. These two developments will be further discussed later on in this work.

2.7 Regulatory Framework in Singapore

Until 2000, engagement with biomedical research ethics has mainly occurred either within highly institutionalised and defined fields of practice, such as clinical trials, or on a 'when necessary' basis, by an *ad hoc* IRB or similar body within academic and healthcare institutions. On the former, the term 'clinical trials' has been defined by legislation to encompass all biomedical research that relates to the testing of a 'medical product' or drug on a human subject.[191] Both regulatory and ethics approval will have to be obtained before a clinical trial may be commenced.

From 2002 onwards, an institutional framework on biomedical research ethics was put in place as a matter of national policy mainly through the efforts of the BAC and the MOH. Although there is an overlap, the BAC's recommendations are directed at the biomedical research community in general, whereas the MOH is primarily concerned with research that either occurs within healthcare premises or conducted by healthcare professionals. This dual approach is due in part to historical factors, particularly since the medical profession and healthcare establishments have traditionally

---

[190] *Ibid*, Section 2.1.
[191] Detailed provisions are set out under the *Medicines (Clinical Trials) Regulations*, which also incorporate and thereby confer regulatory effect on the *Singapore Good Clinical Practice Guidelines* (SGGCP) of 1998.

been closely regulated,[192] whereas researchers and research institutions have not (except for biosafety). In spite of these differences, a governance framework has emerged incrementally and through ever closer connections between the biomedical research and medical communities.

In 2004, the BAC built on the guidelines of the MOH (its National Medical Ethics Committee in particular)[193] and enlarged their application to all human biomedical research conducted in Singapore. Its report on research involving human subjects essentially formalised the requirement for all human biomedical research in Singapore, including research involving human tissue or medical information, to be subject to ethics review by IRBs.[194] The guidelines promulgated in the report built on the existing system of regulations for pharmaceutical trials and human biomedical research conducted by hospitals, private clinics and other healthcare establishments under supervision of the MOH. They also set out the constitution, accreditation and operation of IRBs, as well as their roles and responsibilities, in addition to those applicable to research institutions and individual researchers. In the main, the BAC regards high standards of ethical governance for the protection of life, health, privacy and dignity of human subjects in biomedical research as vital to the progress of biomedical sciences in Singapore. The fundamental responsibility of an IRB is set out as conducting ethics review with the "primary objectives of the protection and assurance of the safety, health, dignity, welfare and well-being of human research subjects".[195] By this formulation, the ethical perimeter appears to be broader than the Belmont principles, although there is continued emphasis on

---

[192] *Private Hospitals and Medical Clinics Act*, Cap 248, 1999 Rev Ed; and *Medical Registration Act*, Cap 174, 2004 Rev Ed.

[193] National Medical Ethics Committee, *Ethical Guidelines on Research Involving Human Subjects*. Singapore: Ministry of Health, August 1997.

[194] Bioethics Advisory Committee, *Research Involving Human Subjects: Guidelines for IRBs*. Singapore: Bioethics Advisory Committee, November 2004.

[195] *Ibid*, at 41, paragraph 5.20.

free and informed consent, respect for privacy and confidentiality, and respect for vulnerable persons. Although the guidelines of the BAC do not have any direct regulatory authority, they have been accepted by the MOH,[196] and by the Agency for Science Technology and Research (A*STAR), the principal public funder of biomedical research in Singapore. Consequently, the medical profession and biomedical researchers who are funded by A*STAR are required to observe these guidelines. In 2007, the MOH issued supplementary guidelines on the day-to-day workings of an IRB, for which the BAC has set out the operating principles. These include guidelines on the composition of an IRB, a more elaborate discussion on the informed consent process, meeting requirements and requirements relating to documentation.[197]

As we have considered earlier, a regulatory framework on hESC research has been established by the BAC's SC Report of 2002, and with the enactment of the *Human Cloning and Other Prohibited Practices Act* in 2004. The ethical implications of cytoplasmic hybrid embryos and other types of human-animal combinations have been considered as part of a broader review undertaken by the BAC in 2007 of its recommendations published in the SC report, along with the related topics of procurement and use of human eggs for biomedical research. The ED Report and HA Report that followed from this review will be discussed in chapters 3 to 6. For the purposes of this chapter, it need only be noted that the creation and use of cytoplasmic hybrid embryos and animal chimeras in research are permitted in Singapore but only on a strictly regulated basis. In its consolidated guidelines published in June 2015, the BAC indicates that the main "ethical hazard lies in the possibility of inadvertently creating an

---

196 Ministry of Health, Directive 1A/2006: *BAC Recommendations for Biomedical Research*, 18 January 2006.
197 Ministry of Health, *Operational Guidelines for Institutional Review Boards*. Singapore: Ministry of Health (Biomedical Research Regulation Division), December 2007, at 8-9, paragraphs 7.10.5, 7.12, Section 10.

animal with human characteristics, especially, but not exclusively, mental attributes".[198] In ethics review, it sets out six relevant factors that should be considered together:[199] proportion or ratio of human to animal cells in the animal's brain, age of the animal, recipient species, brain size of the animal involved, state of integration of human neural cells, and presence of pathologies in the host animal. The BAC further indicates that research using established pluripotent stem cell lines and confined to cell culture or research that involves routine and standard research practice with laboratory animals should be exempted from IRB review.[200] Other ethical requirements set out by the BAC do not differ from those of the AMS, although conscientious objection is maintained in its provision that no clinical or research personnel should be under a duty to conduct or assist in human pluripotent cell research, or research involving human-animal combinations to which they have a conscientious objection. It further requires that no one should be put at a disadvantage only because of her or his objection.[201] This limited regulatory approach in the form of the BAC-MOH framework was the main governance mechanism until the *Human Biomedical Research Bill* was passed in Parliament on 18 August 2015.

The *Human Biomedical Research Act* (HBRA) establishes a regulatory framework for human biomedical research that is in many ways an amalgamation of critical features of a prototype legislation that was proposed by the MOH in 2003,[202] and the BAC-MOH framework centred around IRBs. While the explanatory statement sets out the goals of the HBRA as regulating the conduct of human biomedical

---

[198] Bioethics Advisory Committee, *Ethical Guidelines for Human Biomedical Research*. Singapore: Bioethics Advisory Committee, 2015, at 56, paragraph 7.22.

[199] *Ibid*, at 57. These considerations have been drawn from Mark Greene, *et al.* Moral Issues of Human-Non-Human Primate Neural Grafting, *Science* (2005) 309: 385-386.

[200] *Ibid*, at 57, paragraph 7.24.

[201] *Ibid*, at 59, paragraph 7.31.

[202] *The Regulation of Biomedical Research Bill*, 2003. Public consultation was conducted on this document, but it was never presented in Parliament.

research, regulating tissue banks and tissue banking activities, prohibiting certain types of human biomedical research, and prohibiting the commercial trading of human tissue, most of the legislative provisions are concerned with the first two goals. Whether a research intervention or activity falls within the scope of the legislation is determined in accordance with an inclusion-exclusion criteria prescribed by it. This inclusion-exclusion criteria is not intended to displace the ethics framework, but must be interpreted within it as the legislative intent is to reinforce certain ethical provisions with legal force. For this reason, the definition of 'human biomedical research' has not been as broadly defined as it was in the Draft 2003 Bill or in the BAC-MOH ethics framework, but rather in terms of the type of research that is done on or involving a research participant, or as belonging to a specified category of research.

The first of the two-stage inclusion criteria requires an assessment of the nature of the research, more precisely whether it relates to a specified biological material deemed to be of ethical, cultural or religious sensitivity,[203] or a specified intention that is concerned with:

(a) The prevention, prognostication, diagnosis or alleviation of any disease, disorder or injury affecting the human body;

(b) The restoration, maintenance or promotion of the aesthetic appearance of human individuals through clinical procedures or techniques; or

(c) The performance or endurance of human individuals.[204]

If the research relates to a specified intention, a second-stage assessment is required to ascertain if the intent is actualised in any one of these three forms:

---

203 *Human Biomedical Research Act* 2015. Section 3(3) identifies these materials as human gametes or human embryos, cytoplasmic hybrid embryos, human-animal combination embryo and human stem cells or neural cells.

204 *Ibid*, Section 3(2)(a)-(c).

(a) An intervention that has a temporary or permanent physical, mental or physiological effect on the research participant,

(b) The use of any individually-identifiable human biological material; or

(c) The use of any individually-identifiable health information.[205]

Once it is determined that the research satisfies the inclusion criteria, it must then be determined if it is nevertheless excluded under the Second Schedule, prohibited under the Third Schedule, or restricted under the Fourth Schedule of the legislation. For instance, clinical trials of medicinal products will satisfy the inclusion criteria, but it is a category of research that falls within the exclusion criteria as an item under the Second Schedule.[206] Not surprisingly, ethically more contentious types of research such as those that involve hESCs and HACs are mainly listed on the Third and Fourth Schedules. Under the Third Schedule, the types of prohibited human biomedical research are listed as those that involve:[207]

(1) Development of cytoplasmic hybrid embryos or HAC embryos created in vitro beyond 14 days or the appearance of the primitive streak, whichever is earlier;

(2) Implantation of any human-animal combination embryo into the uterus of an animal or a human;

(3) Introduction of human stem cells (including iPSCs) or human neural cells into the brain of living great apes whether prenatal or postnatal; and

---

[205] *Ibid*, Section 3(2)(i)-(iii).
[206] Other research excluded from the statutory definition of human biomedical research include minimal risk studies and tests that relate to normal human psychological responses and behaviours or measurement of human intelligence, as well as activities that are already governed under a different statutory regime. *Ibid*, Schedule 2, paragraphs 1, 2, 6 and 7.
[207] *Ibid*.

(4) Breeding of animals which have had any kind of pluripotent stem cells (including iPSCs) introduced into them.

On the third prohibition above, Singapore's position on the introduction of human pluripotent or neural cells into the brain of living great apes is more restrictive than the UK or the US. The AMS has, for instance, recommended exercise of additional oversight and stringent control over any proposals for research where there is doubt as to the potential functional effect of modification of the brain in larger animals and NHP.[208] If an experiment is intended to study the effect of incorporating human neurons into the brain of a NHP, it could start with obtaining evidence based on modest neuronal incorporation into rodents at an initial phase. In subsequent phases, measured and gradated replacements in NHPs could then be conducted, provided that they are also supported by a range of tests for assessing different aspects of primate cognition.[209] Such an incremental research approach should be developed at the outset collaboratively among researchers, inspectors and the national expert body (i.e. the ASC). Given the difficulty in predicting the outcome of human-animal chimeric brain experiments in larger animals, the HBRA reflects a more pragmatic stance in a complete ban on research using chimeric human neural tissue on NHPs.

Restricted human biomedical research may only be conducted after requirements set out in the HBRA are satisfied. These includes notification to be provided to MOH, IRB review, appropriate consent having been obtained from the research subject, and/or conduct of the research only by certain specified persons, at certain specified premises and in the specified manner.[210] Such types of research listed on the Fourth Schedule are those that involve:

---

208 Academy of Medical Sciences, *Animals Containing Human Material*. London: Academy of Medical Sciences, 2011, at 50.
209 *Ibid*, at 49.
210 *Human Biomedical Research Act* 2015, Section 31.

(a) Human-animal combination embryos, further elaborated as cytoplasmic hybrid embryos, human-animal combination embryos created by the incorporation of human stem cells (including iPSC), and human-animal combination embryos created in vitro by using human gametes and animal gametes, or one human pronucleus and one animal pronucleus;

(b) Introduction of human stem cells (including iPSC) into a prenatal animal foetus or animal embryo;

(c) Introduction of human pluripotent stem cells (including iPSC) into a living postnatal animal;

(d) Introduction of human stem cells (including iPSC) or human neural cells into the brain of a living postnatal animal; and

(e) Any entity created as a result of the process referred to in sub-paragraphs (b), (c) and (d) above.

While the HBRA does not significantly modify the existing ethics review infrastructure, this re-articulation of regulatory oversight in the legislation is necessary to redraw a governed space so that it could apply uniformly to all human biomedical researchers and research institutions.[211] The legislation also defines what counts as a research institution. As the term suggests, such an entity must be composed of at least two or more persons, and have management and control over human biomedical research that is conducted in Singapore. In order to be legally recognised, the research institution is required to notify MOH and submit a declaration of compliance before it commences operation. Once recognised as such, it is under legal obligation to appoint an IRB to review all research under its supervision and control, and to report any serious adverse events as defined in the legislation. Within what is described as a system of self-accountability, research institutions are recognised to have a central role. The legislation further requires a close relationship between a research

---

[211] *Ibid*, Section 3(5).

institution, and its appointed IRB, primarily because the research institution (RI) assumes responsibility for the research that has been reviewed by its IRB. The legal responsibilities of an IRB are essentially similar to its role within the ethical framework; its primary responsibility being the protection of the safety, dignity and welfare of human research participants.

In its SC Report and its HA Report, the BAC has recommended that a single national body be established to review and monitor all stem cell research involving human pluripotent stem cells or human-animal combinations conducted in Singapore. This national body is likely to be similar to the national entity that has been recommended by the AMS, or a dedicated review process like SCRO or an ESCRO committee. It is still unclear if such a separate and dedicated entity, or a triaging body like the ASC in the UK, will be established. Currently, all such research will require review by an IRB. However, there appears to be a disparity in the additional requirements. Whereas approval from MOH must be obtained if research involving the use of human eggs, human embryos, or 'HAC gamete/embryos' is conducted in a licenced premise (i.e. a hospital or a clinic),[212] only notification is required under the HBRA if such research falls only within this regime.[213] In the light of the legislative provision that reserves for the Minister the power to prescribe additional requirements to be satisfied for restricted human biomedical research,[214] and in the interest of consistency and completeness (particularly in the interface

---

[212] Ministry of Health, *Licensing Terms and Conditions for Assisted Reproduction Centres*, 2011, at paragraphs 9.1 and 10.3. The role of the MOH under this regime is likely to be similar to the HFEA's. Whether this mechanism should be consolidated with the newly established regime under the HBRA is an open question at the time of writing.

[213] *Human Biomedical Research Act* 2015, Section 31(2)(c). Restricted human biomedical research is to be reviewed by an IRB or "such other committee as may be prescribed, comprising members with certain specified qualifications." Hence, at the minimum, restricted human biomedical research must be subject to review by an IRB (which may or may not be a stem cell specific IRB) and notice must also be provided to MOH.

[214] *Ibid*, Section 31(1).

between IRB review and animal ethics review), it seems likely that a dedicated review process will be implemented under the HBRA.

2.8 Pragmatism in Bioethics and in Law

Political liberalism and pragmatism are concepts clearly beyond the scope of this book to develop fully, but they are implicit in the policy work that has gone on around the human embryo in biomedical research. The 14 day limit and its inscription in legislation, along with the regulatory infrastructure that has emerged, could well be interpreted as an expression of the middle-ground view that a human embryo has intermediate moral status. It is also a rather elaborate compromise, as Devolder has argued, that ultimately lacks internal consistency. Its expression in the discarded-created distinction fails as the use of either research or supernumerary embryos encourages the creation of embryos that will be destroyed. The researcher's involvement (referred to as 'agency cost') in both cases is equivalent.[215] The use-derivation distinction (whether with cut-off dates or not) also fails because, embryo destruction is encouraged in using hESCs for research.[216] In this concluding section to the chapter, I want to pick up on where Devolder's discussion left off – on the cost of compromises. She explains that compromising in ethics is almost always pro-blematic due to the epistemic cost entailed. It hampers the formation of correct beliefs because a compromise position is mistakenly taken to have evidential value after some time, which it in fact lacks. Compromise also weakens commitments that are important for epistemic progress.[217]

---

[215] Katrien Devolder, *The Ethics of Embryonic Stem Cell Research*. Oxford: Oxford University Press, 2015, at 75-76.

[216] *Ibid*, at 104

[217] *Ibid*, at 148-151. Devolder refers to these two components of the epistemic cost of compromises as the 'Problem of False Testimony' and the 'Problem of the Erosion of Epistemic Standards'.

To be fair, Devolder makes clear at the end of her work that she is not offering policy advice, and her intent has only been to emphasise the need to clearly distinguish between the correct ethical position and a compromise.[218] It seems to me that what is to be taken as the correct ethical position ultimately depends on the sort of moral status that a human embryo should have, which remains ethically ambiguous. The middle ground viewpoint is an epistemically problematic compromise if one's analytical stance is that an embryo should have full moral status. If people do generally hold the view that an embryo should have some intrinsic value, but not to the extent of fully grown and competent human beings, then the middle ground may well be a reasonable analytical starting point. Returning to our consideration of the policy work on human pluripotent stem cell research, it seems to me that it is quite a different epistemic work-in-progress. From the practices of the advisory or professional bodies (like the Warnock committee, BAC, AMS or NAS) that we have considered, their intent is clearly not directed at resolving first order moral questions. Turning to the BAC in particular, its role is anchored in its repeated emphasis on 'just' and 'sustainable'. And its work has been directed at a more pragmatic goal of devising fair and durable terms of cooperation on an issue that has drawn diverse and irreconcilable ideologies and beliefs. In a general sense, this enterprise is one that challenges all liberal constitutional democracies, and was a central focus in Rawls's *Political Liberalism*.[219] By his analysis, mutual respect and cooperation based on terms that are fair is an indispensable component to any response to this question. Being fair or 'just' is not limited to impartiality, but must be reasonable in an ethical sense, which is a willingness to propose fair terms of

---

[218] *Ibid*, at 152.
[219] John Rawls, *Political Liberalism*. New York: Columbia University Press, 1996. In this work, Rawls queries (at 4) if it is possible "for there to exist over time a just and stable society of free and equal citizens who remain profoundly divided by reasonable religious, philosophical and moral doctrine?".

cooperation and abide by them when others do, as well as to accept the use of public reason rather than to attempt to enforce one's own comprehensive doctrine through law.[220]

In my view, the ideals of political liberalism underscore the policy work on human pluripotent stem cell research we have considered in the earlier sections. As I have also explained, the endeavours have largely been pragmatic;[221] not to be understood in a conventional sense, but rather as akin to a philosophical tradition that is focused on functionality and practice, rather than the search for an *a priori* metaphysical truth. Policy work and its epistemology are recognised to be fallible and revisable. Often undertaken with an experimental mind-set, it need not be entirely committed to empiricism (as in the case of the BAC's approach). Pragmatism also underscores the work of regulatory authorities like the HFEA, as the following passage illustrates:[222]

> Our laws cannot reflect the sheer variety of moral customs and beliefs held by the population. In general, then, the law enforces what might be termed the lowest common denominator of morality: the Millian principle, which states that freedom should be curtailed only where there is risk of harm to others. This is what the current regulatory framework seeks to do, while recognizing the challenges inherent in identifying and defining what constitutes risk. Clearly, this is not identical with everyone's perception of morality, but – in theory at least – differing value systems can operate with this legal context, without necessarily being enforced by it. Accordingly, the law around fertility treatments avoids proscriptions based on moral assumptions ... Rather, the most basic kind of risk-avoidance strategy is adopted.

---

[220] *Ibid*, at 54.

[221] Philip Kitcher, *Preludes to Pragmatism: Toward a Reconstruction of Philosophy.* Oxford: Oxford University Press, 2012.

[222] Ruth Deech and Anna Smajdor, *From IVF to Immortality: Controversy in the Era of Reproductive Technology.* Oxford: Oxford University Press, 2007, at 177-178.

It is also animated in the English Court of Appeal's decision in *R (on the application of Quintavalle) v Human Fertilisation and Embryology Authority*, which demonstrates an attempt to manage normative indeterminacy within a structure that is established for this purpose, and essentially on the basis that the judgment offers a fair and reasonable forward in the public sphere.[223] Arguably, the policy and regulatory practices that have emerged around human pluripotent stem cell research reflect a broader civic epistemology, which may have some semblance to Rawls's notion of a reasonable comprehensive doctrine.[224] This is a topic we shall return to in Chapter 7. We first consider specifically how professional and public bodies like the BAC have drawn on bioethics and law to constitute this civic epistemology, as well as its artefacts.

---

[223] [2003] 3 All ER 113.
[224] John Rawls, *Political Liberalism*. New York: Columbia University Press, 1996, at 36.

3

Comparison as Bioethical Practice

3.1 Introduction

Comparison in the form of comparative tables is ubiquitous in bioethics and taken for granted. Legal and non-legal norms are regarded as effectively similar, thereby lending support to the argument of Hans Kelsen that differences are mainly attributable to a variety of analytical or prescriptive standpoints. To a large degree, this phenomenon could be seen as a result of theoretical syllogism supported by pre-existing normative discourses and frameworks. On a levelled normative platform, comparison becomes functional in terms of relating problem to goal, and incommensurability is overcome. It is argued that comparison is not merely functional, but also relational and reflexive. Comparison creates normative positionality, which arises from the making of associative claims. This exercise is closely related to reputational standards (e.g. perceptions of 'ethically sound research practices') and has often been strategically deployed to advance certain policy agendas. However, positionality necessitates reflexivity, so that the ordering and internalisation entailed in comparison is also interpretive sense-making, which could make a profound impact on the comparatist 'self'. In addition, comparison could instil a sense of solidarity. This in turn confers a degree of durability on the relations drawn, and blurs the distinction between technique and epistemology in comparison.

Annelise Riles provides an intriguing account of Henry Wigmore's idiosyncratic "parade of oddities" that ranges from facsimiles of the American Declaration of Independence to an eight-foot-tall copy of the stone bearing the Hammurabi Code.[225] Even more so is the parallel that she draws between Wigmore's collection with a diverse array of curios collected by Ming and Qing emperors from different civilisations, cultures and historical episodes. Whether in treasure boxes or on display stands, these collections tell us some things about the time and place from which the objects were drawn, or at least their imputed meanings. For Henry Wigmore and perhaps for these emperors of Imperial China, the experiences that these collections invoke are arguably similar to what one would gain from a reflective visit to say, the British Museum. Although one can never quite fully understand the stories, beliefs, practices, mind-sets or cultures surrounding the collections, they could confer on one a sense of the place that Britain has (and has had) in the world. One could further imagine that in studying a French tea cup in his collection, a Qing emperor better appreciates Chinese tea culture through contrast with French upper class sensibilities in tea appreciation.[226] In other words, the objects in the emperor's collection confer a self-understanding by mapping the place of Chinese civilisation in the world. This knowledge of self comes not only from the constituent artefacts in the collections, but from the collections in their entirety.

The office of the BAC Secretariat is relatively modest in size when compared with the offices of similar bodies such as the Danish Council of Ethics. However, not far from the main door and just outside the meeting room is an in-built cabinet that stretches from ceiling to floor and across the entire west wall. Behind the sliding doors that conceal the cabinet shelves are rows of neatly aligned

---

[225] Annelise Riles, Wigmore's Treasure Box: Comparative Law in the Era of Information. *Harvard International Law Journal* (1999) 40, 1: 221-283, at 258.
[226] *Ibid*, at 268 and 277.

folders, marked and segregated by country. Within each clearly labelled folder are documents on laws, regulations and policies on topics of bioethical concern in different countries. Placed alongside these folders are publications of different bioethics bodies, similarly segregated by jurisdiction. At certain parts along the shelves, one would find souvenir-like objects, either from visitors to the Secretariat or from visits overseas. This impressive display is not unlike museum collections or collections of the Ming and Qing emperors. But unlike the artefacts of the Imperial household, many of the folders and publications constitute the Secretariat's tools of trade. These materials both enable and arise from comparative work that the Secretariat actively engaged in. In fact, it is difficult to think about policy work without some form of comparison being undertaken. In the course of preparing materials and documents for consideration at meetings of the BAC and its Working Group, as well as for meetings with their consultation parties, one of my key responsibilities with the Secretariat was to determine comparatively how other jurisdictions were addressing similar bioethical concerns. There appeared to be a common mind-set among policy-makers, scientists and interested members of the public alike that there was not only a shared understanding of these concerns, but also some common response to them. Hence a genuine interest in relevant international responses and developments was evident in all quarters. More importantly, these bioethical concerns were both understood and responded to relationally, and in some instances, collaboratively.

This chapter considers the rationales and techniques by which comparative projects for the BAC's reports on human oocyte donation and research involving human-animal combination have been carried out. In particular, I attempt to explicate the comparative mentality, comparative law-as-technocratic practice, and their epistemological and relational significance. Although policy work is a critical state function, it operates beyond the nation-state as policy workers have to "reach 'upwards' to the international level, 'sideways' to business groups and non-governmental organisations, and 'downwards' to local communities and social groups."[227] This aspect of policy work is perhaps most evident in the comparisons that appears to me to be near ubiquitous in the policy environment. As we shall see, comparisons undertaken by the BAC cuts across all these domains. At the international level, many transnational documents and organisations continue to exert significant influence over how 'ethical' conduct should be understood and practiced. There is indeed significant effort, spearheaded by international organisations such as CIOMS, UNESCO and WHO, to harmonise and operationalise certain standards pertaining to biomedical research. In recent years, this agenda has taken an increasingly institutional form around the globe. As a policy body, the 'upwards' reach of the BAC has always been influenced by interests 'sideways' and 'downwards'. Comparison creates relationality that is both discursive (at the level of narratives) and political (among jurisdictions, commonly referred to as 'benchmarking'). Such relationality could in turn provide a justification for change.[228] In the comparative projects of the BAC, any such change that comparative relationality invokes would not find sufficient legitimacy unless also supported at some level by interests 'sideways' and 'downwards'. This is due in part to the discursive emphasis in bioethics on giving due regard to 'local' conditions. In considering comparative law-as-technocratic practice and mind-set, the 'upward' reach has a normative character and procedural form, as the sections that follow should hopefully make clear.

---

[227] Hal K Colebatch, Robert Hoppe and Mirka Noordegraaf, Understanding Policy Work. In Hal K Colebatch, Robert Hoppe and Mirko Noordegraaf (eds.), *Working for Policy*. Amsterdam: Amsterdam University Press, 2010, pp 11-25, at 21-22.

[228] In her study, Annelise Riles observes that comparative argument presented in graphical form to show a lack of 'global standards' is commonly used in many documents of the Japanese government to advance law reform projects. As we shall see, such comparative argument is also commonly utilised in the policy environment of Singapore. Annelise Riles, *Collateral Knowledge: Legal Reason in the Global Financial Market*. Chicago: University of Chicago Press, 2011, at 206-207.

3.2 Enabling Comparison through De-Juridification

Women were delineated as a particular group of research subjects because oocytes can only be obtained from them. This delineation was not a difficult one to make, unlike an artefact like human-animal combinations. Whereas the delineation between men and women on the basis of oocyte production reinforced a categorical (and biological) conceptualisation of 'women', human-animal combinations were regarded as fudging the delineation between human beings and non-human animals (especially primates). Hence the decision to split the draft into two consultation papers arose in part from the recognition that egg donation would not give rise to subject matter complications in a way that human-animal combinations were expected to. This assessment turned out to be correct in that the subsequent categorical definition of 'women' in both the ED Consultation Paper and ED Report did not attract any opposition or serious contention, not even from women-interest groups that have voiced concerns over reductionist conceptualisation of women's roles and rights in society. Another reason for the ready acceptance of this delineation was circumstantial. The scandal revolving around Professor Hwang Woo-Suk brought public attention to the very real risk that women could be exploited for research. Hence the introduction of measures to safeguard the interests of women in stem cell research – and any delineation to that effect – was a welcomed development.[229] The delineation and constitution of 'women' as a special class of research subjects will be discussed later on in the dissertation. Here, we consider the contribution of comparative law as a technocratic tool to the problematisation and comprehension of oocyte donation in stem cell research, as well as of human-animal combination, and their resolution.

---

[229] Interestingly, even a number of key organisations concerned with women's welfare did not think they have any significant role to play in the public consultation. Fieldnotes, 7 November 2007.

The 'problematisation' of women as potential donors of oocytes for research entailed a reasoning process that seems to me quite like conventional legal analysis, in that it encompassed thinking through a series of questions. We first asked whether oocyte donation should be allowed at all. If this was to be prohibited, it would be necessary to consider alternatives in view of the fact that oocytes are required to advance SCNT. However, if oocyte donation was to be allowed, public concerns over possible ethical infractions similar to those witnessed in South Korea would have to be addressed. Research was undertaken by the Secretariat to determine, through comparison, the policy and regulatory responses of leading scientific jurisdictions.

In 2007, only a limited number of jurisdictions had specifically considered oocyte donation for the purposes of stem cell research. And even for these jurisdictions, the central concern has been with human fertility and artificial reproduction. Furthermore, there was significant divergence in regulatory responses to the procurement, use and disposal of oocytes, as well as fertility treatment for women. This could be an outcome of what the authors of the 2007 Surveillance report of the IFFS consider to be a struggle between the requirements of good medical practice and societal values (such as human dignity) on human procreation.[230] Although primarily concerned with ART, the 2007 Surveillance was an important document for at least four reasons. First, it was a source of information on "why and what society is trying to achieve by its monitoring of ART".[231] More importantly for the Secretariat, this information also related to the legal or regulatory

---

[230] Jean Cohen, Howard Jones Jr., Ian Cooke and Roger Kempers (eds.), IFFS Surveillance 07. *Fertility and Sterility* 87 Suppl. 1: S1-S67. The struggle between 'good medical practice' and societal values has been explicitly set out in the Federation's 2010 Surveillance: "The great variations in the details of what can and cannot be done under legislation and guidelines from country to country suggest that influences are at work other than the goal of good medical practice." See Howard Jones Jr., Ian Cooke, Roger Kempers, Peter Brinsden and Doug Saunders (eds.), *IFFS Surveillance 2010*. Mount Royal, NJ: International Federation of Fertility Societies, September 2010, at 11.

[231] 2007 Surveillance: *Ibid* at S5.

constructions of oocytes and embryos. Second, it offered valuable insights on how the medical profession viewed, and contributed to, these constructions. Third, there was breadth of coverage and a policy orientation that rendered the information more accessible and useful, even though it was not otherwise detailed or adequately referenced to the respective sources. Fourth, the tabular analysis of comparative information in relation to countries with statutes or laws on ART and on donation of gametes provided inspiration on the type of analysis that could be deployed. Indeed, the comparative tables set out in the BAC's ED Consultation Paper and ED Report[232] on regulatory approaches to egg donation are broadly similar to the tabular analysis of the IFFS on donation of gametes.[233]

Apart from the IFFS 2007 Surveillance, a report by the European Commission on reproductive cell donation (EC RCD Report) was similarly helpful.[234] This comparative project was undertaken to determine the extent to which European Union member states have implemented the Directive on human tissues and cells,[235] and to address concerns over reports that some Romanian women have been exploited for eggs.[236] The EC RCD Report provided more substantial information and was more rigorous in its analysis than the IFFS 2007 Surveillance given the ability of the European

---

[232] Bioethics Advisory Committee, *Donation of Human Eggs for Research*. Singapore: Bioethics Advisory Committee, 7 November 2008, at 18-19, and at A-19-A-20.

[233] Jean Cohen, Howard Jones Jr., Ian Cooke and Roger Kempers (eds.), IFFS Surveillance 07. *Fertility and Sterility* 87 Suppl. 1: S1-S67, at S29-S30.

[234] European Commission. *Report on the Regulation of Reproductive Cell Donation in the European Union: Results of Survey*. Brussels: European Commission, February 2006.

[235] European Parliament and European Council. Directive 2004/23/EC of the European Parliament and of the Council of 31 March 2004 on setting standards of quality and safety for the donation, procurement, testing, processing, preservation, storage and distribution of human tissues and cells, Article 12 (on compensation).

[236] European Commission. *Report on the Regulation of Reproductive Cell Donation in the European Union: Results of Survey*. Brussels: European Commission, February 2006, at 2.

Commission to obtain relatively detailed information from many of its 27 member states and its narrower focus on essentially four concerns pertaining to reproductive cells (being informational privacy, compensation, consent and cross-border dealings).[237] Similar to the IFFS 2007 Surveillance, the EC RCD Report sets out comparatively the four different regulatory responses that member states have adopted:

(1) Explicit regulation through law or government rules that are legally binding,

(2) National or international guidelines that are binding,

(3) National or international guidelines that are not binding, and

(4) No regulation.[238]

A jurisdiction-by-jurisdiction tabular presentation of the regulatory responses to and sources (where available) of three of the four main concerns was also provided to substantiate the conclusions derived.[239] In contrast, the IFFS devised three categories of regulatory responses:

(a) Legally binding law, regulation or guidelines,

(b) Guidelines that are binding although not necessarily of a legal or regulatory nature, and

(c) No regulation.[240]

---

[237] In contrast, the 2007 IFFS Surveillance covered ART practices in 57 countries. The number of countries covered increased to 162 in the 2010 IFFS Surveillance.

[238] European Commission. *Report on the Regulation of Reproductive Cell Donation in the European Union: Results of Survey.* Brussels: European Commission, February 2006, at 7-8.

[239] *Ibid,* at 10-17.

[240] Jean Cohen, Howard Jones Jr., Ian Cooke and Roger Kempers (eds.), IFFS Surveillance 07. *Fertility and Sterility* 87 Suppl. 1: S1-S67, at S9. In the 2007 Surveillance, a separate table (at S11) provided information on whether a statute-covered country has a licensing body, the manner in which clinical surveillance has been conducted and the penalty for non-compliance. In the 2010 Surveillance,

Under this scheme, a country would be (in relation to donation of gametes for instance) 'Covered by statute', 'Covered by guidelines' or 'Not covered by statute or guidelines'.

Given the breadth of the 2007 IFFS Surveillance, the authors indicated that their classificatory scheme was devised to provide a very general overview of the regulatory landscape for ART and to facilitate discussion. They recognised that "the classification is admittedly arbitrary in that some part of an ART programme may be subject to national legislation, whereas other parts and perhaps the major part are covered by guidelines".[241] Although the simplicity in approach presented a very general level of commonality, subtle distinctions have not been properly accounted for. A negative implication of this could be a greater risk of misunderstanding or that the classification might itself be rendered inaccurate. For instance, the classification of Singapore as a 'guidelines' country in the 2007 IFFS Surveillance is itself problematic.[242] While the reference source was not explicitly indicated, the relevant 'guideline' would be a set of directives issued by the Ministry of Health on assisted reproduction services,[243] under which oocyte donation is permitted provided that certain requirements are observed. [244] However, as the binding authority of the directives is derived from the *Private Hospitals and Medical Clinics Act*, [245] it would have been more appropriate to

---

both tables (on regulatory responses and licensing body) were merged into a single table: Howard Jones Jr., Ian Cooke, Roger Kempers, Peter Brinsden and Doug Saunders (eds.), *IFFS Surveillance 2010*. Mount Royal, NJ: International Federation of Fertility Societies, September 2010, at 13-15.

[241] Jean Cohen, Howard Jones Jr., Ian Cooke and Roger Kempers (eds.), IFFS Surveillance 07. *Fertility and Sterility* 87 Suppl. 1: S1-S67, at S8.

[242] *Ibid*, at S9.

[243] Ministry of Health, *Licensing Terms and Conditions for Assisted Reproduction Centres*, 2011.

[244] The IFFS has correctly indicated this in a table on donation of gametes: Jean Cohen, Howard Jones Jr., Ian Cooke and Roger Kempers (eds.), IFFS Surveillance 07, *Fertility and Sterility* 87 Suppl. 1: S1-S67, at S30.

[245] Cap. 248, amended 2008.

categorise Singapore as a 'statutes' country instead. It may be that as there is no legislation that specifically addresses ART, this linkage between the directives and its originating legislation was missed out. Also omitted in the 2007 IFFS Surveillance was the *de facto* role that the Ministry performed as the licensing body of ART clinics under the same legislative framework.[246] In comparison to the UK for instance, Singapore could be interpreted as a 'guidelines' country as it does not have a specific legislation on ART and a specific licensing body (whereas the UK did in the form of the Human Fertilisation and Embryology Authority). Relative to the US however, Singapore should properly qualify as a 'statutes' country as it has a regulatory framework that is constituted under legislation and operates on a licensing system. Interestingly, the IFFS revised its categorisation in 2010, listing Singapore as a 'statutes' country *with* a licensing body,[247] when there have been no major changes to the regulatory framework from 2007. Curious enough, Singapore remains categorised as a 'guidelines' country in the tabular analysis of donation of gametes, even in its 2013 report.[248]

A key component in comparative analysis is the de-contextualisation and generalisation that are entailed. Continuing with our analysis of Singapore, legislation is usually intended to create a general framework within which more substantive provisions are set out in regulation (under a variety of names such as directives, rules or guidelines). This is especially true of those that are directed at technological matters (including biomedical sciences), as the law is

---

[246] Jean Cohen, Howard Jones Jr., Ian Cooke and Roger Kempers (eds.), IFFS Surveillance 07. *Fertility and Sterility* 87 Suppl. 1: S1-S67, at S11-S12.

[247] Howard Jones Jr., Ian Cooke, Roger Kempers, Peter Brinsden and Doug Saunders (eds.), *IFFS Surveillance 2010*. Mount Royal, NJ: International Federation of Fertility Societies, September 2010, at 15.

[248] *Ibid*, at 50; IFFS, *IFFS Surveillance 2013*. Mount Royal, NJ: International Federation of Fertility Societies, October 2013, at 20.

often viewed as slow to change and hence lagging behind.[249] There are exceptional statutory responses that arise from time to time, such as the *Human Cloning and Other Prohibited Practices Act*,[250] but even then, it is not prescriptive as to procedural details and it was enacted under relatively unusual circumstances.[251] The very process of de-contextualisation and generalisation began from the initial stages of the research in the attempt to understand and concisely describe the regulatory positions of different jurisdictions on the subject of oocyte donation and the salient concerns that they addressed. As the authors of the 2007 IFFS Surveillance observed, a number of countries made this task a formidable one.[252] Among the 'core' common law jurisdictions, Australia, India and the United States were such countries. At that time, these three jurisdictions did not have any national legislation that addressed ART, but have relied on a less direct form of control. In India, ART clinics are accredited by state-level accrediting authorities. A state authority is 'regulatory' in that it could order the closure of a clinic within its jurisdiction or levy fines. The guidelines that the state regulatory authorities implement are prescribed by the Indian Ministry of Health and Family Welfare,

---

[249] Interview with Associate Prof Terry Kaan, 16 June 2009. The reasons underlying this view are varied and complex. On the one hand, statutory laws are regarded by some policymakers as embodiment of social consensus or values. Consequently, laws are not to be readily adopted, revised or repealed. Others consider any changes to or repeal of laws to undermine their institutional credibility. Still others, particularly the bureaucracy, adopt this view in order to keep laws general and so secure for themselves maximum operational flexibility. This view is further discussed in a later chapter.

[250] Cap. 131B, 2005 Revised Edition.

[251] I have considered the unique circumstances leading up to its enactment elsewhere. See Calvin Ho, Governing Cloning: United Nations' Debates and the Institutional Context of Standards. In Benjamin J Capps and Alastair V Campbell (eds.), *Contested Cells: Global Perspectives on the Stem Cell Debate*. London: Imperial College Press, 2010, pp 121-154.

[252] Jean Cohen, Howard Jones Jr., Ian Cooke and Roger Kempers (eds.), IFFS Surveillance 07. *Fertility and Sterility* 87 Suppl. 1: S1-S67, at S8.

and are hence 'national' standards.[253] The exact legal status of the guidelines is unclear but as they are issued by the central government, state regulatory authorities would be expected to implement them, particularly since India is a unitary state. For federalist jurisdictions of Australia and the United States, ART clinics fall within the almost exclusive purview of their constitutive states. In Australia, ART practices in the state of Victoria are strictly regulated by state legislation.[254] While the situation is similar in the United States, the federal government exerts some degree of control over ART research through the Food and Drug Administration (FDA). For instance, embryology laboratories and implantation of gametes (falling within the definition of tissue transplantation) must meet regulatory requirements of the FDA.[255]

Unlike the IFFS Surveillances, no caveat or indication of categorical ambiguities has been reported in the EC RCD Report. Greater confidence on the part of the EC in categorisation of regulatory approaches or responses may be attributable to its narrower issue focus and reliance on the Directive as an interpretive framework. A helpful aspect of the EC RCD Report was its brief descriptions of regulatory positions (including sources), as supplementary information to the comparative analysis. This issue-specific country-by-country analysis was adopted by the BAC Secretariat in conducting its background work. Information produced was presented within an interpretive framework developed based on key 'markers' or considerations

---

[253] Government of India (Ministry of Health and Family Welfare) and National Academy of Medical Sciences (Indian Council of Medical Research), *National Guidelines for Accreditation, Supervision and Regulation of ART Clinics in India.* New Delhi: S. Narayan & Sons, 2005.

[254] The relevant state statutes are *Assisted Reproductive Treatment Act* 2008, *Research Involving Human Embryos Act* 2008 and *Prohibition of Human Cloning for Reproduction* Act 2008.

[255] Under the US Code of Federal Regulations (CFR) 21 Part 1271 on *Human Cells, Tissues, and Cellular and Tissue-based Products*, facilities that perform IVF treatments are required to register with the FDA.

derived from ethical, legal and regulatory literature. With growing interest in stem cell technology and the scandal around Professor Hwang, there was a sizeable literature on the subject. These key 'markers' were drawn from regulatory provisions relating to oocyte donation for non-treatment purposes, consent requirements, payment and unexpected occurrences from the donation. Once substantiated, this interpretive framework was re-formulated as an overview of regulatory positions pertaining to oocyte donation for research. Table 3.1 is a segment of this overview.[256] To facilitate discussions in meetings, this tabular display was re-formulated to focus on critical issues that require specific attention, such as payment for oocyte donation. Table 3.2 is an excerpt from a more comprehensive table that was circulated for discussion at meetings.[257]

An improvisation that was devised to circumvent the difficulty of categorising countries such as the US was to raise the analysis to a normative level through de-juridification. This came about when my initial insistence in clearly distinguishing the ethical standards of national organisations from standards prescribed by regulation or statute was regarded as either being excessively pedantic or

---

[256] Fieldnotes, 20 August 2007. Since 2007, a number of the countries considered, have revised and updated their regulatory positions. In India, a new set of guidelines have been issued in 2013: Indian Council of Medical Research, Department of Health Research and Department of Biotechnology, *Guidelines for Stem Cell Research*, 2013. Under Section 13.2, donation of eggs is allowed but subject to oversight by an ethics committee, as well as consent requirements. In Singapore, the guidelines on assisted reproduction services of 2006 has been replaced by the *Licensing Terms and Conditions for Assisted Reproduction Centres* of 2011. In the UK, the Human Fertilisation & Embryology Authority has similarly updated its requirements following the amendment of the HFEA in 2008: Human Fertilisation and Embryology Authority. *Code of Practice.* London: Human Fertilisation and Embryology Authority, 2009 (October 2015, 8th Edition).

[257] Fieldnotes, 21 August 2007. The regulatory provisions in Japan has been updated in 2014. See: Ministry of Education, Culture, Sports, Science and Technology of Japan, *Guidelines for the Derivation of Human Embryonic Stem Cells*, 2014; and Ministry of Education, Culture, Sports, Science and Technology of Japan, *Guidelines for Distribution and Utilization of Human Embryonic Stem Cells*, 2014. See also footnote to Table 3.1, and discussions in Chapters 2 and 6.

Table 3.1. Regulatory Landscape in Select Jurisdictions on Egg Donation (as at 2007)

Country/ Organisation	Women Not Undergoing Fertility Treatment as Oocyte Donors for Research	Consent Requirements	Payment/ Compensation/ Reimbursement	When Unexpected Event Occurs	Comments/Other Requirements
China Ministry of Health and Ministry of Science and Technology Guidelines	Not specified	Written informed consent required	Selling or/and buying of human gamete, zygote or embryo prohibited	Information not available	Privacy of donor protected; IRB responsible for approval and supervision of the research.
India Indian Council of Medical Research (ICMR) Department of Biotechnology, Ministry of	Allowed (Para. 11.4)	Informed consent required Minimum information provided in the Guidelines The attending physician responsible for the infertility treatment and the investigator deriving	No commodification of human egg, sperm or embryo or somatic cells for use in SCNT, by way of payment or services, except for reimbursement of reasonable expenses incurred by the	Research subjects who suffer physical injury as a result of their participation are entitled to financial or other assistance to compensate them equitably for any temporary or permanent impairment	IRB and IC –SCRT to review and approve the process of procurement of gametes, blastocysts or somatic cells for the purpose of generating new hES cell lines, including procurement of blastocyts in excess

Table 3.1. *(Continued)*

Country/ Organisation	Women Not Undergoing Fertility Treatment as Oocyte Donors for Research	Consent Requirements	Payment/ Compensation/ Reimbursement	When Unexpected Event Occurs	Comments/Other Requirements
Science and Technology (DBT)		or proposing to use hES cells preferably should not be the same person.	person {amount to be decided by the Institutional Committee for Stem Cell Research and Therapy (IC-SCR)/ National Apex Committee for Stem Cell Research}.	or disability. In case of death, their dependents are entitled to material compensation [ICMR, Ethical Guidelines for Biomedical Research on Human Subjects, 2000 (p.21, Section V).]	of clinical need from infertility clinics.
Singapore *Guidelines for Private Healthcare Institutions providing Assisted Reproduction Services:* Regulation 4 of the *Private*	Allowed (AR Directives 8.6)	Explicit consent required Comprehensive information to be provided When consent is taken, there should be no coercion, inducement or undue influence. The principal physician and	Commerce and sale of donated materials prohibited.	In the event of any significant injury, the subject must be entitled to receive compensation regardless of whether there may or may not have been legal negligence or legal liability on any other basis. Where no provision for	IRB and MOH approval required for all research involving human embryos and oocytes. Clinic performing the oocyte retrieval must be licensed by the MOH. Potential oocyte donors, who are not undergoing any

(Continued)

Table 3.1. (Continued)

Country/Organisation	Women Not Undergoing Fertility Treatment as Oocyte Donors for Research	Consent Requirements	Payment/Compensation/Reimbursement	When Unexpected Event Occurs	Comments/Other Requirements
Hospitals and Clinics Regulations 2006 (Cap 248, Rg 1) NMEC, *Ethical Guidelines on Research involving Human Subjects*		embryologist in charge of the patient's AR treatment must not be the principal investigator of the research team working on the same oocyte and/or resulting embryo obtained from his/her patient.		compensation has been made, this fact ought to be disclosed to the research subjects before the initiation of the study. [NMEC *Ethical Guidelines on Research involving Human Subjects*, Section 3.3.2]	fertility treatment, must be interviewed by a panel. The panel must be satisfied that the prospective donor is of sound mind, has clear understanding of the nature and consequences of the donation and has given explicit consent without coercion or inducements.
UK HFE Act, 1990 HFEA Code of Practice, 6th Edition, 2003	Not allowed [HFEA Code of Practice – section 5.8 (ii)] Currently the sources of	Voluntary - No pressure or undue influence and sufficient time allowed for decision to be made	From 1 April 2006, donors may be reimbursed for reasonable expenses incurred within the UK in connection	"Reasonable expenses incurred by an egg donor who becomes ill as a direct result of donating, may also be reimbursed by the	The objective of the research should satisfy one or more of the purposes listed in the HFE [Research

Table 3.1. *(Continued)*

Country/Organisation	Women Not Undergoing Fertility Treatment as Oocyte Donors for Research	Consent Requirements	Payment/Compensation/Reimbursement	When Unexpected Event Occurs	Comments/Other Requirements
	human eggs for research are eggs that failed-to-fertilise during IVF cycles or eggs donated from women undergoing sterilisation. In May 2006, the HFEA announced that it will be preparing a consultation programme on egg donation for research. This is to address the range of strong	Written consent required beforehand for any observers' presence during examination, treatment or counselling Donors may specify the conditions for the use of their oocytes Withdrawal of consent allowed up till the time the oocyte is used Consent for oocyte donation to be taken: After counselling and sufficient and appropriate information (oral + written) provided	with the donation and be compensated for loss of earnings (but not for other costs or inconveniences) in connection with the donation, up to a daily maximum of £55.19 but with an overall limit of £250 for each course of sperm donation or each cycle of egg donation. There is no restriction on the value of other benefits but these are limited to treatment services in the course of the	treatment centre" (HFEA COP 4.3)	Purposes) Regulations 2001 Person responsible for the infertility treatment and the research should not be the same person. Suppliers of gametes or embryos who are not individual donors may be given and may receive money or other benefits for that supply subject to the conditions. The most that they may be given or receive is enough money or money's worth to reimburse reasonable expenses. The supplier may take

(Continued)

Table 3.1. (*Continued*)

Country/ Organisation	Women Not Undergoing Fertility Treatment as Oocyte Donors for Research	Consent Requirements	Payment/ Compensation/ Reimbursement	When Unexpected Event Occurs	Comments/Other Requirements
	and contrasting views among professionals on this issues as well as international concern.	In advance i.e. beore the fertility treatment starts Where genetic research is to be carried out on identifiable samples, explicit consent must be obtained after sufficient information is provided.	donation cycle unless there is a medical reason why they cannot be provided at that time (i.e. centres are no longer permitted to offer sterilisation as a benefit in kind).		into account all costs, including out-of-pocket expenses connected directly with the particular supply.

Table 3.2. Re-formulated Comparative Table with Focus on Payment (as at 2007)

Country/Organisation	Donation of Human Oocytes for Research	Compensation / Reimbursement
China (Hong Kong) *Human Reproductive Technology Ordinance*	Oocytes may not be donated to create embryos for the purpose of research. (Section 15, (1))	No payment may be made or received for the supply of, or for an offer to supply, oocytes. (Section 16, (1))
China *Ethical Guiding Principles on Human Embryonic Stem Cell Research* (2003)	Oocytes may be voluntarily donated.	The buying and selling of oocytes is prohibited.
India Indian Council of Medical Research - *National Guidelines For Stem Cell Research and Therapy* (2006)	The donation of oocytes for research, including donations from healthy women not undergoing treatment, is permitted. (Paragraph 11.4)	Commodification of oocytes by way of payment or services is prohibited, except for reimbursement of reasonable expenses incurred by the person. (Paragraph 11.3)
Japan *Guidelines for Derivation and Utilization of Human Embryonic Stem Cells* (2001)	Oocytes may not be donated to create embryos for the derivation of embryonic stem cell lines. (Article 6)	
Singapore *Directives for Private Healthcare Institutions Providing Assisted Reproduction Services*, Revised Mar 2006 (AR Directives) *Human Cloning and Other Prohibited Practices Act* 2004 (Human Cloning Act)	The donation of oocytes for research, including donations from healthy women not undergoing treatment, is permitted. (AR Directives, Paragraph 8.5)	The commercial trading in oocytes is prohibited, but the reimbursement of any reasonable expenses incurred by a person in relation to the supply of oocytes is permitted. (Human Cloning Act, Section 13) The buying and selling of oocytes shall not be carried out in any AR Centre. (AR Directives, Paragraph 4.11.2i)

(Continued)

Table 3.2. (*Continued*)

Country/Organisation	Donation of Human Oocytes for Research	Compensation / Reimbursement
UK HFEA Statement on Donating Eggs for research, 21 February 2007 (HFEA Statement) Directions Given under the HFE Act 1990, Giving and receiving money or other benefits in respect of any supply of gametes or embryos, Ref. D.2006/1 (HFE Directions 2006/1)	The donation of oocytes for research, including donations from healthy women not undergoing treatment, is permitted. (HFEA Statement)	A donor may be reimbursed reasonable expenses which he or she has incurred, in connection with the donation. Donors may be compensated for loss of earnings (but not for other costs or inconveniences) up to a daily maximum of £55.19 but with an overall limit of £250 (or the equivalent in local currency) for each course of sperm donation or each cycle of egg donation. There is no restriction on the value of other benefits which may be given to the donor, but the only benefits which may be offered for this purpose are treatment services. These services should be provided to the donor in the course of the donation cycle unless there is a medical reason why they cannot be provided at that time. (HFEA Directions 2006/1)

scrupulous. For instance, the ethical recommendations of the NAS would not formally amount to the 'national' position of the US as they do not have any formal legal or regulatory effect. I came to understand, from my colleagues first and then from meetings with key stakeholders, that the formal distinction between law and non-law prescriptions was not important as the practical consequences of violation were considered to be equally punitive. It was at this normative stratosphere that the recommendations (including proposed best practices and guidelines) of key national organisations (and, in the case of the US, key states such as California also) were taken to represent the 'national' position of a jurisdiction, particularly in the absence of a clear regulatory or statutory stance. This is arguably neo-positivist in orientation, as it is justified on the basis that the biomedical research and medical communities do not draw a clear distinction between law and ethics in practice, and they regard legal and ethical standards to be equally binding.[258] A further reason was an interest in general 'data' that would address policy (rather than legal or academic) concerns.[259] Whereas a guideline was considered to be too particular for comparison, its normative under-pinning made explicit through de-juridification was not. Within this expanded interpretive framework, the position of the US on payment for oocyte donation was presented in the form of Table 3.3 (excerpt).[260]

Table 3.3. Payment for Egg Donation in the USA (as at 2007)

Organisation	Donation of Human Oocytes for Research	Compensation/ Reimbursement
The Medical and Ethical Standards Regulations of the CIRM	Donation is allowed but informed consent required. The physician attending to any donor and the Principal Investigator shall not be the same person unless exceptional circumstances exist and with IRB approval.	Donors should receive no payment beyond reimbursement for permissible expenses. § 100100. Informed Consent Requirements, (b) (3) (D) (vii)

(Continued)

---

[258] My fieldwork data suggests that many doctors and researchers, even some policy-makers and regulators, have this broad normative mind-set towards ethical and legal requirements. This aspect of my research and its implications are further discussed below.

[259] Such an approach has been applied in comparative law: Anne Meuwese and Mila Versteeg, Quantitative methods for comparative constitutional law. In Maurice Adams and Jacco Bomhoff (eds.), *Practice and Theory in Comparative Law.* Cambridge: Cambridge University Press, 2012, pp 230-257.

[260] Fieldnotes, 21 August 2007. The regulatory landscape in the USA at the time of publication of this book is discussed in Chapter 2.

Table 3.3. (*Continued*)

Organisation	Donation of Human Oocytes for Research	Compensation/ Reimbursement
The Ethics Committee of the American Society for Reproductive Medicine - Financial Compensation of Oocyte Donors, Fertility and Sterility, E-pub 18 April 2007	Donation is allowed but informed consent must be taken before the collection of oocytes. Physicians should secure consent with a witness present and then place the consent form in a confidential file.	Compensation should be structured to acknowledge the time, inconvenience, and discomfort associated with screening, ovarian stimulation and oocyte retrieval. Compensation should not vary according to the planned use of the oocytes, the number or quality of oocytes retrieved, the number or outcome of prior donation cycles, or the donor's ethnic or other personal characteristics Total payments to donors in excess of $5,000 require justification and sums above $10,000 are not appropriate.
National Research Council and the Institute of Medicine of The National Academies - *Guidelines for Human Embryonic Stem Cell Research*, 2005, Amended 2007	Donation is allowed provided that written informed consent has been obtained. Minimum information to be provided before consent could be given. In addition, confirmation of consent required before research use and donors have right to withdraw consent before use.	Oocyte donors may be reimbursed only for direct expenses incurred as a result of the procedure, as determined by an Institutional Review Board. No cash or in kind payments should be provided for donating oocytes for research purposes. (Recommendation 16)
Bedford Stem Cell Research Foundation *Guidelines for Research with Human Eggs and Egg Donor Time Commitment*	Donation is allowed provided that consent is voluntary and informed.	Compensation provided for effort, travel and childcare expenses. Donor reimbursement ranged from US$560 to US$4,004, depending on expenses incurred and the stage of completion.

Regressing a regulatory requirement to its normative source corresponds well with the jurisprudence of Hans Kelsen. In Kelsen's view, law is a normative system which operates on the basis of normative imputation.[261] It is within this 'personifying fiction' that the notions of 'state' and 'person', among others, serve as a unifying point of imputation of norms.[262] More important for our analysis is his view that there is no specific system of norms that is distinctively or exclusively 'legal'. For Kelsen, differences between norms in law and those of other normative systems such as religion and ethics arise from differences in analytical or prescriptive standpoints.[263] Whereas Natural Lawyers have attempted to anchor substantive normative content in Reason, he considered basic norms to be relative (as they arise from different points of view), contingent and dependent on social practice.[264] A legal system, or indeed any system of norms, must be adhered to and put into action in order for it to be regarded as valid.[265] In other words, a basic norm could only be considered to be valid if it is 'efficacious'.[266] This is in turn dependent on certain social

---

[261] Hans Kelsen (tr. Michael Hartney), *General Theory of Norms.* Oxford: Clarendon Press, 1991, at 24.

[262] Jochen von Bernstorff and Thomas Dunlap, *The Public International Law Theory of Hans Kelsen: Believing in Universal Law.* Cambridge: Cambridge University Press, 2010, at 51.

[263] This does not mean that legal norms and moral norms are one and the same. Kelsen points out that in law, there is an essential connection between the norm commanding certain actions and the sanction-decreeing norm in most circumstances, whereas in morality, the latter is secondary to the former in all circumstances. Hans Kelsen (tr. Michael Hartney), *General Theory of Norms.* Oxford: Clarendon Press, 1991, at 143.

[264] Andrei Marmor, The Pure Theory of Law. *The Stanford Encyclopedia of Philosophy* (Spring 2016 Edition), Edward N Zalta (ed.). Available at: http://plato.stanford.edu/archives/spr2016/entries/lawphil-theory/.

[265] Hans Kelsen (tr. Michael Hartney), *General Theory of Norms.* Oxford: Clarendon Press, 1991, at 28. Kelsen argues that the validity of a norm is its existence: "That a norm 'is valid' means that it exists."

[266] Hans Kelsen (tr. Anders Wedberg), *General Theory of Law and State.* Cambridge MA: Harvard University Press, 1945, at 29. Hans Kelsen makes this observation on the outcome of normative imputation: "There is no such thing as responsibility in natural reality. Responsibility is constituted by a normative order such as

facts that constitute the content of the basic norm. Such 'social facts' are arguably similar to what Herbert Hart regards as 'Rules of Recognition'.[267]

Even if the validation of norms may be dependent on their social subscription, Kelsen follows David Hume in rejecting the viability of a linkage between the descriptive ('is') and the normative ('ought'). Indeed, his 'Pure Theory of Law' proposes law as an entirely normative construct, premised upon a hypothetical foundational norm that is both descriptive and prescriptive, and from which all other normative statements could be derived.[268] This is the famous basic norm (or *Grundnorm*), which – for Kelsen – is the only means by which objective validity of all resulting norms could be established through theoretical syllogism.[269] For the purposes of the comparative work I was involved in, the critical take-away point is that norms constitute a scheme of interpretation.[270] By Kelsen's analysis, legal norms are similar to (perhaps even the same as) ethical norms once the action commanding norm is dissociated from the sanction-decreeing norm.[271] It becomes possible, consequently, to place legal

---

morality or law ... This concept has not the negative meaning that the human will is not causally determined, but the positive meaning that human will, and consequently the human behavior caused by this will, is the end point of a normative imputation." See Hans Kelsen, *What is Justice? Justice, Law and Politics in the Mirror of Science*. Berkeley, Los Angeles and London: University of California Press, 1971, at 345.

[267] H L A Hart, *The Concept of Law*. Oxford: Clarendon, 1961, at 105.

[268] Hans Kelsen (tr. Max Knight), *Pure Theory of Law*, Berkeley and Los Angeles: University of California Press, 1967, at 8-9.

[269] Hans Kelsen (tr. Michael Hartney), *General Theory of Norms*. Oxford: Clarendon Press, 1991, at 252-254.

[270] Hans Kelsen (tr. Max Knight), *Pure Theory of Law*, Berkeley and Los Angeles: University of California Press, 1967, at 3-4.

[271] Kelsen points out that while law need not be moral or otherwise rely on moral justification, it can be part of morals when legal norms are consistent with moral norms: Hans Kelsen (tr. Max Knight), *Pure Theory of Law*, Berkeley and Los Angeles: University of California Press, 1967, at 62-63.

norms on the same analytical plane as ethical norms for the purpose of constructing an interpretive grid or framework. As noted earlier, most policy-makers, researchers and the public assume that legal norms are part of a broader system of moral norms. Almost all BAC members similarly hold this view (that legal norms are generally moral), even though they recognise the possibility of immoral laws.[272]

While Kelsen does not quite say what the *Grundnorm* is, if one considers it to be something like: 'Everyone is to observe the law, or suffer sanction for disobedience', this could be formulated in the context of biomedical research as: 'The procurement and provision of oocytes for biomedical research are to be done ethically'. From this fundamental premise, different values and approaches could be gathered in substantiating the different meanings of 'ethically'. The comparative table was thus constructed as a normative (interpretive) framework to 'fit in' different legal and ethical positions (and the jurisdictions they represent) on oocyte donation. Normative generality further enables the inclusion of regional and international standards in the analysis. The table would now present 'national' positions on par with regional and international standards on a common subject-specific normative platform in order to enable comparison. Relating this back to Kelsen, his 'Pure Theory of Law' similarly encompasses an international dimension. In his analytical scheme, international law was conceptualised as a formalised structure that normativised not only the relationship between states as equal subjects, but also between the state and its citizens. By this structure, an international normative order could be constituted

---

[272] The past and present BAC members whom I have interviewed were asked how they considered law to be different from ethics and morality. They were generally of the view that morality relates to personal values whereas ethics is concerned with shared values. Morality and ethics differ from law in that they are not explicitly backed by the state through sanction.

above states, so that "a norm of international law determined the spatial and temporal sphere of validity of state legal orders" that delimit "the material validity of state legal orders" as well as "regulate any human conduct through the instrument of the treaty".[273] Immediately apparent is the sublimation of context and circumstance in order to attain logical consistency. This de-contextualisation leads to a situation where:

> the relationship of both the state to the citizen and of the order of international law to the state were merely normative linkages between legal subjects that were themselves nothing more than the personified entity of a derived complex of rights and obligations ... [and that] the object of legal norms was, in the final analysis, always the conduct of individuals.[274]

To be sure, contemporary approaches have tended to rely less on formalistic construction of a universal normative order. They invariably exhibit sensitivity to cultural differences and substantive justice requirements. Take for instance Richard Evanoff's bioregional perspective on 'global ethics', where significant convergence of cultural values and norms is considered to be necessary to promote ecological sustainability, achieve social justice and maximise human wellbeing.[275] In addition, his approach encompasses not only the ideological (i.e. society and self), but also the material

---

[273] Jochen von Bernstorff and Thomas Dunlap, *The Public International Law Theory of Hans Kelsen: Believing in Universal Law.* Cambridge: Cambridge University Press, 2010, at 94 and 118. Kelsen's intent is to construct a 'world state' or civitas maxima, which requires neutral institutions to implement and enforce a system of universal law. See Hans Kelsen (tr. Max Knight), *Pure Theory of Law*, Berkeley and Los Angeles: University of California Press, 1967, at 328-347.

[274] von Bernstorff and Dunlap: *Ibid*, at 72.

[275] Richard Evanoff, *Bioregionalism and Global Ethics: A Transnational Approach to Achieving Ecological Sustainability, Social Justice, and Human Well-being.* New York and London: Routledge, 2011, at 37.

(i.e. ecological).[276] A motivation for developing a 'global' framework arises from a recognition of the limited explanatory power of both 'possibilism' (or 'localism') and 'determinism',[277] and the need to avoid any suggestion of a 'global monoculture', arising from the concept of 'global villages' and Wallerstein's notion of 'world system'.[278] With these sensibilities in mind, Table 3.4 constructed in the course of my work included the following regional and international standards on a single analytical platform.[279]

This simple, albeit deceptively straightforward, approach was quite immediately recognised as an important means of conveying information to the public. While interested members of the public would be keen to know how any position on oocyte donation proposed for Singapore would compare with other countries, they were unlikely to be interested in intricate details and discursive subtleties. For those who might be interested in such details, primary and secondary sources relied upon in the construction of the interpretive framework have been set out in the list of reference of the ED Report. The broad interpretive framework also helped policy-makers gain a sense of where Singapore's position was in relation to other countries. Within this framework, the position of different jurisdictions could be 'fitted in'. The 'fitting in' of jurisdictions is perhaps most clearly illustrated in this early version of a tabular display (see Table 3.5).[280]

However, this simple table of 'fitted' jurisdictions was not ultimately used in either the ED Consultation Paper or the ED Report as it was felt to be informationally inadequate. Instead, using the same interpretive framework, an informationally richer tabular display

---

276 Evanoff elaborates Dieter Steiner's "human ecological triangle": *Ibid*, at 34.
277 *Ibid*, at 172-173.
278 *Ibid*, at 13.
279 Fieldnotes, 21 August 2007. The 2016 guidelines of the ISSCR are discussed in Chapter 2.
280 Fieldnotes, 15 August 2007.

Table 3.4.   International Standards on Payment for Human Eggs (as at 2007)

Regional/International Organisation	Donation of Human Oocytes for Research	Compensation/Reimbursement
Bulgaria, Croatia, Cyprus, Czech Republic, Estonia, Greece, Hungary, Iceland, Lithuania, Moldova, Poland, Portugal, Romania, San Marino, Slovenia, Turkey *Convention for the Protection of Human Rights and Dignity of the Human Being with regard to the Application of Biology and Medicine: Convention on Human Rights and Biomedicine* (Oviedo, 4.IV.1997)	Oocytes may not be donated to create embryos for the purpose of research. (Article 18)	The human body and its parts shall not, as such, give rise to financial gain. (Article 21)
European Society of Human Reproduction and Embryology (ESHRE) ESHRE Task Force on Ethics and Law 12: Oocyte donation for non-reproductive purposes - Human Reproduction (March 2007)	Donation allowed subject to informed consent.	Oocyte donation for research should be a primarily altruistic act motivated by the wish to contribute to the advancement of science and medicine. However, oocyte donors should receive reimbursement for all direct and indirect costs of the procedure and should receive a compensation for the time lost and inconvenience suffered during the treatment. The compensation should be fair and in proportion to the amounts currently paid to research subjects. To prevent undue inducement and disproportional recruitment among vulnerable groups, illiterate and poor women should be excluded as donors.

Table 3.4. (*Continued*)

Regional/International Organisation	Donation of Human Oocytes for Research	Compensation/Reimbursement
International Federation of Gynecology and Obstetrics *Ethical Guidelines on the Sale of Gametes and Embryos*	Donation allowed subject to informed consent.	The donation of genetic material should be altruistic and free from commercial exploitation. Reasonable compensation for legitimate expenses is appropriate.
ISSCR *Guidelines for the Conduct of Human Embryonic Stem Cell Research* (21 December 2006)	Donation allowed subject to informed consent.	Where reimbursement for research participation is allowed, there must be a detailed and rigorous review to ensure that reimbursement of direct expenses or financial considerations of any kind do not constitute an undue inducement. Financial considerations of any kind should not be based on the number or quality of the oocytes themselves that are to be provided for research. There must be monitoring of recruitment practices to ensure that no vulnerable populations, for example, economically disadvantaged women, are disproportionately encouraged to participate as oocyte providers for research. (Section 11.5b)

of jurisdictional positions on the issues of concern was developed. The 'constructed' nature of the tabular display entitled "Regulatory Approaches of Selected Countries to Human Egg Donation" ultimately published in the ED Report was acknowledged in a number of qualifications presented alongside.[281] Regional and international normative standards have not been included in the table in order to avoid public confusion. In the public mind, international standards

---

[281] Bioethics Advisory Committee, *Donation of Human Eggs for Research*. Singapore: Bioethics Advisory Committee, November 2008, at 19, table references (1) to (4).

Table 3.5. 'Fitted' Table on Egg Donation (as at 2007)

Oocyte Donation is Prohibited	Oocyte Donation from IVF Fertility Patients is Permitted	Oocyte Donation from Healthy Participants Permitted	Embryos May Not Be Created for Research	Reimbursement Permitted	Compensation Permitted
	Australia	Australia		Australia	
	Canada	Canada		Canada	
				Czech Republic	
			Finland	Finland	Finland
			France		
			Hong Kong	Hong Kong	
			Iceland		
	India	India		India	
			Ireland		
			Italy		
Norway					
	Singapore	Singapore		Singapore	
	Sweden	Sweden			
			Switzerland		
	UK	UK		UK	UK

could be seen as universal norms that should be observed by all jurisdictions. If so, the juxtaposition of national standards with those labelled as 'international' could undermine the legitimacy of the former.

For the comparative table on oocyte donation that was put together, abstraction and interpretive application to the issues under consideration from the policy standpoint of Singapore was explicitly acknowledged.[282] It was further noted that while many jurisdictions

---

282 The IFFS similarly acknowledges reductionism in its approach. Howard Jones Jr., Ian Cooke, Roger Kempers, Peter Brinsden and Doug Saunders (eds.), *IFFS Surveillance 2010*. Mount Royal, NJ: International Federation of Fertility Societies, September 2010, at 11.

have regulatory or professional governance frameworks to ensure that ART practices are properly carried out, donation of oocytes for research might not have been specifically addressed. In the absence of explicit provision, it was assumed that "many countries that allow egg donation for assisted reproduction would generally allow a similar donation to research that is concerned with reproduction".[283] Hence what we witness here is not only a translation of different relations of governance (be they ethical, regulatory or statutory in nature) to a more generic normative template, but also the re-definition of essentially medical concerns (i.e. in ART) to research interests. In other words, if egg donation for assisted reproduction is allowed, the implication would be that such donation should be allowed for research directed at improving ART. However, such an implication could not be extended to oocyte donation for SCNT, which might be regarded as morally repulsive or sensitive. Where such information was unavailable, this was duly indicated in the table as 'NI'. In addition, it was made clear that the table was not concerned with reproductive or therapeutic cloning even though oocytes would be obtained for this technological application. The ethical, legal and social implications of this technology have been considered in an earlier report.[284] Instead, the table is primarily concerned with the permissibility of oocyte donation for the purposes of research (stem cell research in particular) and with payment where such donation is permitted. The two components of payment (an issue we will discuss further later on) – being compensation and reimbursement – are reiterated. Although the table is intended to be instructive, the information presented is not a precisely accurate representation of the regulatory approaches of foreign jurisdictions. To a large extent, this is due to limitations in

---

283 Bioethics Advisory Committee, *Donation of Human Eggs for Research*. Singapore: Bioethics Advisory Committee, November 2008, at 19, table reference (4).
284 Bioethics Advisory Committee, *Ethical, Legal and Social Issues in Stem Cell Research, Reproductive and Therapeutic Cloning*. Singapore: Bioethics Advisory Committee, June 2002.

the construction process itself, especially with problems of interpretation and translation. The basis on which countries were selected
for consideration was also explained as including "availability of
information (in English), availability of legislation and guidelines
(both legally binding and non-binding) on the issues considered, and
the extent that these issues have been deliberated on and debated in
those countries."[285] The table ultimately published in the ED Report is
in the form of Table 3.6.[286]

Table 3.6. Published Comparative Table on Egg Donation (as at 2007)

Country	Egg Donation for Assisted Reproduction (AR)	Payment for Egg Donation for AR	Egg Donation for Research	Payment for Egg Donation for Research
Austria	✗	na	✗	na
Australia (Commonwealth)	p	R	p	R
Belgium	p	C	p	NI
Brazil	p	NI	p	R
Canada	p	R	p	R
China	✗	na	p	R
Czech Republic	p	R	p	R
Denmark	p	C	p	NI
Estonia	p	R	p	R
Finland	p	R	p	R
France	p	R	p	R
Germany	✗	na	NI	NI
Greece	p	✗	p	✗
Hong Kong	p	C	p	C

285 Bioethics Advisory Committee, *Donation of Human Eggs for Research*. Singapore:
Bioethics Advisory Committee, November 2008, at 19, table reference (2).
286 *Ibid*, at 18-19. The footnote references have been edited out of the table in the
interest of conciseness.

Table 3.6. (*Continued*)

Country	Egg Donation for Assisted Reproduction (AR)	Payment for Egg Donation for AR	Egg Donation for Research	Payment for Egg Donation for Research
Hungary	p	C	p	C
India	p	C	p	R
Israel	p	NI	NI	NI
Italy	✕	na	NI	NI
Japan	✕	na	p	R
Korea (South)	p	R	p	R
Netherlands	p	R	p	R
New Zealand	p	R	p	R
Norway	✕	na	✕	na
Singapore	p	R	p	R
Slovenia	p	R	NI	NI
South Africa	p	R	p	R
Spain	p	C	p	C
Sweden	p	R	p	R
Switzerland	✕	Na	NI	NI
Taiwan	p	C	NI	NI
Turkey	✕	Na	NI	NI
United Kingdom	p	C	p	C
USA (Federal)	p	C	p	C

Table Legend

✕   Prohibited

p   Allowed

C   Compensation allowed

R   Reimbursement of expenses allowed

na   Not applicable

NI   No information that directly addressed the issue was found or the position on the issue was unclear

In summary, diverse relations of governance vis-à-vis oocyte donation have been rendered comparable through at least two levels of generalisation. By redefining regulatory and statutory relations as norms (through de-juridification), they were rendered comparable to ethical standards. By evaluating both medical treatment and bio-medical research under the broader purpose of achieving reproductive conception, two different sets of technique were rendered comparable (or at least, complementary). Through these generalisations, the comparative table ultimately constructed could be regarded as a normative epistemic framework, within which the different relations of governance on oocyte donation could be related one to another. Their positionality *inter-se* would in turn prescribe a certain value and credibility. What the comparative table obscures however is its own situatedness in the standpoint of Singapore (although, as indicated earlier, a footnote reference admits to this).

3.3 Translational Extension of the Normative Framework

A similar approach was adopted in analysing the governance of research involving human-animal combinations. Focusing on norma-tive content, the interpretive framework within which comparison was undertaken enabled different jurisdictions to be placed on a single scale, regardless of the different degrees of formalisation. For instance, the guidelines of the NAS, where applicable to human-animal combinations, have been taken to be the 'national' position of the US for a number of reasons, including the absence of federal legislation or regulation on the subject, and its treatment as such by researchers, policy-makers and international organisations. As we have con-sidered, the guidelines of the NAS on human-animal combinations served as a model for the regulatory framework in the state of California and for the ISSCR. In constructing a comparative table on the subject (see Table 3.7), it was again acknowledged that the information presented:

need not necessarily be a complete representation of the regulatory approach of the specified country ... [and that the selection of jurisdictions are] based on several factors including availability of information (in the English language), availability of legislation and regulatory guidelines (both legally binding and non-binding), and the extent that these issues have been deliberated on and debated in these countries.[287]

Table 3.7. Comparative Table on Chimeras and Cybrids (as at 2010)

Country	Animal Chimeras	Cytoplasmic Hybrid Embryos
Japan *The Law Concerning Regulation Relating to Human Cloning Techniques and Other Similar Techniques*, 2001 *Guidelines for the Handling of a Specified Embryo*, 2001 *Guidelines for the derivation and distribution of human embryonic stem cells*, 2009 (drawn from Caulfield T *et al*, "Stem cell research policy and iPS cells", *Nature Methods*, 7(2010): 28-33) *Guidelines for the utilization of human embryonic stem cells*, 2009 (drawn from Caulfield T *et al*, "Stem cell research policy and iPS cells", *Nature Methods*, 7(2010): 28-33)	The creation of animal chimeric embryos is allowed, with approval from the Ministry of Education, Culture, Sports, Science and Technology (MEXT) is required (Article 2(1) of the 2001 Guidelines, and Article 6 of the 2001 Law). The transfer of such embryos into a human or non-human uterus is prohibited (Article 3 of the 2001 Law). Research involving the production of germ cells from pluripotent stem cells (whether from human embryonic stem cells or iPS cells) should be allowed under strict oversight, but fertilisation using these derived gametes should be prohibited. In addition, research involving the grafting of human iPS cells into animal embryos is allowed, although implantation of such embryos into an animal uterus is prohibited (2009 Guidelines).	The creation of cytoplasmic hybrid embryos is prohibited. (Article 2(1) of the 2001 Guidelines, and Article 2(1)14 of the 2001 Law). (Further reference: Taupitz J and Weschka M (eds.). *CHIMBRIDS – Chimeras and Hybrids in Comparative European and International Research.* Heidelberg: Springer, 2009. p. 1029)

(Continued)

---

[287] Bioethics Advisory Committee, *Human-Animal Combinations in Stem Cell Research*. Singapore: Bioethics Advisory Committee, September 2010, at A26. The caveat on incomplete representation was not repeated with the table published in the ED. Report (at 27).

Table 3.7. (*Continued*)

Country	Animal Chimeras	Cytoplasmic Hybrid Embryos
Science Council of Japan, *Guidelines for Proper Conduct of Animal Experiments*, 1 June 2006	There are no specific regulations or guidelines on the creation of animal chimeric foetuses or post-natal human chimeras for research. There are guidelines on the use of animals in research.	
Singapore *Human Cloning and Other Prohibited Practices Act*, 2004 *Animal & Birds (Care and Use of Animals for Scientific Purposes) Rules*, 2004 National Advisory Committee for Laboratory Animal Research, *Guidelines on the Care and Use of Animals for Scientific Purposes*, 2004	There are no specific regulations or guidelines on the creation of animal chimeras for research. There are guidelines on the use of animals in research.	It is unclear if the creation of cytoplasmic hybrid embryos is regulated under the Act.
United Kingdom *Human Fertilisation and Embryology Act* 2008 *Animals (Scientific Procedures) Act*, 1986	There are no specific regulations or guidelines on the creation of animal chimeras for research, apart from those that relate to the welfare of laboratory animals.	The creation of cytoplasmic hybrid embryos is allowed only if under licence from the HFEA. (Sections 1(2) and 4(2) of the Act). Development of such embryos beyond 14 days or after appearance of the primitive streak, whichever is earlier, and implantation into a woman or an animal, are prohibited (Sections 4(2)(1), 4(3) and 4(4) of the Act).

Table 3.7. (*Continued*)

Country	Animal Chimeras	Cytoplasmic Hybrid Embryos
United States of America National Academy of Sciences (NAS) , *Guidelines for Human Embryonic Stem Cell Research*, 2005, amended 26 May 2010 National Institutes of Health (NIH), *Guidelines for Research Using Human Stem Cells*, 2009 *Animal Welfare Act*, amended 1990 State law varies significantly, with a number of states that allow nuclear transfer research and a number that do not.	There is no provision under Federal law for the creation of animal chimeras for research, although the use of certain animals in research is regulated by law. Under the NAS Guidelines, the creation of animal chimeras for research is allowed, after additional review and approval by an Embryonic Stem Cell Research Oversight (ESCRO) committee (Paragraphs 1.3(a), 1.3(b)(ii) and 1.3(b)(iii)). Animals into which human embryonic stem cells have been introduced such that they could contribute to the germ line should not be allowed to breed (Paragraph 1.3(c)(iii), NAS Guidelines; Part IV (B), NIH Guidelines). However, the introduction of human embryonic stem cells into non-human primate embryos should not be conducted at this time (Paragraph 1.3(c)(ii), NAS Guidelines)/is ineligible for funding (Part IV (A), NIH Guidelines).	There is no provision under Federal law for the creation of cytoplasmic hybrid embryos for research. Under the NAS Guidelines, the creation of cytoplasmic hybrid embryos is allowed. Development of such embryos beyond 14 days or appearance of the primitive streak, whichever is earlier, and implantation into a human or non-human uterus are prohibited (Paragraph 4.5). When hES cell lines are to be derived from cytoplasmic hybrid embryos, the approval of an ESCRO will have to be obtained (Paragraph 4.4, NAS Guidelines).

In addition, for reasons discussed in Chapter 5, the sub-categorisation of human-animal hybrids as 'true hybrids' and 'cytoplasmic hybrids' in the HA Consultation Paper was subsequently reduced to a single category of 'cytoplasmic hybrid embryos'. As illustration, an excerpt showing the regulatory approaches of Japan (with regulatory provisions), Singapore (no specific provision), the UK (with statutory provision for cytoplasmic hybrid embryos) and the

US (with comprehensive non-regulatory guidelines) from the table published in the HA Report is set out in Table 3.7.[288]

3.4 Positional Relationality in Comparative Tables

Comparative tables bear some resembles to a *huanghuali* yoke-back chair (黄花梨官帽椅) in classical antique Chinese furniture dating back to the Ming dynasty (about 14th to 17th century). In Ming dynasty China (and indeed, much of late Imperial China), comfort and convenience in the design and construction of a chair were secondary to considerations of the hierarchy and status of its user. The location and the type of chair that a person sits on should accurately reflect her social position determined based on factors that include title, seniority and gender. At significant events, a chair may be embellished with exquisite textile and its placement must be precise.[289]

Comparative tables in a variety of forms and applications have been ubiquitous throughout the course of my fieldwork. They were common not only in the projects, but also in the documents of different government agencies and policy bodies (local and foreign) that I dealt with. Their use and placement within documents play a critical role in determining the character and function of these documents. While comparative tables are informative in themselves,

---

[288] See full table at: Bioethics Advisory Committee, *Human-Animal Combinations in Stem Cell Research*. Singapore: Bioethics Advisory Committee, September 2010, at 27-34. See also discussion in Chapter 2. The regulatory provisions in Japan has been updated in 2014. See: Ministry of Education, Culture, Sports, Science and Technology of Japan, *Guidelines for the Derivation of Human Embryonic Stem Cells*, 2014; and Ministry of Education, Culture, Sports, Science and Technology of Japan, *Guidelines for Distribution and Utilization of Human Embryonic Stem Cells*, 2014.

[289] Sarah Handler, *Ming Furniture: In the Light of Chinese Architecture*. Berkeley and Toronto: Ten Speed Press, 2005, at 108. More generally, certain types of chairs, such as the folding stool, were a prestigious seat and a symbol of dignity and power in ancient China, Egypt, Greece and Rome. By the late 6th century, they appeared in tombs of the wealthy. See Florence de Dampierre, *Chairs: A History*. New York: Abrams, 2006, at 37.

they have important symbolic significance. They communicate relationality, due diligence and hence legitimacy. I was myself responsible
for the creation of some of these tables, and ultimately in their
publication in the ED and HA Reports. In the paragraphs that follow,
I will first attempt to explicate my sense of what comparative tables
'do', as well as to elaborate on the ways in which epistemologically
self-contained comparative tables are constructed.

A key responsibility of the BAC has been to ensure that ethical
standards for biomedical research conducted in Singapore are consistent with 'international standards'.[290] Operationally, the 'problem'
was conceived as determining the ethical benchmark by which
research goals and methods could be determined to be 'ethical'.
Although there was a ready supply of ethical principles and norms,
there was no immediate correlation between these principles and
norms to the varied research and regulatory practices adopted by
different jurisdictions. Comparison was undertaken, much by way of
comparative law, to uncover what were generally perceived as 'issues'
in relation to oocyte donation and human-animal combinations, and
possible 'solutions' to them. This comparative approach to problem-
solving entails generalisation that is consistent with an observation
that a purpose for undertaking comparison is the promotion of
universalism at every level.[291] Apart from this problem-solving
modality, other purposes that have contributed to my comparative
endeavours are similar to those set out by Gerhard Dannemann as (to
a very limited degree) unifying law, applying foreign law, facilitating
choice between legal systems, to gain understanding and enhance

---

[290] Interview with Professor Lim Pin, 27 April 2009; Fieldnotes (correspondence 16
    June 2010).
[291] Annelise Riles, Introduction: The Projects of Comparison. In Annelise Riles (ed.),
    Re-thinking the Masters of Comparative Law. Oxford and Portland: Hart Publishing,
    2001, pp 1-18, at 12.

knowledge.[292] However, the primary motivation behind comparative work undertaken in my work was problem-solving through understanding foreign governance approaches and to 'apply' foreign laws or regulations that are suited to 'local' goals and conditions. This was indeed one message that the comparative tables sought to communicate.

However, this notion of comparison glosses over the constructive (and contributive) dimension of comparative work. Indeed, a legally-trained contact who was indirectly involved in my work has this to say about the comparative work:[293] "Singapore is good at taking the best practices from other people. We should definitely continue to look at what leading countries are doing and then adopt those practices that are suitable for us." The assumption underlying this remark is that there are easily adaptable ethical or governance practices 'out there' that can be acquired, much like shopping for an item after price and quality comparisons are made. My experience in the field has been that there were no such ready-made standards and practices to be 'found'. Rather, the purpose behind developing a comparative table as a normative interpretive framework and determining an appropriate 'fit' is very much a concern with building positional relationality. As we have seen, comparability was achieved through the creation of a normative 'map', generated through a process of abstraction and translation of different approaches to governance of oocyte donation or human-animal combinations. It may be argued that positioning a jurisdiction at a certain location on this normative map is to also prescribe to that position a certain normative content. Sharing the mind-set of early modernist comparative lawyers, these acts of

---

292 Gerhard Dannemann, Comparative Law: Study of Similarities or Differences? In Mathias Reimann and Reinhard Zimmermann (eds.), *The Oxford Handbook of Comparative Law*. Oxford and New York: Oxford University Press, 2006, pp 383-419, at 402-406.
293 Fieldnotes, 20 October 2010, ShB.

mapping and attributing positions are intended to be relational.[294] The 'commonalities' that are thereby derived through generalisation are primarily intended to establish normative positions.[295] Much in the way that your seating position presents your social standing in late Imperial China, positionality in comparison tables enables a claim to normative identity through drawing relations with some other occupants of this locality. This claim is a normative one, and often understood as 'standards' in a policy environment. Take for instance the table on oocyte donation.[296] In allowing donation for research, Singapore is shown to share a similar position with key jurisdictions like Australia, China, Japan, the UK and the US. On the issue of payment however, the position proposed for Singapore is mid-way between Australia, China and Japan on the one hand (where only reimbursement of expenses is allowed), and the US on the other (where relatively substantial compensation may be provided).

The current statutory position in Singapore is that there should be no payment for the donation of oocytes other than for reimbursement of certain expenses. On the grounds of fairness, the BAC has proposed for compensation to be provided to healthy donors for loss of time and earnings. However, this compensation is likely to be a limited one given the overarching concern with inducement that amounts to

---

294 As Riles observes: "the early modernist comparative lawyer is best understood ... as a kind of independently operating bureaucrat ... [the comparatists'] ideas create world – they don't just "reflect" or 'influence' it. The relation between knowledge and social facts is literal, not just metaphorical". Annelise Riles, Introduction: The Projects of Comparison. In Annelise Riles (ed.), *Re-thinking the Masters of Comparative Law*. Oxford and Portland: Hart Publishing, 2001, pp 1-18, at 13.

295 Later on, Riles observes: "This bureaucratic mode of scholarship ... gravitates toward particular kinds of arguments and claims. It is much better suited to demonstrating (or rather, negotiating) underlying commonalities (common cores) than to challenging or critiquing paradigms". *Ibid*, at 17.

296 The BAC introduces the comparative table as "a summary of the laws and guidelines of various countries on whether egg donation is allowed, and if so, whether compensation may be provided." Bioethics Advisory Committee, *Donation of Human Eggs for Research*. Singapore: Bioethics Advisory Committee, 7 November 2007, at 17, paragraph 4.20.

undue influence. Hence, while the comparative table accurately reflects the current position of Singapore on the subject of payment (in allowing reimbursement only), it does not accurately represent the BAC's proposed position. As noted earlier, the BAC was not free to choose any position it desired, as it had earlier committed to a position against all forms of commercialisation of the human body. This immediately rules out the option of allowing substantial payment (as in the US) and other financial arrangements that could have this effect (such as the egg-sharing scheme in the UK). The political message from this comparative project is that while Singapore is prepared to relax its 'conservative' stance on non-payment, it is not prepared to embrace fully the 'economic liberalism' of the UK or the US. This was in fact the message that the Press wanted to make explicit, and did so.[297] As we have also seen, there was a broader political agenda behind this shift in stance. A similar motivation directed the comparative work on human-animal combinations. The construction of commonalities among key jurisdictions was intended to show that human-animal combinations are not as 'novel' as people think and that there already are regulatory approaches to address some key concerns arising from the research. But as we have also seen, comparison reveals the limits of regulation and the impossibility of bridging all differences.

Another way of considering relationality is to think of comparison as a heuristic activity, and comparative tables as heuristic devices. Comparative tables served as interpretive frameworks that set out normative options for policy-makers. On the subject of oocyte donation, they could well be seen as resembling a 'scale', limited at

---

[297] For instance, the issue of payment was the focus of new reports on the release of the BAC's consultation paper on donation of oocytes for research in November 2007, followed by its recommendations in November 2008. See Chen Huifen, Payment for women's eggs being mulled. *The Business Times*, 8 November 2007; Serene Luo, Human egg donation: No payment for pain, risks. *The Straits Times*, 6 November 2008; Chen Huifen, Panel favours compensating women who donate eggs for research. *The Business Times*, 4 November 2008.

one end by jurisdictions or organisations that preclude donation altogether, and those that allow the donation at the other end. Intermediate positions would include jurisdictions or organisations that only allow purely altruistic donations and those that allow substantial payment to be provided for the donation. This 'sliding scale' is arguably similar to those developed by Mitchel Lasser in his comparative analysis of the different degrees of formalism and transparency among the highest judicial institutions in France, the European Union and the US.[298] Lasser identifies two fundamental questions that guided the construction of his 'sliding scales':[299]

(1) What is to be used as, and included in, the objects of comparison?

(2) With regard to what attributes are these objects to be compared?

He relies on a claim of typicality in justifying the choice of the European Court of Justice (ECJ), the *Cour de Cassation* and the US Supreme Court for analysis and comparison.[300] This typification is both determined by and also shapes, through articulation, the discursive characters of these institutions: radical bifurcation (between the *Cour* and the *Magistrats*) in the French system, soft bifurcation (between the formal, deductive, magisterial and univocal discourse of judicial decisions in contrast to the more personal, open-ended and insecure opinion of the Advocate-General) of the ECJ, and discursive integration in the US (where facts and reasoning are

---

[298] Mitchel de S-O-l'E Lasser, *Judicial Deliberations: A Comparative Analysis of Judicial Transparency and Legitimacy*. New York and Oxford: Oxford University Press, 2004, at 241-268.

[299] *Ibid*, at 242.

[300] Lasser provides this explanation: "What makes the French judicial system French, the European (EU) system European, and the American (U.S.) system American are discursive and conceptual attributes that manifest themselves throughout those judicial systems, attributes that surface again and again despite the obvious variation in the parties, the subject matter, the legal issues, and the like handled by the assorted courts in question." *Ibid*, at 297 (see also 271).

all reflected in the judgment).[301] An important contribution of this constructed scale is, as Lasser explains, the revelation that:

> [While] traditional American comparative accounts have always stressed the radical formalism of French judicial decision-making, ... [he] also wanted to underline the similarly radical openness of the professional discourse of the French haute magistrature. The scale representation ... offers a visual depiction of this characteristic French double radicalism.[302]

When 'degree of formality' is replaced with 'extent of disclosure' as the scalar variable, the ECJ has been found to be more transparent whereas the *Cour de Cassation* was the least.[303]

The didactic nature of comparative tables as 'sliding scales' of sorts is similarly evident in those generated by the IFFS and the BAC. In its reports of 2007, 2010 and 2013, the IFFS's 'sliding scales' were the basis by which policy developments on IVF have been assessed. For instance, it considered major changes in Italy to be 'retrogressive'.[304] Since 2004, ART has been limited to adult heterosexual couples who are married or living together, after medical certification of sterility or infertility, and subject to a requirement that a maximum of three oocytes can be fertilised and implanted as embryos, regardless of its quality and the age of the future mother. These stringent require-ments are premised on a religious belief that human 'personhood' begins at conception, which the IFFS considers to be a 'cultural bias' and hence not 'good medical practice'.[305] It further noted that Costa

---

301 *Ibid*, at 256.

302 *Ibid*, at 257-258 (emphasis in original).

303 *Ibid*, at 260.

304 Jean Cohen, Howard Jones Jr., Ian Cooke and Roger Kempers (eds.), IFFS Surveillance 07, *Fertility and Sterility* 87 Suppl. 1: S1-S67, at S8.

305 The IFFS indicates: "The great variations in the details of what can and cannot be done under legislation and guidelines from country to country suggest that influences are at work other than the goal of good medical practice. Italy can be used as an example. Italian law limits insemination to no more than three oocytes and requires that all fertilized oocytes be transferred. This is not good 21st

Rica is a country where IVF is prohibited,[306] presumably due to a similar 'cultural bias'. Hence the 'scale' becomes not only a basis of assessment, but also a definition of what amounts to 'good medical practice'. The comparative tables of the BAC similarly create interpretive 'scales' that facilitate policy choices by setting out a broad spectrum of possibilities. By choosing a position within the limits of the scales, policy positions are rendered more defensible in a sense that it is not an anomaly. Certain locations on the scale might be all the more desirable if they are shared with jurisdictions of interest or influence. Hence claims to consistency with 'best international standards' are very often matters of positioning on some normative interpretive 'scale'. This is also a reason for the centrality of comparative tables in many aspects of policy work.

3.5 Open-Endedness in Relational Solidarity

Although the comparative tables resemble Lasser's sliding scales, the motivations behind their construction are of a different character. Lasser's goal was to provide a more open and accommodating approach to understanding another legal system. He was critical of the restrictive approach of a generation of American comparative jurists that sought to evaluate the French legal system through an essentially American standpoint by focusing only on French appellate judgements. While judicial decisions have been central to the legal process in common law jurisdictions, they have a more limited role in the French legal system, which operated on a different master narrative directed at securing different socio-political goals. Lasser considers that:

> The comparativist must not only gather and convey detailed information about procedural structures, institutional forms,

---

century medicine and reflects the cultural bias of the national legislative body." Howard Jones Jr., Ian Cooke, Roger Kempers, Peter Brinsden and Doug Saunders (eds.), *IFFS Surveillance 2010*. Mount Royal, NJ: International Federation of Fertility Societies, September 2010, at 11.

306 *Ibid.*

professional organisations, discursive practices, methodological approaches, conceptual frameworks, and the like; she must also decode and explain the interaction between them. This intricate work demands a good deal of ideological reconstruction: what is the dominant underlying logic and self-understanding according to which, for example, the work performed by judges and other important institutional players is felt to be legitimate?[307]

In contrast to Lasser's comparative agenda, there was less immediate interest in uncovering the dominant logic embedded in master narratives of the different jurisdictions considered in the comparative work of the ED Report and the HA Report. Instead, the focus has been on mapping out the range of policy options in relation to the issues on hand, and the means to secure legitimacy for a policy stance when one is adopted. In a policy environment, norms are not viewed in a rigid and inflexible manner but are malleable, particularly where there is a diversity of norms. Norms are thereby both resource and tool directed at achieving particular social and political agendas. To be sure, this is not to say that policy makers are disinterested in the dominant logic of the systems compared, but the desired social and political objectives tend to colour the understanding and choice of jurisdictions.

The instrumental and pragmatic nature of the comparative projects I was involved in appears like what Annelise Riles has observed to be the different focus (and lack of communication) between comparative lawyers and socio-legal scholars.[308] Evaluating

---

[307] Mitchel de S-O-l'E Lasser, Transforming Deliberations. In Nick Huls, Maurice Adams and Jacco Bomhoff (eds.), *The Legitimacy of Highest Courts' Rulings: Judicial Deliberations and Beyond*. The Hague: TMC Asser Press, 2009, pp 33-53, at 37.
[308] Annelise Riles, Comparative Law and Socio-Legal Studies. In Mathias Reimann and Reinhard Zimmermann (eds.), *The Oxford Handbook of Comparative Law*. Oxford and New York: Oxford University Press, 2006, pp 775-813, at 783-785. Elsewhere, Riles notes: "The field of comparative law is populated by three disparate groups of scholars: first, 'traditional' comparative lawyers; second, specialists in particular bodies of non-Western law such as Japanese or Chinese

my own frame of mind in making comparison as a bioethical concern, it was not dissimilar to the comparative work that I undertook while in legal practice. In this respect, I am inclined to think of comparative work of the Secretariat as being similar in orientation to that of 'comparative lawyers'. As we have earlier considered, the approach adopted was essentially normative, applying an almost Weberian definition of law, or 'law on the books'. This orientation should not be surprising as the BAC was appointed by the state to provide it with advice, and the relevance of policy responses by other countries to similar issues is taken-for-granted. As a field, 'bioethics' tends to be construed normatively (much like Kelsen's concept of law), no less so by the BAC and policy-makers. There is also some ambivalence in the treatment of social context, as there has not been a clear or consistent rationale as to the inclusion of some social factors or considerations, but not others. On the whole, a socio-legal scholar is likely to find the legal and social analyses to be 'amateurish', but not in a disparaging sense of the word.[309] Riles explains that while John Henry Wigmore's comparative legal scholarship could be considered amateurism in its presentation of "a heap of raw material" composed of text that leaves glaring analytical gaps and without any attempt at analytical output,[310] she explains that these peculiarities are best understood as

---

law; and third, younger scholars working under the banner of so-called 'new approaches'". Annelise Riles, Wigmore's Treasure Box: Comparative Law in the Era of Information. *Harvard International Law Journal* (1999) 40, 1: 221-283, at 225.

[309] Annelise Riles, Encountering Amateurism: John Henry Wigmore and the Uses of American Formalism. In Annelise Riles (ed.), *Re-thinking the Masters of Comparative Law*. Oxford and Portland: Hart Publishing, 2001, pp 94-126, at 98. Indeed, Riles argues (at 125) that "... if amateurism is defined as a failure to analyze, then comparative law is inherently amateuristic", as it is this particular characteristic that sets it apart from comparative socio-legal scholarship.

[310] *Ibid*, at 114. Riles adds (at 121): "The texts used in American law schools in Wigmore's time, as today, are, as their name implies, 'materials' – collections of essays and documents. The idea is that the very absence of answers to the text's open-ended questions will stimulate a response from the student and spark a dynamic discussion in class; they are tools for creating a moment."

the influences of American (Langdellian) legal formalism, where "the text does not stand for the self in the way it does for the academic, nor does the textual debate stand for the community in which the self is constituted. This is because for the formalist, the relevant site of academic relationality is not the text but the classroom."[311] Hence the analytical gaps in Wigmore's comparative works are intended to enable contingency. Where the ED Report and the HA Report are concerned, the relevant site of relationality resides not in these documents, but in the political and bureaucratic domains. In many instances, it would not be necessary to offer so comprehensive an analysis as to dictate a definite policy trajectory. Indeed, a number of more 'targeted' recommendations of the BAC have not been 'operationalised' as they were felt to be difficult to implement or of a lower priority in the political agenda.[312] A more open-ended presentation of materials and analysis creates gaps that enable flexibility in policy definition and implementation. In other words, analytical gaps in comparison make room for political and bureaucratic contingencies. The presence of gaps should not lead to the assumption that no or inadequate analysis was done. The reports of the BAC, while relatively brief, have been effective in securing legitimacy through the production of cogent arguments and through (as we have seen) positional solidarity in ethical or policy stance with leading jurisdictions. Analysis in the backroom has been very comprehensive but very little substantive materials and analytical outputs are ultimately published in the reports. This is perhaps reminiscent of the French judicial system, where decision-making procedures of the French high courts are designed to generate extensive internal judicial debates, which are not reflected in the published judicial decision.[313] Like the French judicial institution, the

---

[311] *Ibid*, at 122.

[312] Fieldnotes, 2 August 2010, MH.

[313] Mitchel de S-O-l'E Lasser, Transforming Deliberations. In Nick Huls, Maurice Adams and Jacco Bomhoff (eds.), *The Legitimacy of Highest Courts' Rulings: Judicial Deliberations and Beyond*. The Hague: TMC Asser Press, 2009, pp 33-53, at 41.

BAC is not composed (with the exception of one or two members in certain terms of appointment) of elected representatives. However, the brevity of its report and the relatively open-endedness of its recommendations is not so much a matter of safeguarding republicanism (as Lasser attributes to the French judicial system), than practical concerns of accessibility to policy-makers and the public alike, and of securing policy flexibility and implementability.

3.6 Functionality in Open-endedness

Law in practice has often been viewed as essentially parochial. The lead counsel in an international transaction will nevertheless have to rely on the opinions of local counsels to ensure the legality of the deal's local components. However, in the absence of an appropriate or clear answer to the issues on hand, Lord Bingham observes that foreign authority may be significant or decisively influential.[314] He goes further in acknowledging the importance of foreign influences,[315] especially in the resolution of shared issues in an increasingly connected world.[316]

There is a sense of *praesumptio similitudinis* in Lord Bingham's argument for the relevance of foreign laws, in that legal systems of foreign jurisdictions are considered to encounter the same problems. Even if different solutions are applied, similarly just results are desired.[317] Outside of an adjudicative setting, this presumption has been similarly applied in my comparative work as a heuristic principle. Gerhard Dannemann suggests that while the presumption

---

[314] Thomas H Bingham, *Widening Horizons: The Influence of Comparative Law and International Law on Domestic Law*. Cambridge: Cambridge University Press, 2010, at 8.

[315] Lord Bingham considers English law as "a mongrel, gaining in vigour and intelligence what it has lost in purity of pedigree." *Ibid*, at 5-6.

[316] *Ibid*, at 3.

[317] Konrad Zweigert and Hein Kötz, *An Introduction to Comparative Law* (tr. Tony Weir). Oxford: Clarendon Press, 1998 (Revised 3rd ed.), at 40.

appears to find broad application in encouraging one to discover similarities in foreign laws and legal systems, it is in fact limited to those areas of substantive private law which are not culturally or politically sensitive (thereby excluding all of public law, criminal law, procedural law and even family and inheritance law).[318] In bioethics, power over processes of life,[319] and commonality of the struggle against death and dying, are perhaps the basis of unification into a single shared problem that different civilisations have attempted to address through a variety of social institutions, including religion and law.[320] Under this rubric, different legal systems become comparable by their social function. As a key functionalist methodology, this rationale grounded in 'common problems' was among the rationales deployed in the construction of comparative tables for the ED and HA Reports.

In critique of this approach, Richard Hyland points out that the 'common problems' approach is only possible at a generic level. As illustration, he observes that although everyone in every society has to eat, no society or legal system has to confront food-related problems in this generic form.[321] The obscurity or fiction of generality

---

[318] Gerhard Dannemann, Comparative Law: Study of Similarities or Differences? In Mathias Reimann and Reinhard Zimmermann (eds.), *The Oxford Handbook of Comparative Law*. Oxford and New York: Oxford University Press, 2006, pp 383-419, at 395.

[319] Marilyn Strathern points out a critical detachment from the stability of 'nature' as a given with the various interventions into life that science and technology now enable. Marilyn Strathern, *After Nature: English Kinship in the Late Twentieth Century*. Cambridge: Cambridge University Press, 1992, at 195.

[320] Jack Goody, for instance, points to similarities in human cultures, common situations (structural), common development of social evolution, the logic of the situation and inherent potentialities, that enable meaningful comparisons to be made. Jack Goody, Globalization and the Domestic Group. In Max Kirsch (ed.), *Inclusion and Exclusion in the Global Arena*. New York: Routledge, 2006, pp 31-41, at 33 and 36.

[321] Richard Hyland, *Gifts: a study in comparative law*. New York: Oxford University Press, 2009, at 70.

is the result of abstraction, which is inevitable in rendering commensurability. In addition, abstraction enables functionalists to extricate law from society, so that legal norms can be applied as tools to implement social goals. However, Hyland questions the correctness of this view in his observation that:

> Very often, the law does not work that way. The norm comes first, and only then is a particular functionality ascribed to it ... If the law were functional in the way legal functionalists assume, it would demonstrate two characteristics. First, we would know the purpose for which our legal norms are promulgated. Second, we would be able to determine the social consequences of applying the norms. Yet neither characteristic describes the legal systems examined here.[322]

Hyland considers that both the purpose and consequence of a norm are indeterminate, and it is impossible to find purpose in a legal norm.[323]

It is questionable if this strong Realist stance is defensible in every situation. Even if there is no inherent purpose to a legal norm and its attributed purpose is continuously reformulated, it does not mean that this purpose lacks any measure of durability for a time. As earlier considered, an effect of objectification through law is meaning creation, and this has been found to be relatively durable. In addition, the work of the BAC on oocyte donation and human-animal combinations suggests that different communities have been working at different levels to secure a range of possible readings, if not a specific reading, of relevant ethical and legal norms. These communities – whether regulatory, scientific or ethical – take these norms to be the *Tertium Comparationis* by which 'common problems' could be addressed and resolved. It is more difficult to tease apart

---

[322] *Ibid*, at 74. Hyland describes the viewpoint of functionalists as: "They see society as a house in need of repair. We are the general contractors; the legal norms are our tools. The social problems come first. Legal norms are crafted to solve the problems."

[323] *Ibid*.

norms from problems. These reports of the BAC suggest that norms did play a significant part in shaping the nature and character of both the problem and its solution(s), but there did not appear to be a perceived need to know if the norms gave rise to the problems or *vice versa* (I return to this problem-solution nexus shortly). A reason for this could be the focus on shared or common principles. Not surprisingly, debate over whether such principles may be said to be found or are matters of social construction continues. Regardless of foundational basis, ethical principles have been an important means of initiating dialogue and achieving consensus amidst vast diversity. They have in turn provided inspiration of a universalist heritage, where different laws may in fact be based on the same principles due to differences in circumstances, values and cultures.[324] As no circumstance is ever exactly alike, James Gordley points to the centrality of principles in establishing commonality in comparative law.[325]

3.7 Similitude through Framing in Bioethics

I want to return to an earlier point relating to the normative shaping of problem and solution. Composed of individuals with different ideological and discursive backgrounds and lineages, the meeting point has often been on practical functionality of normative governance systems, including law.[326] Pre-existing bioethical discourses

---

[324] James Gordley, The universalist heritage. In Pierre Legrand and Roderick Munday (eds.), *Comparative Legal Studies: Traditions and Transitions*. Cambridge: Cambridge University Press, 2003, pp 31-45, at 40-41.

[325] *Ibid*, at 44-45. Gordley seems to suggest that socio-legal comparison begins where comparative law ends.

[326] Ralf Michaels considers Lasser's approach in *Judicial Deliberations* to be a functional method in that although Lasser sets out to compare judicial styles as a cultural analysis of mentalities, he explains different styles of legal systems as equivalent regarding the functions they serve, i.e. transparency, judicial accountability and control. See Ralf Michaels, The Functional Method of Comparative Law. In Mathias Reimann and Reinhard Zimmermann (eds.), *The Oxford Handbook of Comparative Law*. Oxford and New York: Oxford University Press, 2006, pp 339-382, at 341-342.

have been influential in advancing a sense of *praesumptio similitudinis*. For instance, universalism is apparent in the principled-basis by which Ezekiel Emanuel analysed shifts in paradigms of medical ethics. [327] Where beneficence as determined by physicians was regarded as the dominant principle of medical ethics prior to the 1950's, he considers self-determination to be encouraged by the courts and legislatures in the 1980's. This in turn contributed to a plurality of values with no hierarchy in the medical ethics of today.[328] The situation may not be as amorphous as Emanuel sets out in his analysis. In Singapore, medical law continues to place considerable emphasis on beneficence, or acting in the best interests of patients.[329] As for biomedical research, the 'founding principles' of bioethics (i.e. autonomy, beneficence, non-maleficence and justice) continue to hold sway in the minds of researchers, research administrators and regulators.[330] This could perhaps be said in very general terms across the jurisdictions of my study, although there will undoubtedly be some exceptions. In fact, my initiation into the lifeworld of bioethics could be described as encounters with complex inter-play of principles.

Let me try to give a 'snapshot' of bioethical knowledge that applies in the day-to-day operation of a policy body. There is now a general expectation that any decision of a bioethics body or an IRB be grounded in one or more ethical requirements set out in a number of key documents. Some documents are specific to particular types of

---

[327] Ezekiel Emanuel, The Evolving Norms of Medical Ethics. In Ronald M Green, Aine Donovan and Steven A Jauss (eds.), *Global Bioethics: Issues of Conscience for the Twenty-First Century*. Oxford: Clarendon Press, 2008, pp 53-76, at 54.

[328] *Ibid*, at 65-66, and 74.

[329] See for instance the *Ethical Code and Ethical Guidelines* of the Singapore Medical Council, which has regulatory force under the *Medical Registration Act*, Cap. 174 of Singapore.

[330] Fieldnotes dated 17 January 2008 (meeting with IRB administrators and researchers), 12 August 2008 (meeting with regulators), and 26 May 2009 (meeting with researchers).

biomedical science and technology, such as UNESCO's *Universal Declaration on the Human Genome and Human Rights.*[331] The principles set out in these documents may overlap, and the extent of their relevance often depends on the specific circumstances of each case. Key principles include justice,[332] respect for human health, welfare and safety (or beneficence),[333] respect for the human body, religious and cultural perspectives and traditions (i.e. a broader reading of beneficence),[334] respect for free and informed consent (or autonomy),[335] respect for vulnerable persons (autonomy and justice) and respect for human dignity.[336] Apart from the international domain, there are also important normative documents by regional and professional bodies.[337] The diversity and complexity of ethical structures that have arisen from these principles led some to conclude that there are different 'models' to policy decision-making in

---

[331] United Nations Educational, Scientific and Cultural Organization, *Universal Declaration on the Human Genome and Human Rights*, 1997.

[332] National Commission for the Protection of Human Subjects of Biomedical and Behavioral Research, *The Belmont Report: Ethical Principles and Guidelines for the protection of human subjects of research*, 18 April 1979 (the 'Belmont Report').

[333] Nuremberg Military Tribunal. *Trials of War Criminals before the Nuremberg Military Tribunals under Control Council Law* No 10, Vol 2. Washington, DC: US Government Printing Office, 1949, pp 181-182 (the "Nuremberg Code"), Articles 4 and 5.

[334] See documents of the United Nations General Assembly: *Universal Declaration of Human Rights* 1948 (Article 26), *International Convention on Economic, Social and Cultural Rights* (Articles 1.1, 2.2 and 15), and *International Convention on the Elimination of All Forms of Racial Discrimination* 1965 (effective from 1969). See also UNESCO's *Declaration on Race and Racial Prejudice* 1982, Articles 1 and 5.

[335] World Medical Association, *Declaration of Helsinki – Ethical Principles for Medical Research Involving Human Subjects*, 2013 (as amended), at paragraphs 25-32.

[336] See Articles 1, 2, 6, 10, 11, 12 and 15 of the UNESCO's *Universal Declaration on the Human Genome and Human Rights* 1998.

[337] Those that are commonly referred to include Council of Europe's *Convention for the Protection of Human Rights and Dignity of Human Beings with respect to the Application of Biology and Medicine* 1997, and the *International Ethical Guidelines for Biomedical Research Involving Human Subjects* (1982; 2002 updated) of the Council for International Organizations of Medical Sciences (CIOMS).

biomedical research,[338] and calls for greater harmonisation by key international organisations such as the World Health Organization.[339] The strong normative linkage between research ethics and medical ethics (and medical law) cannot be omitted, as the latter has been an important source of ethical content and aspirations. The upshot of this intricate display of pervasive ethical superstructures is to highlight the basis of 'commonality' by which comparisons are made in bioethics. Indeed, any comparative law project relating to biomedical science and technology will very likely be seriously wanting in propriety and legitimacy unless it has been under-taken with an appreciation of these ethical superstructures and their influence on key actors that include bioethicists, research administrators, biomedical research regulators and policy-makers, researchers and physicians.

The most direct implication of these ethical superstructures is in constituting a framework within which certain actions are determined to be ethical or unethical. As the 'fit' among these various structures is not seamless,[340] there is a significant number of 'grey areas' where the ethical acceptability of certain actions remains unclear (for instance, the provision of compensation for participation in clinical trials remains a controversial subject). Nevertheless, the construction of 'ethical' within such a framework is arguably similar to the way in which arbitrage serves as a framework in Hirokazu Miyazaki's study.[341] Within the 'framework' of arbitrage, transactions

---

[338] Bartha M Knoppers, Emily Kirby and Rosario Isasi, Genetics and Stem Cell Research: Models of International Policy-making. In John M Elliott, W Calvin Ho and Sylvia SN Lim (eds.), *Bioethics in Singapore: The Ethical Microcosm*. Singapore: World Scientific, 2010, pp 133-163.

[339] Alex Capron, American Law and the Governance of Research Ethics: Time for International Change (2010) *Singapore Academy of Law Journal* 22: 769-784.

[340] It is even more difficult to say whether different ethical structures could come together as a coherent system as some structures are opposed, with no clear prospect of reconciliation. See Isaiah Berlin, *The Crooked Timber of Humanity*. Princeton: Princeton University Press, 1990, at 12.

[341] Hirokazu Miyazaki, Between arbitrage and speculation: an economy of belief and doubt. *Economy and Society* (August 2007) 36 (3): 396-415, at 402.

that are speculative in character have been perceived to be risk-free up to a point. As we have seen, comparative projects are concerned with navigating through different frameworks of ethical norms, with a clear view to map specific relationalities and create particular meanings. Not surprisingly, we have already observed that the BAC has its own distinct framework of ethical principles, which has served to carve out a distinct decisional space.

3.8 Overcoming Incommensurability

I go further by arguing that it is within a broad normative framework that comparison made sense in these comparative projects. The construction of a framework seemed obviously necessary as a first step to effecting comparison. More precisely, it enables the application of what has appeared to me to be syllogistic logic – a mode of reasoning that Geoffrey Samuel considers to be quite possibly one of the most evident techniques (in combination with analogy) in legal method and legal reasoning.[342] The central logic to this technique and device relates not only to the construction of a genus (i.e. the major normative premise) and a species (the minor descriptive premise), but also the association between the two that generates concrete experience, such as in the division between things *in genere* and *in specie*.[343]

The application of syllogistic reasoning in law towards the construction (more often perceived as 'derivation' in a policy setting)

---

[342] Roman jurist Alfenus was said to have deployed this technique in addressing issues like: "Does a boat actually exist or is it simply a matter of individual planks? Does society exist or are there only individual men and women?" This technique has contributed to the development of analytical devices in law such as subrogation, fundamental to current legal understanding of risk substitution and transfer. See Geoffrey Samuel, Comparative Law and the Legal Mind. In Peter Birks and Arianna Pretto (eds.), *Themes in Comparative Law: In Honour of Bernard Rudden*. Oxford and New York: Oxford University Press, 2002, 35-47, at 37-38.

[343] *Ibid*, at 44.

of a rule or canon characterised by generality and normative weight in my comparative work is intended in part to overcome claims of incommensurability. As the caveats to the comparative tables on oocyte donation and human-animal combinations make clear, the BAC's interest is not to cross 'epistemological boundaries'.[344] Unlike superstructures such as the shared legal framework of the European Union, these comparative tables, while directed at producing some rule of similitude, are not directed as harmonisation.[345] But as we have seen, such ethical superstructures have been drawn upon in the BAC's comparative tables for the more limited purpose of creating a standard that not only defines a space for action locally, but also justifies these actions, if taken globally. In other words, the intermediatory role of the BAC is closely linked to the substantive purpose of its comparative projects. However, the extent to which ethical superstructures are drawn upon and incorporated into local policies and standards depends on situational and political factors.

There is another critical role that ethical superstructures have played in the comparative projects of the BAC. Within a principled framework, the purposes behind policy actions of foreign jurisdictions are discoverable (or imputable). It is on this basis that James Whitman argues that the burden of incommensurability should not completely overwhelm comparative efforts.[346] Referring to Max

---

344 Construction in comparison is implied in Pierre Legrand's argument that "even the most sophisticated comparative analysis originating from one tradition will, ultimately, fail to cross epistemological boundaries". Pierre Legrand, Alterity: About Rules, For Example. In Peter Birks and Arianna Pretto (eds.), *Themes in Comparative Law: In Honour of Bernard Rudden*. Oxford and New York: Oxford University Press, 2002, 21-33, at 22. He considers there to be an essentially irreconcilable difference between the common law and civil law systems. In relation to his 'rule model', the civil law is understood to operate on an 'if-then' basis whereas the common law adopts an 'as-therefore' approach (at 28).

345 Pierre Legrand, The same and the different. In Pierre Legrand and Roderick Munday (eds.), *Comparative Legal Studies: Traditions and Transitions*. Cambridge: Cambridge University Press, 2003, 240-311, at 294.

346 Whitman considers over-emphasis of incommensurability to be an excess of Romanticism. Hence he disagrees with Pierre Legrand's views on

Weber, he indicates that human action is not only purposive
(*zweckrational*), but also consistent with large normative commitments (*wertrational*), concerned with upholding tradition
(*traditional*) or emotional and primordial (*affektuell*) commitments.
Hence human actions are always accessible to our understanding.
He proposes for the focus to be on action, rather than worry about
how we understand persons, texts or cultures.[347] Referring to the
hermeneutic approach of Hans-Georg Gadamer in addressing the
problem of 'understanding' the 'other',[348] he encourages comparatists
to direct their attention on *Vorverständnis* (or pre-understanding, the
unarticulated, taken-for-granted assumptions that underlie the law),
which may be inarticulate and difficult to communicate, but not
impossible. In his view, this understanding need not be 'total' as the
concern of comparison is not in explaining the total culture, but in
normative justifications and tacit assumptions.[349]

Indeed, my sense has been that incommensurability is not usually
a concern for comparative work in bioethics, conceived as a broad
ethical framework or a network of frameworks sharing a common

---

[347] *Ibid*, at 323-324.
[348] Hans-Georg Gadamer (tr. & rev. Joel Weinsheimer and Donald G. Marshall), *Truth and Method*. London and New York: Continuum, 2004.
[349] Whitman argues: "'Law' is not best thought of as a rooted set of cultural facts that can be 'understood' only in cultural context. 'Law' is best thought of as an activity that aims at normative justification of certain human acts and of the exercise of the authority of some humans over others. Different societies unquestionably offer different normative justifications for different acts; moreover, different societies work with different sorts of tacit Vorverständnis that bear on the operation of their 'law'...Nevertheless, a set of normative justifications and tacit assumptions is not the same thing as a total 'culture'." See James Q Whitman, The Neo-Romantic Turn. In Mathias Reimann and Reinhard Zimmermann (eds.), *The Oxford Handbook of Comparative Law*. Oxford and New York: Oxford University Press, 2006, pp 312-344, at 343-344.

non-transplantability, and refers to the spread of sexual harassment law into Continental Europe as illustration. See James Q Whitman, The Neo-Romantic Turn. In Mathias Reimann and Reinhard Zimmermann (eds.), *The Oxford Handbook of Comparative Law*. Oxford and New York: Oxford University Press, 2006, pp 312-344, at 336-339.

core. While the importance of social, cultural or historical differences is almost always recognised, they are not taken as amounting to incommensurability. In fact, the general mind-set of many bioethicists and policymakers that I have encountered does not appear to be dissimilar from the *common core approach* in comparative law. This approach has been traced to the Cornell Hypothesis, which postulates that there is a common core of legal concepts and precepts shared by some or even most of the world's legal systems. On incommensurability, the authors of *Schlesinger's Comparative Law* agrees with Whitman that claim of 'incomparability' or unbridgeable differences should not be assumed, as deconstruction of legal ontology (such as abstract legal categories like 'contract', 'tort' and 'unjust enrichment') often leads to the discovery of fundamental analogies hidden behind apparently irreconcilable differences.[350]

The constructivist essence of the common core approach has been an important basis for the comparative projects of international organisations and academic institutions, whose works (as we have seen) have had a significant impact on the BAC. Take for instance, the IFFS surveillance reports. Governance systems on ARTs are regarded as open and complex aggregates of laws and pseudo-legal elements, with the surveyors themselves serving as geographers in tentative area-by-area survey or as zoologists dealing with the problem of classifying legal systems.[351] Arguably, the presence of ethical principles and superstructures have inspired and driven a comparative mind-set in the study of bioethical issues. There is also a sense of what Mark Freedland refers to as a belief in "the possibility and importance of legal solidarity and community".[352] This mind-set

---

[350] *Ibid*, at 99. A similar deconstruction is considered necessary when comparing professionalised with less professionalised law (at 97).

[351] *Ibid*, at 177 and 214. Classifying is seen as the ultimate purpose of comparative work (at 258-260).

[352] Mark Freedland makes this remark in relation to the personal preference of the comparer in realising legal solidarity and community within the European region. Mark Freedland, Introduction: Comparative and International Law in the Courts.

and belief encourages one, when faced with a problem, to look beyond the self and to deliberate on the other as an equal or perhaps even an example. The effect could perhaps be taken to be similar to the way in which the European Union's *Product Liability Directive* encouraged courts in the UK, France and Germany to examine through comparison the substantive and procedural aspects of contaminated blood transfusion.[353] Referring to European Union law more generally, Guy Canivet observes that fundamental principles embedded within the legal framework have been intrinsic to the actualisation of the European order by French courts through the gradual internalisation of common values.[354] This was said to be similarly the case in Italy.[355]

In more practical terms, a belief in solidarity and a comparative mind-set incentivises social interaction and discursive engagement. Expressing a view similar to Lord Bingham's, Guy Canivet indicates that legal cultures are influenced by factors external to them, even if such influences are moderated or subtle.[356] It is critical not to

---

In Guy Canivet, Mads Andenas and Duncan Fairgrieve (eds.), *Comparative Law Before the Courts*. London: The British Institute of International and Comparative Law, 2004, pp xv-xxvi, at xxv.

[353] Michael Brooke QC and Ian Forrester QC, The Use of Comparative Law in A & Others v National Blood Authority. In Guy Canivet, Mads Andenas and Duncan Fairgrieve (eds.), *Comparative Law Before the Courts*. London: The British Institute of International and Comparative Law, 2004, pp 57-83.

[354] Guy Canivet, The Use of Comparative Law Before the French Private Law Courts. In Guy Canivet, Mads Andenas and Duncan Fairgrieve (eds.), *Comparative Law Before the Courts*. London: The British Institute of International and Comparative Law, 2004, pp 181-193, at 184-185. See also Roger Errera, The Use of Comparative Law Before the French Administrative Law Courts. In Guy Canivet, Mads Andenas and Duncan Fairgrieve (eds.), *Comparative Law Before the Courts*. London: The British Institute of International and Comparative Law, 2004, pp 153-163.

[355] Aldo Sandulli, The Use of Comparative Law Before the Italian Public Law Courts. In Guy Canivet, Mads Andenas and Duncan Fairgrieve (eds.), *Comparative Law Before the Courts*. London: The British Institute of International and Comparative Law, 2004, pp 165-178.

[356] Guy Canivet observes: "The French private law judge is no longer – if he ever really was – considered as the 'mouth that produces the words of the law' (in the famous words of Montesquieu). He is commissioned to adjust law to the values of his

underestimate this belief in solidarity, which I find to be pervasive in biomedical research, healthcare and bioethics communities. It is a basis of sociality and defines the respective worldviews in communal terms where no researcher, physician or bioethicist considers herself or himself as acting alone. This is perhaps the strongest argument against any claim of incommensurability in a strong sense. Indeed, when I attempted to explain my concern with incommensurability in the comparative projects of the BAC, it was either politely dismissed or met with various expressions of incomprehension.[357] Comparison as a social activity is communicative. And as Patrick Glenn explains, human communication precludes any strong claim to incommensurability.[358]

Even if we should reject incommensurability in many instances, one should be wary not to confuse the drawing of relationality with *carte blanche* discursive displacement. It is often difficult to pinpoint the exact extent of borrowings or influences from external sources. Wholesale transplantation of biomedical research regulatory practices or mind-set has not and is unlikely to occur. However, external factors and pre-existing norms have been sufficiently influential to displace any strong-form notion of autopoiesis.[359] What

---

society...local and foreign legal cultures constantly interact... *no legal culture is exclusively inward-looking...*" Guy Canivet, The Use of Comparative Law Before the French Private Law Courts. In Guy Canivet, Mads Andenas and Duncan Fairgrieve (eds.), *Comparative Law Before the Courts*. London: The British Institute of International and Comparative Law, 2004, pp 181-193, at 182-183 (emphasis added).

[357] Fieldnotes, 20 August 2008, Secretariat.

[358] H Patrick Glenn, *Legal Traditions of the World: Sustainable Diversity in Law*. Oxford and NY: Oxford University Press, 2007 (3rd ed.), at 45.

[359] Although Cotterrell appears to be critical of Alan Watson's notion of legal transplants as too simplistic, since the importation of legal ideas and practices into a legal system tends not to be as 'easy' as Watson seems to suggest, it is unlikely that Cotterrell would agree with Pierre Legrand's application of autopoiesis in a strong sense, where legal or other institutional cultures are impenetrable as a normatively self-sufficient discourse. See Pierre Legrand, European Legal Systems are not Converging, (1996) 45 *International and Comparative Law Quarterly* 52; Roger Cotterrell, Comparatists and Sociology. In

remains clear, at least from my research, is the lawyer as techno-scientist, operating within a problem-solving modality and accompanying engineering mentality where "social ends could be accommodated ... by a highly rationalised, technical means-ends framework that would calibrate law according to changing social conditions."[360] It is realistic, functional and practicable; and not directed at political critique or philosophical contemplation. In other words, where anti-formalism holds sway in comparisons undertaken within academia,[361] formalism (or Kennedy's 'right-wing' anti-formalism)[362] appears to dominate comparative work in the policy environment. Of course, neither the BAC nor its Secretariat would think of their work as apolitical. Rather, they do not consider politics to be the business of the BAC, which has after all been constituted by the government to provide *expert* advice. Hence the *technocratisation* of comparative projects is a means by which the BAC distantiates itself from immediate political interests. It is also a way of attaining 'objectivity', which in turn advances the legitimacy of its recommendations with both the government and the public.

The constructivist nature of functional comparison directed at undermining differences and at system building provides a simple explanation for this lack of regard for the 'social'. Thinking further however, the 'social' has always been there, but not apparently so.

Pierre Legrand and Roderick Munday (eds.), *Comparative Legal Studies: Traditions and Transitions*. Cambridge: Cambridge University Press, 2003, pp 131-153, at 146-150.

[360] Annelise Riles, Property as Legal Knowledge: Means and Ends (2004) *Journal of the Royal Anthropological Institute* 10:775-795, at 785.

[361] David Kennedy observes that anti-formalism became mainstream from the 1950's, although within this camp, there was a distinction between those who emphasised technical characteristics and universal or shared features, as opposed to those who emphasised cultural characteristics and differentiatedness. David Kennedy, The methods and the politics. In Pierre Legrand and Roderick Munday (eds.), *Comparative Legal Studies: Traditions and Transitions*. Cambridge: Cambridge University Press, 2003, pp 345-433, at 403-406.

[362] *Ibid*, at 417. However, 'right-wing' anti-formalists here are less likely to view the law as autonomous, going by the features that Kennedy attributes to this camp.

Comparative projects are important means by which policymakers 'make sense' of the policy terrain. This policy terrain is the social totality that becomes the substrate for technocratic structuration. As we have seen, both the policy issues and responses are extricated from the same social bedrock. Structuration renders definition and confers meaning. It further enables association to be made, thereby creating a sense of solidarity and legitimacy. Hence an expression of 'making sense' is making comparison, and in respect of which ethics and law are the tools by which social structuration is achieved. Amidst social construction, the tools are most evident, and brackets out the 'social'.

3.9 Relationality in Comparative Tables as Policy Devices

As a matter of approach, the comparative projects that culminated in the comparative tables on oocyte donation and human-animal combinations do not fit neatly into Dannemann's three major stages of comparative enquiries; these being selection (of what will be compared), description (of the law and its context in the legal systems under consideration), and analysis.[363] The assemblage of 'relevant' jurisdictions could be broadly regarded as 'selection' but not in the sense of a formal quantitative sampling. This 'selection' through abstraction is a matter of construction that deploys ethical and legal knowledge as resource and tool. More importantly, the 'selection' process is not simply a matter of grouping things together based on certain characteristics, but it has been a relational exercise from the start.

Relationality occurs at various levels. First, 'selection' involves correlating relations of governance at the level of jurisdictions to a broader ethical superstructure, most apparent in the body of

---

[363] Gerhard Dannemann, Comparative Law: Study of Similarities or Differences? In Mathias Reimann and Reinhard Zimmermann (eds.), *The Oxford Handbook of Comparative Law*. Oxford and New York: Oxford University Press, 2006, pp 383-419, at 406.

international and transnational normative documents on bioethics (including medical ethics). In fact, the term 'correlation' is surprising appropriate as it suggests co-production in the association between these relations of governance within a broader ethical framework, although it is rarely the case that one wholly defines the other in multi-factorial analysis. This association further suggests the reason for appeal to universalism and foundationalism in many comparative projects on bioethical policy, quite unlike a strict Weberian statist approach for instance (although this aspect is nevertheless present).[364] Second, 'selection' is also a matter of relationality among the jurisdictions compared. In a policy environment, this could be described as 'benchmarking', so that where Singapore's position is said to be shared with Countries X and Y, for instance, a generally common ethical standard is seen to apply in all three jurisdictions. It is further crucial to recognise that this association cannot be simply claimed, but must be substantiated in order to have credibility. In some sense, it is like a currency peg, whereby an exchange rate of a country is closely tied to that of another. Once the association is made, the ethical policies of Countries X and Y will continue to have influence, although the extent may vary depending on a variety of factors. This aspect of relationality is perhaps most evident at the third level of relations between the ethical standards producer and those upon whom these standards apply. At a meeting between the BAC and researchers, a Japanese researcher queried if bioethical policies in Singapore are too 'western'.[365] I was similarly asked by a regulator if the BAC is being too 'westernised' in putting emphasis on the principle of autonomy in requiring specific consent for certain types of research.[366] On further enquiry, I discovered that these sentiments arose from the relationality that has been established between

---

[364] Ahmed White, Max Weber and the Uncertainties of Categorical Comparative Law. In Annelise Riles (ed.), *Re-thinking the Masters of Comparative Law*. Oxford and Portland: Hart Publishing, 2001, pp 40-57, at 43.

[365] Fieldnotes, 26 May 2009.

[366] Fieldnotes, 26 July 2010, MT.

bioethical policies in Singapore with those of key 'western' countries, especially the UK and the US. Another colleague in bioethics from Taiwan told me that he appreciated what appeared to him to be a more open and less hierarchical bioethical setup in Singapore owing to 'the British influence'. To some degree, there is some truth to these perceptions that there is in general a strong association between ethical policies in Singapore with those in the UK, for instance. There is a clear policy rationale for this stance, but it would be misleading to think of Singapore's policies as being entirely as one with those of the UK (or any other country).

I want to elaborate on positional relationality at the level of jurisdictions that the BAC's comparative projects establish. While these projects could explain differences and similarities with a view to 'learn' from other jurisdictions as a more conventional purpose usually attributed to comparative work, this was not the most important purpose. Instead, comparative tables are intended to be devices that generate relationality through comparison. We have considered this in the manner that comparison constructs and attributes positionality. In addition, comparative tables create the normative standards that govern oocyte donation and human-animal combinations. Lorraine Daston describes an instructive encounter with the Ware Collection of Blaschka Glass Models of Plants (or Glass Flowers) at the Harvard Museum of Natural History. She asks:[367]

> What kind of things are the Glass Flowers? Much of their fascination derives from their unclassifiability – itself a paradox, since they were made and are still displaced in order to demonstrate post-Darwinian phylogenetic botanical classification. They are at once undeniably artificial and flawlessly natural ...

---

[367] Lorraine Daston, The Glass Flowers. In Lorraine Daston (ed.), *Things That Talk: Object Lessons from Art and Science*. New York: Zone Books, 2004, pp 223-254, at 225.

Daston then observes that while possessing some degree of mass appeal, these flowers are neither valued by botanists nor artists.[368] She concludes that these constructs have a representational meaning over and above their physical form, but what exactly the meaning is has not been articulated.[369]

Like the Blaschka Glass Flowers, comparative tables are unlikely to satisfy the 'superior people' (to borrow Daston's language) of comparative law or socio-legal scholarship. As with other comparative tables, they classify through categorisation, but defy any meaningful categorisation themselves. Whereas Daston considers this to be some form of non-reductionist aesthetic communication, I understand this as an 'inner logic' that the comparative tables possess. They were developed for the specific purpose of constructing, correlating and communicating relationalities within the broad narrative of 'bioethics'. The representations that they encapsulate have been taken to be 'standards' that (co-)relationalities generate. However, the specificity in function of these tables precludes their broader application as 'generalisable knowledge' and further renders them non-representational. In this sense, comparative tables are akin to Annelise Riles's 'collaterals' in her study of financial derivatives in Japan. Riles provides as illustration a scenario whereby a trader at Paribas Bank agrees with a trader at Sanwa Bank to swap a certain amount of currency at a certain price in a year's time, pursuant to a swap agreement.[370] As assurance that Sanwa Bank will be able to meet its future obligation, Sanwa Bank would provide Paribas Bank with collateral. Sanwa's collateral will "precisely stand for, be the measure of, the extent to which it [Paribas Bank] can compel Sanwa to act as

---

368 *Ibid*, at 252: "The fact that thousands of tourists come to gawk at the models every year does not improve their standing in the Republic of Letters. Superior people do not visit the Glass Flowers."
369 *Ibid*, at 254.
370 Annelise Riles, Collateral Expertise: Legal Knowledge in the Global Financial Markets. *Current Anthropology* (December 2010) 51 (6): 795-818, at 801.

promised", [371] and thereby lower the greater information needs ('messy details') that Paribas Bank would otherwise be faced with. In ethnographic terms, Riles argues that the collateral is:

> an explicit modality of (temporary delineated) politics [and has] the same kind of political instability and ambiguity that characterizes the debt-like relations of the swap. [372]

She adds that a collateral is then:

> both a technology and a political problem, both a means to an end and a special kind of relationality [which] ... raises a problem of an attenuated, seemingly interminable (albeit ultimately finite) present of mutual entanglement. [373]

The BAC's comparative tables share a similar kind of political instability and ambiguity in the instrumental relationalities that they draw. As a technology and a political problem, I would prefer to think of these characteristics as manifestations of an inner logic. In policy process, the inner logic of comparative tables is a crucial means by which external information, values and material factors are translated into a policy environment and internalised. This logic confers on comparative tables the capacity to be utilised as normative tools in public policy.

As Wittgenstein observes, it is easy to assume that comparison produces 'objective' (or generally applicable) knowledge on the subjects compared rather than knowledge that is most immediately useful only for the comparatist. [374] His critique provides the occasion

---

[371] *Ibid*, at 802.
[372] *Ibid*.
[373] *Ibid*.
[374] Ludwig Wittgenstein (edited by Rush Rhees and translated by A C Miles), *Remarks on Frazer's Golden Bough*. Swansea: The Brynmill Press, 1979. Wittgenstein argues (at 5e): "Even the idea of trying to explain the practice – say the killing of the priest-king – seems to me wrong-headed. All that Frazer does is to make this practice plausible to people who think as he does. It is very queer that all these

to reflect further on what the BAC's comparative tables do in a policy environment. We have seen that these comparisons create rela-tionalities within a broader narrative (or perhaps varied and fragmented narratives) of 'bioethics'. Taken in isolation, these albeit hypothetical (as yet unproven causal) explanations advanced through comparison could be instructive as a form of general knowledge. In policy work, they are not only means of self-knowledge (through mapping of relationalities, as we have seen), but embody as well as perpetuate a composite form of rationalities. Consistent with the observation of Hal Colebatch and others, policy work is largely concerned with solving problems and the application of known techniques of governing to areas of concern.[375]

As public policy, the communicative character in the overarching goal of linking interaction and discourses in ways that enhances inter-subjective space is evident. Whether this inter-subjective space amounts to 'new' knowledge is, as we have discussed, an ancillary concern at best. More critical for our purpose are the non-instrumental rationalities that compose this shared space. In specifically incorporating, for instance, an 'ethical' dimension to the funding and practice of science, rationalisation based on values, tradition and (to a lesser extent) emotions are re-invigorated, at times countering a scientific instrumental rationalism that Weber regards as unstoppable.[376] The BAC's work could be viewed as a re-calibration of weightage in motivational rationalities, given that many contra-dictions that we witness in the politics of biomedical science arise from the interplay of different rationalities taken from standpoints that could be economic or political, ethical or aesthetic. This could also

practices are finally presented, so to speak, as stupid actions ... Frazer cannot imagine a priest who is not basically an English parson of our times with all his stupidity and feebleness."

375 Hal K Colebatch, Robert Hoppe and Mirka Noordegraaf, Understanding Policy Work. In Hal K Colebatch, Robert Hoppe and Mirko Noordegraaf (eds.), *Working for Policy*. Amsterdam: Amsterdam University Press, 2010, at 6.

376 Max Weber, Science as a vocation. In Wolfgang Schirmacher, *German Essays on Science in the 20th century*. New York: Continuum, 1996, at 223-237.

be seen as a form of communicative resistance to the disenchantment of scientific (instrumental) rationality, bearing in mind that 'ordering' and rationalising through issues in public policy could never be entirely value neutral. And again, what is value-based could nevertheless have an instrumental character. Formal rationalisation in terms of logical consistency in ethical content and systems through the application of rules or procedures has an instrumental character as it seeks to regularise certain actions so that they are always goal oriented and purposeful.

3.10 Comparison in Bioethics

Comparison was undertaken as a means of immersion into a discursive environment on human stem cell research, particularly where it relates to egg donation and human-animal combinations. Where legal and regulatory provisions were concerned, reaching 'upward' necessitated de-juridification to lift policy concerns to a sufficiently general normative platform that enabled comparison. Arguably, this exercise is no different from an approach in comparative law that involves detailed analysis of (albeit 'law on the books') regulatory and policy positions of different countries. From a jurisprudential standpoint, this manner of abstraction and generalisation appears to follow a Kelsenian tradition, where legal norms are essentially derivatives of foundational moral and social norms. This could well be the basis by which legal scholars have argued for a more open-ended approach to comparative law, and to include components and considerations that are beyond the 'legal' in a formalistic sense.[377] Despite my involvement (as someone who is legally trained), the comparative tables produced for both the ED and HA Consultation Papers and Reports to address specific bioethical

---

[377] See for instance: Maurice Adams and John Griffiths, Against 'comparative method': explaining similarities and differences. In Maurice Adams and Jacco Bomhoff (eds.), *Practice and Theory in Comparative Law*. Cambridge: Cambridge University Press, 2012, pp 279-301.

concerns would not have been significantly different from those produced exclusively by comparative lawyers. These tables are instrumental and pragmatic, even if somewhat 'amateurish'. But this approach was useful as a technocratic skill directed at 'making sense' of issues in the context of bioethics and figuring out viable options. This is a constructivist process, inherently communicative and functional (i.e. qualities that are arguably more amenable to policy generation than conceptual critique). In addition, it was directed at overcoming incommensurability in a strong sense.

While technocratic comparison could be viewed as comparing relations of governance in an 'objective' non-relational way, the comparative tables appear to work very much in the opposite direction. Comparison was needed to gain a degree of self-awareness in order to establish solidarity with other 'like-minded' jurisdictions. As we have seen, such self-awareness does not often tell us anything more about the comparatist. The most practical benefit of this exercise is that the solidarity achieved confers legitimacy on a policy if other jurisdictions that share this position are held in high regard. In normative terms, solidarity through positional association becomes the basis of standards, or 'international best practices'. These standards are by no means uniformly adopted or shared by every jurisdiction. Standards are normative platforms that enable communication across different discursive and social context, essentially by undermining and supplanting discursive and situational differences, and by focusing on particular problems and functions (thereby operating somewhat like Mitchel Lasser's 'sliding scales'). Such a 'constructivist' approach is again conducive to a policy environment as not every issue is (fundamentally or expediently) resolvable or reconcilable in the political domain or as a first-order concern. Differences are undermined through the drawing of normative and functional equivalence through syllogistic reasoning and analogy, which are techniques commonly used by comparative lawyers, but not exclusively so.

Making comparisons and evidence to that effect – especially in the form of comparative tables – are critical symbols of policy due diligence. Whether in internal discussions or for meetings with researchers, religious group leaders, policy-makers or other stakeholders, comparative positions have always been provided. Comparative tables, as devices that create associations, would usually be the subject of discussion. Interestingly, while comparative tables are relational and communicate through typification, they are themselves difficult to typify.

At the commencement of my fieldwork, documents were being prepared for meetings. Among these documents, comparative tables on human oocyte donation and human-animal combinations were circulated ahead of the meeting for consideration and specifically marked for discussion. No explanation was needed as it was generally assumed that policy positions from outside of Singapore were available and relevant. This *praesumptio similitudinis* could be justified on at least two bases discussed in some detail above. First, certain international events contributed to the harmonisation of issue-framing across jurisdictions. Second, there already exists a number of substantive bioethical viewpoints on stem cell research and human-animal combinations at the time of my fieldwork. Taken together, a discursive space broadly regarded as 'bioethics' enabled the artefact of human-animal combinations to be bracketed out and problematised in terms of a number of essentialised concerns, which I term 'focal points'. We next evaluate the nature and dynamics of this space and the focal points that animate it.

4

Scripting Bioethics from the Bottom Up

4.1 Starting from the Top

During the 56th Session (2001 to 2002) of the United Nations General Assembly (UNGA), France and Germany tabled a proposal for the promulgation of a legally binding treaty or convention to prohibit reproductive cloning of human beings. The original French-German proposal[378] was essentially directed at reproductive cloning and did not assume a firm position for or against SCNT. However, France and Germany subsequently amended their proposal to recommend that a moratorium be imposed on the conduct of SCNT immediately following the completion of negotiations on the reproductive cloning convention.[379] This amendment was made to reflect the growing number of delegations concerned with the practice of SCNT. With this amendment, France and Germany were able to retain a majority of countries supporting their proposal. These included countries that did not have a position on SCNT, but supported the proposal so that reproductive cloning could be prohibited at the international level.

---

[378] See A/C.6/57/WG.1/CRP.1.

[379] See A/C.6/57/L.8 (hereinafter, the 'French-German proposal'). The list of sponsors is set out in A/C.6/57/L.8/Corr.1.

Although the proposal was adopted by consensus at the 56th UNGA, contention arose when the United States, Spain, and the Holy See-led coalition sought a ban on SCNT along with reproductive cloning.[380] The basic premise for the position held by this coalition was that there could be no distinction made between SCNT and reproductive cloning, as both involved the use of a common technological process. Clarity in the simplicity of this formulation proved attractive to many countries (especially those with a predominantly large Catholic population) without having first arrived at a national position on the subject. Various alternative proposals were put forward, including one from Mexico to impose a ban on reproductive cloning and a moratorium on SCNT, so as to allow the latter to be debated while resolving the former. This proposal was supported by the Netherlands, Australia, and various Latin American and African countries.

When the UNGA reconvened for the 57th session in the fall of 2002, the discussions were largely grounded in emotive rhetoric. As Singapore has a national position on the subject, one of the goals of the Singapore delegation was to deploy this as a basis for advancing the French-German proposal. Despite already having legislation that disallowed SCNT, France and Germany were prepared to work with countries adhering to different views on SCNT in order to secure a legally binding treaty prohibiting reproductive cloning. They were motivated by a belief that human reproductive cloning was an imminent threat, and prompt response on the part of the international community would be politically expedient. Hence, they took the pragmatic approach to focus only on reproductive cloning. In opposition, strong US support for a comprehensive ban on all forms of cloning could have been due in part to the need to play up to the

---

[380] The Ad Hoc Committee on an International Convention against the Reproductive Cloning of Human Beings was formed through the UNGA's resolution 56/93 of 12 Dec 2001. It was tasked to "consider the elaboration of a mandate for the negotiation of such an international convention, including a list of the existing international instruments to be taken into consideration and a list of legal issues to be address in the convention."

domestic religious and pro-life lobby, and partly by the desire not to lose its scientific and commercial lead to other countries that did not face similar political obstacles. Other countries that supported the US-Spain proposal were driven by ideological positions on the sanctity of life and the rights of the embryo. In addition, arguments advanced in support of a comprehensive ban on all forms of cloning included the following concerns:[381]

(1) If SCNT is not prohibited, it creates a loop-hole which prevents effective enforcement of prohibition against the implantation of that cloned embryo into the uterus of a woman;

(2) 'Slippery slope' argument in that once scientists are allowed to carry out SCNT, there would be little to prevent them from going one step further and engage in reproductive cloning;

(3) SCNT is against human dignity because it involves the killing of a life when stem-cells are extracted from the cloned embryo thereby destroying it. The killing of this nascent life cannot be justified for any reason, even if it is to save other lives;

(4) Adult stem cell research, which is not ethically objectionable, will yield just as much benefit as embryonic stem cell research, including SCNT;

(5) SCNT will lead to exploitation of women, especially in poor countries, as there will be illicit trade in eggs for profit;

(6) Chances are remote that developing countries can avail themselves of the potential benefits that might be derived from SCNT research; and

(7) There are more pressing concerns facing developing countries (such as malaria), and the resources that would be poured into SCNT research would be better utilised on these areas of pressing concern.

---

[381] These arguments are consolidated based on the author's interviews with some members of the Malaysia and Singapore delegation at the 57th UNGA.

Only a minority of countries that included Australia, Belgium, China, Israel, Singapore, South Africa, Sweden, Switzerland and the United Kingdom were fervent in keeping the door to SCNT open. When it eventually became clear that no agreement could be arrived at between the two factions, the discussions were adjourned to a year later.[382]

At the 58th Session in 2003, countries remained divided along roughly similar lines. Costa Rica now led a group of sixty-eight states with the most stringent proposal which recommended criminal sanctions and extradition of any person involving in any form of cloning.[383] The French-German position could not be sustained after strong domestic political pressure from the German legislature and public resulting in the withdrawal of Germany's support for its own proposal.[384] Belgium took over the initiative in the French-German proposal as it was consistent with its domestic policy of banning reproductive cloning as a matter of urgency. Following this development, the Belgian proposal gained the backing of the original supporters of the French-German proposal, in addition to a number of Nordic states.[385]

In the course of the debates, both sides actively engaged with smaller states that did not have any immediate interest in cloning technology. When it seemed likely that the Costa Rican proposal would carry the day, the delegation of Iran, on behalf of the member States of the Organisation of the Islamic Conference, moved to adjourn the debate on the agenda item until the 60th Session of the UNGA in September 2005. The motion was passed by a narrow margin with

---

[382] UN Doc. A/57/569 (2002) at 7.

[383] UN Doc. A/58/73 (2003).

[384] Nigel M de S Cameron and A V Henderson. Brave New World at the General Assembly: The United Nations Declaration on Human Cloning. *Minnesota Journal of Law Science and Technology* 2008; 9: 145-238, at 169 and 189-191.

[385] UN Doc. A/C.6/58/L.8 (2003), About a week before debate was resumed at the UNGA, the German government announced that it would no longer sponsor the French-German proposal, but would instead support the Belgian proposal: *Ibid* at 190.

80 countries having voted in favour, 79 countries having voted against and 15 countries having abstained.

The 59th session of the UNGA reconvened for general debate on 21 September 2004, with an address by US President George W Bush that included a call on member states to ban all forms of cloning. Cloning remained an issue in US domestic politics as the nation prepared for its Presidential election in November that year. The position of the US federal government on embryonic stem cell research and SCNT was not shared by all of its constituents. In March 2004, 70 members of Congress wrote to President Bush to relax his ban of federal funding for research on embryonic stem cells created after 9 August 2001.[386] These legislators threatened to push for legislation to achieve this goal if the President failed to act. This followed from the confirmation by the National Institutes of Health that, of the 78 embryonic lines that qualify for federal funding, only 17 are actually ready for research. In addition, private institutions announced that they would push ahead in human embryonic stem cell research with private funds. Later in the year, voters in the state of California approved of Proposition 71 on 2 November. This initiative established a $3 billion bond measure to fund stem cell research in the state through the California Institute for Regenerative Medicine (CIRM).

Despite strong lobbying on both sides, no consensus was reached either by the UNGA or by the Sixth Committee when it met on 21 October 2004.[387] By that time, motivation in pushing for a legally binding treaty significantly waned. In February 2005, a draft non-binding declaration initially prepared by Italy and subsequently revised as a proposal by Honduras was submitted.[388] It was the

---

[386] Brian Vastag. Private Efforts Pick Up Stem Cell Slack, *Journal of the American Medical Association* 2004; 291 (17): 2059.

[387] *Report of the Sixth Committee – Addendum*, UN Doc. A/59/516 Add. I (2004). 71 states voted in favour, with 35 states voting against, and 43 states abstaining.

[388] UNGA, Sixth Committee Working Group. 2005. *Report of the Working Group Established Pursuant to General Assembly Decision 59/547 to Finalize the Text of a*

amended proposal from Honduras that was subsequently adopted by the UNGA on 8 March 2005.[389] While the UN *Declaration on Human Cloning* recommended legal prohibition of reproductive cloning, no agreement was reached on the issue of whether a human embryo could also qualify as a 'person' upon whom (or indeed, which) fundamental rights would attend. The lack of consensus ultimately resulted in a declaration, regarded by many to be without moral or legal authority, aside from saying nothing about cloning or human dignity.[390]

Ironically, the UN initiative had a catalytic effect on a number of member states interested in SCNT. The threat of being subsumed into a disagreeable discourse motivated these states to articulate a national position that would be useful in at least two ways. First, it served as a discursive barrier against an allegation of condoning unethical scientific practices in exchange for some form of (often economic) benefit. Bioethics has become an intrinsic component to a member state's reputation of doing 'good science', which in turn influences the flow of, as well as its claim over, scarce resources and talent. Second, it enabled solidarity in that like-minded member states came into alliance with one another to amplify their political clout.

In this chapter, we consider 'bioethics' as a discursive policy space within which the artefacts of human stem cell science and technology are embedded, and how it has been produced, received and consumed. I propose the emergence of a bioethical account on human stem cell

---

United Nations Declaration on Human Cloning. U.N. Doc. A/C.6/59/L.27/Rev.1. 23 Feb.

[389] UNGA Resolution 59/280 (2004) incorporates the *United Nations Declaration on Human Cloning.*

[390] The *Human Cloning Declaration* is set out as A/Res/59/280, 23 Mar 2005. I have considered the unique circumstances leading up to its enactment elsewhere. See Calvin Ho, Governing Cloning: United Nations' Debates and the Institutional Context of Standards. In Benjamin J Capps and Alastair V Campbell (eds.), *Contested Cells: Global Perspectives on the Stem Cell Debate.* London: Imperial College Press, 2010, pp 121-154.

research and application in the form of a global script, with mixed epistemological qualities of revolutions, rivalries and co-operations that mirror to different degrees the three main accounts of globalisation (i.e. imperialism, transplantation and assemblage). As Peer Fiss and Paul Hirsch observe, the notion of 'global' is also a process by which the meaning of events is socially constructed and negotiated.[391] Sense-making is enabled within the frames of meaning that constitute interpretive spaces.[392] I advance four observations about the global script. First, the 'global' script arose out of events that were essentially local. Analysing the development of stem cell policies from the standpoint of the BAC, the key triggering event that led to the formalisation of guidelines for embryonic stem cell research could be traced to then US President George W Bush's decision to stop federal funding of such research. Second, the normative content of the global script is not merely drawn from one 'local' script, but several. As there are important differences among the various 'local' scripts, the 'global' script could be seen as broadly overlapping consensus of ethical and policy positions rooted in distinct and possibly incommensurable conditions, ideologies and goals. Consequently, the 'global' script is itself an incomplete account and carries, in a number of instances, inconsistencies and contradictions that in turn add to its own discursive dynamism. Third, the 'global' script draws on a number of other local and transnational scripts, especially those relating to notions of the 'common good' and 'dignity', among others. Finally, it

---

[391] Peer C Fiss and Paul M Hirsch. The Discourse of Globalization: Framing and Sense making of an Emerging Concept, *American Sociological Review* (2005) 70, 1: 29-52.

[392] Sense-making is distinguished from framing in its emphasis on "the internal, self-conscious process of developing a coherent account of what is going on, while framing emphasizes the external, strategic process of creating specific meaning in line with political interests ... If framing focuses on *whose* meanings win out in symbolic contests, sense-making shifts the focus to understanding *why* such frame contests come into being in the first place, as well as how they are connected to 'hard' structural changes, and over which territory they are fought". *Ibid*, at 31 (emphasis in original).

reflects different relationships (and relationalities) among states and international organisations that cannot be adequately accounted for by a single dominant discourse on globalisation, be it imperialism, transplantation or assemblage. Arguably, the relationships entailed in the 'global' script have been more participatory than directive, and the relationalities more subtle.

We first consider the creation of a 'local' script in the guidelines for stem cell research issued by the NAS. This script was endorsed, with some important qualifications, by the State of California, and could be taken together as the US script. It acquired transnational influence when it was substantively adopted by the ISSCR. The US script (and its internationalised version) has been influential on the AMS, which was instrumental in steering the policy direction of the UK government on the subject, including the incorporation of critical changes to the legislative framework on some aspects of stem cell research. These changes in the UK could be surmised as another 'local' script that has parallel but different concerns from those of the US. Separately, the DCE and the EU generated their own scripts on hybrids and chimeras in stem cell research. The US and UK scripts were considered, but did not otherwise have pervasive conceptual influence over their European or Japanese counterparts. Nevertheless, the deliberative outcomes of the DCE and the special project group of the EU and did not significantly differ from those of the US and UK. In the deliberation of the BAC, the commonalities in the various 'local' scripts could be consolidated into a 'global' script, particularly when related to other globalised discourses on the common good and human dignity. While there is strictly speaking no formal 'global' script as such, these commonalities are embedded in the policy documents of the various bodies or institutions considered here. Documents embody social phenomena through various modes of objectification. These documents create 'focal points' by which a particular social phenomenon is (or could be) linked or related to a broader system of reference. Referencing is a means by which organisation is achieved, so that the artefacts of eggs, chimeras and hybrids acquire epistemological form that enables comprehension.[393] This is analogous to the way in which the facts of a particular case are (re)organised so that they are focused around a legal reference point like 'unconscionability' in order for *meaningful* legal recourse to be sought in the law of restitution.[394] In the same way a judgment uses documents as mediation technology to confer meanings on social phenomena. It is through this drawing of relations that a subject gains conceptual coherence as object. This chapter considers the ways in which the 'focal points' developed in a variety of 'local' scripts have been important in the shaping of 'focal points' in the HA Report. These 'focal points' are broadly synonymous with what is more commonly known as 'bioethical issues' or 'ethical, legal and social issues'. Later in this work, we will consider how these 'focal points' relate to the concept of juridification.

The careful study of foreign policy documents by the BAC illustrates the transnational character of policy work. It is perhaps not often appreciated that there is a certain communicative rationality among policy-makers. After all, the study of policy documents entails an inquiry into some aspect of the institutional authors. However, one should be wary of jumping to the conclusion that policy-makers and policy bodies are intimately connected *inter se* (as perhaps a notion of

---

[393] I borrow this reference from Thomas Schelling, who used this term to refer to points of reference that coordinate expectations in the absence of prior agreement. Thomas Schelling, *The Strategy of Conflict.* Cambridge: Harvard University Press, 1960, at 54-58. In addition, the term 'focal points' are akin to 'fixed points' in legal reasoning, where statutes, judicial decisions and *travaux préparatoires* serve as boundaries to constrain deliberation and enable the production of an outcome or closure. See Aleksander Peczenik, Justice in legal doctrine. In Guenther Doeker-Mach and Klaus A Ziegert (eds.), *Law, Legal Culture and Politics in the Twenty First Century.* Stuttgart: Franz Steiner Verlag, 2004, pp 197-211.

[394] In the US, see the decision of Justice Wright in *Williams v. Walker-Thomas Furniture Co.*, 350 F.2d 445 (D.C. Cir. 1965); in the UK, the decision of Lord Denning in *Lloyds Bank Ltd v Bundy* [1975] QB 326.

legal or regulatory transplantation may suggest). The institutions in my study neither acted in concert nor in isolation. They operate under very specific socio-political conditions and the documents that they produce were intended to address the cognitive and broader needs of their particular circumstance. Instead, these institutions appear to be associated in loose networks. Their association is neither purely a methodological construct as Marcus indicates[395] nor as structured as the 'global forms' of Stephen Collier and Aihwa Ong.[396] While these documents have been produced for specific audiences, they are, like legal rules, open textured. Arguably, these networks are embodiments of intersubjective space that these institutional authors unconsciously created. Hence this chapter also discusses documents as an institutional technology of mediation and social relations, although the latter is admittedly more ambiguous in intent and application. We begin by considering key institutions and their scripts.

4.2 The National Academy of Sciences

In 1999, the US NBAC, appointed by President William J Clinton, published a report on hESC research.[397] A recommendation of the NBAC was for the DHHS to establish a National Stem Cell Oversight and Review Panel. A set of guidelines was developed by the Human Pluripotent Stem Cell Review Group of the NIH in 2000,[398] which reflected many of the recommendations of the NBAC. Both the report of the NBAC and the NIH guidelines were closely studied when crafting

---

395 George E Marcus. *Ethnography Through Thick and Thin*. Princeton NJ: Princeton University Press, 1998, at 195.
396 Stephen J Collier and Aihwa Ong, Global Assemblages and Anthropological Problems. In Aihwa Ong and Stephen J. Collier, *Global Assemblages: Technology, Politics, and Ethics as Anthropological Problems*. Singapore: Blackwell Publishing, 2005, pp 3-21 at 11.
397 National Bioethics Advisory Commission, *Ethical Issues in Human Stem Cell Research*. Rockville, MD: U.S. Government Printing Office, 1999.
398 National Institutes of Health, Guidelines for Research Using Human Pluripotent Stem Cells. Federal Register 65 (166, 25 August 2000): 51975.

the SC Report. However, by the time the SC Report was published in 2002, US federal policy on hESC research changed drastically. The guidelines of 2000 were superseded in 2001 following an executive order issued by President George W Bush to limit the scope of federally funded hESC research to cell lines derived prior to 9 August 2001.[399] But in the absence of federal law, hESC research can be carried out in the US with private funding provided that it was not otherwise prohibited by state law. In 2005, a comprehensive ethical framework was proposed by the NAS for hESC research that was not federally funded.[400] With the foreclosure of access to public funds, the research community was unable to look towards governmental bodies, particularly the NIH, for ethical or regulatory guidance. It turned to Dr Bruce Alberts, a biochemist and at that time the President of the NAS, and the Editor-in-Chief of the illustrious journal *Science*. Recognising the desire of the stem cell research community to avoid being perceived as mavericks, the NAS met the cost of developing its 2005 guidelines out of its own funds.[401]

The NAS' leadership role in championing science as a profession seems imbued in the very building that houses it. From Galileo's star

---

[399] The NIH then developed a set of criteria based on the limitations imposed by President Bush. National Institutes of Health, *Notice of Criteria for Federal Funding of Research on Existing Human Embryonic Stem Cells and Establishment of NIH Human Embryonic Stem Cell Registry*. 7 November 2001.

[400] National Academy of Sciences: National Research Council and Institute of Medicine. *Guidelines for Human Embryonic Stem Cell Research*. Washington, DC: National Academies Press, 2005. This version of the NAS Guidelines is accompanied by a detailed explanatory text that is not reproduced together with subsequent revisions.

[401] Interview with Dr Fran Sharples, Director, Board on Life Sciences, National Academy of Sciences, 21 July 2011. Dr Sharples explained that the Board of Life Sciences is part of the National Research Council, which is a private non-governmental body. However, its work has essentially been funded by way of federal contracts. This showed that human embryonic stem cell research was considered to be a very important area for the NAS to fund the development of guidelines. Subsequent amendments to the 2005 guidelines continued to be funded mainly by the NAS, although some funding was also obtained from charities, such as the Howard Hughes Institute.

map of 1610 to Thomas Edison's incandescent light bulb patented in 1884, these images etched onto the left wall of its marble lobby suggest a continuum in human inventions. The NAS is a prestigious society of distinguished scholars engaged in scientific and engineering research. It was signed into being on 3 March 1863 by President Abraham Lincoln with a mandate in its Act of Incorporation to "investigate, examine, experiment, and report upon any subject of science or art" whenever called upon to do so by any department of the government.[402] The NAS expanded to include the National Research Council in 1916, the NAE in 1964 and the IOM in 1970. As such, the NAS and its constituents are sometimes referred to as the National Academies. The NAS is governed by a council of 12 members and is reported to have approximately 2,100 members and 380 foreign associates, of whom nearly 200 have won Nobel Prizes.[403]

The first version of the *Guidelines for Human Embryonic Stem Cell Research* issued in 2005 was prepared by an expert committee co-chaired by biochemist Richard Hynes and bioethicist Jonathon Moreno, and supported by a secretariat that was headed by Dr Fran Sharples. These guidelines were subsequently amended on three occasions; in 2007,[404] in 2008 to include iPSC technology,[405] and again in 2010 to reflect changes made by the NIH under the Obama Administration.[406] Taken together, the NAS Guidelines (the 2005

---

[402] Rexmond C Cochrane. *The National Academy of Sciences: The First Hundred Years 1863-1963.* Washington DC: National Academy of Sciences, 1978, at 596. Cochrane indicates the NAS' most famous and long-lived ancestor as England's Royal Society, which received its charter from Charles II in 1662.

[403] The data is drawn from the website of the NAS: www.nasonline.org.

[404] National Academy of Sciences: National Research Council and Institute of Medicine, *2007 Amendments to the National Academies' Guidelines for Human Embryonic Stem Cell Research.* Washington, DC: National Academies Press, 2007.

[405] National Academy of Sciences: National Research Council and Institute of Medicine, *2008 Amendments to the National Academies' Guidelines for Human Embryonic Stem Cell Research.* Washington, DC: National Academies Press, 2008.

[406] National Academy of Sciences: National Research Council and Institute of Medicine, *Final Report of the Human Embryonic Stem Cell Research Advisory*

Guidelines, as amended in 2007, 2008 and 2010: the 'NAS Guidelines') recommend the establishment of an ESCRO committee for the review of any research involving hES cells or human iPS cells. This is regardless of the source from which such cells are derived (i.e. whether from a human embryo or from SCNT).[407] While it may share some members with an IRB, an ESCRO committee is not a subcommittee of, or a substitute for, the IRB. Its purpose is to provide an additional level of review and scrutiny due to complex issues raised by hES cell research.[408] As for the standard of review, the NAS Guidelines present three categories:

(a) Research that does not require additional review by the ESCRO committee,

(b) Research that requires additional review and approval by the ESCRO committee, and

(c) Research that should not be conducted at this time.[409]

Most research involving human-animal chimera or cytoplasmic hybrids falls into the second category. As such, the research will have to be reviewed by the IRB, IACUC, Institutional Biosafety Committee and the ESCRO committee.[410]

The NAS Guidelines limit experimentation on a human embryo or embryo-like constructs (such as cytoplasmic hybrids) to 14 days of

---

Committee and *2010 Amendments to the National Academies' Guidelines for Human Embryonic Stem Cell Research*. Washington, DC: National Academies Press, 2010. Amendments were mainly introduced to reflect President Barack Obama's Executive Order 13505: *Removing Barriers to Responsible Scientific Research Involving Human Stem Cells*, which was issued on March 9, 2009. The Executive Order states that the Secretary of Health and Human Services, through the Director of NIH, may support and conduct responsible, scientifically worthy human stem cell research, including human embryonic stem cell research, to the extent permitted by law.

[407] *Ibid*, Guideline 1.1(a).
[408] *Ibid*. See Guideline 2.
[409] *Ibid*. Guideline 1.3.
[410] *Ibid*, Guideline 1.3(b)(i) and (ii).

development. It further recommends the prohibition of the implant-tation of such hybrids into a uterus.[411] Even with the breakthrough of iPSC technology, cytoplasmic hybrids (and SCNT more generally) is still valued as a research tool to facilitate understanding of the reprogramming process of somatic nuclei. In incorporating a new set of guidelines that relate specifically to iPSC technology,[412] the orientation of the NAS reflects that of the NBAC in treating the subject of pluripotency in a more generic manner. As for animal chimeras, the NAS considers experiments incorporating hES cells into postnatal animals to be an essential form of preclinical testing, similar to standard testing of drugs, transplants, and medical devices in animals before human clinical trials.[413] Concerns over such experiments mainly pertain to the possibility of the hES cells or neural derivatives conferring 'higher-order' brain functions in the animal, or of human cells arising in non-human germline.[414] It observes that the issue regarding the potential for contribution to brain function is not easily resolved and should be explored through animal experiments. In addition, due care is required in conducting experiments that create such possibilities.[415] Concerns have also been expressed over germline modifications, but these could be more easily addressed by disallowing the chimeric animals to breed. In summary, the degree of ethical concern over incorporation of hES cells into an animal will vary with its stage of development.[416]

---

[411] *Ibid,* Guideline 4.5.

[412] *Ibid,* Guideline 7 (Recommendations for research use of non-embryo-derived human pluripotent stem cells).

[413] National Academy of Sciences: National Research Council and Institute of Medicine, *Guidelines for Human Embryonic Stem Cell Research.* Washington, DC: National Academies Press, 2005, at 39.

[414] *Ibid,* at 40.

[415] *Ibid.*

[416] National Academy of Sciences: National Research Council and Institute of Medicine. *Guidelines for Human Embryonic Stem Cell Research.* Washington, DC: National Academies Press, 2008, Guideline 6.

The proposed prohibitions in the third category (i.e. experiments involving the incorporation of hES cells into other species at the embryonic stage) similarly apply to non-embryo-derived human pluripotent stem cells. The NAS maintains the position that the following types of research should not be permitted at this point of time:[417]

(a) Experiments that involve transplantation of human pluripotent stem cells into human embryos; and

(b) Research in which human pluripotent stem cells are introduced into nonhuman primate embryos, pending further research that would clarify the potential of such introduced cells to contribute to neural tissue or to the germline.

In addition, the NAS continues to express caution over the use of human neural stem cells[418] and potential germline modification.[419]

On 9 March 2009, President Barrack Obama removed restrictions on hES cell research imposed by President Bush.[420] Following this, a new set of guidelines was issued ·by the NIH.[421] In the creation of human-animal chimeras, these guidelines reflect the position of the NAS in that research involving the following will not be eligible for funding:[422]

(a) The introduction of hES cells or human iPS cells into nonhuman primate blastocysts; and

---

[417] *Ibid*, Guideline 7.3(c)(iii).

[418] *Ibid*, Guideline 7.4.

[419] *Ibid*, Guideline 7.5.

[420] Barack Obama (2009). *Removing Barriers to Responsible Scientific Research*. Executive Order 13505. For a discussion of some developments following this reversal of policy, see Mary A Majumder and Cynthia B Cohen, Future Directions for Oversight of Stem Cell Research in the United States: An Update. In *Kennedy Institute of Ethics Journal* (2009) Vol. 19 No. 2, pp 195-200.

[421] National Institutes of Health, *Guidelines for Research Using Human Stem Cells*. *Federal Register* 74, 128 (7 July 2009): 32170-32175.

[422] *Ibid*, at 32175, Guideline IV.

(b) The breeding of animals where the introduction of hES cells or iPS cells may contribute to the germline.

But unlike the NAS Guidelines, the NIH denies funding for research "using hESCs derived from ... somatic cell nuclear transfer, partheno-genesis, and/or IVF embryos created for research purposes".[423] Consequently, research involving the derivation of stem cells from a cytoplasmic hybrid embryo will not be eligible for NIH funding. This position is more conservative than that proposed by the NBAC of the Clinton administration.

Although the NAS is not a conventional standards-setting government body like the NIH, the circumstance under which the first version of the guidelines on stem cell research was produced rendered the NAS a surrogate of the NIH and the *de facto* standards body in the US.[424] The relationship between the NAS and the NIH is often not as straightforward as it may seem. Dr Sharples explained that the NAS could be regarded as a client of the NIH in that it has received substantial funding of about US$10 million in grants. However, there has always been some tension between funding that the NIH provided to the NAS and funding that it could otherwise provide directly to investigators. In the current climate of tight budget constraints, the NIH was expected to scrutinise the projects that the NAS conducts. To quote Dr Sharples: "NIH has less money, we get less money".[425] She further observed that with Dr Francis Collins as Director, the NIH may have a preference for obtaining advice directly from the scientific community rather than to go through the NAS. However, she also indicated that it could be appropriate to exclude the government in discussions on certain issues in order to have a

---

[423] *Ibid*, Guideline V.

[424] Cohen and Majumder argue for a more uniform, authoritative and participatory approach, with NIH taking the lead. Cynthia B Cohen and Mary A Majumder, Future Directions for Oversight of Stem Cell Research in the United States. In *Kennedy Institute of Ethics Journal* (2009) 19, 1: 79-103, at 89-90.

[425] Interview with Dr Fran Sharples, Director, Board on Life Sciences, National Academy of Sciences, 21 July 2011.

'safe forum' or not have the authorities 'breathe down your neck'. This was a reason for not consulting the government when the NAS guidelines were revised from 2007 onwards. As a practical matter, it appears clear that the NAS guidelines have been taken to be the *de facto* governance standards for the US, and the key features of the ethical framework proposed by the NAS are largely reflected in the ethical rules of the ISSCR and the CIRM, a statutory body established by the State of California to fund stem cell research. We consider each of them in turn.

4.3 International Society for Stem Cell Research

The ISSCR was formed in 2002 as an international professional organisation of stem cell scientists. It meets annually, mainly in North America, and has co-organised regional meetings. The ISSCR has been presided by well-established stem cell researchers like Irving Weissman, who served as the immediate past President.[426] In 2007, it launched the journal *Cell Stem Cell* as a high-end forum for stem cell biology. A year later, experts in law and public policy were involved in its 'Global Forum' series, and a Global Advisory Council was formed to help the ISSCR set a strategy for advancing stem cell research and public education.[427] Nancy Witty observed that since its founding:

> [The ISSCR] remains the only international membership society that embraces researchers, clinicians, ethicists and policymakers, industry representatives, civic leaders, and patient advocates. This broad constituency both motivates and enables the ISSCR to present a united voice for the continued global support of stem cell research and the exchange of scientific information.[428]

---

[426] George Q Daley, Letter from the President, *Cell Stem Cell* (2008) 3: 151-152.
[427] George Q Daley, Heather M Rooke and Nancy Witty, Global Forum Discusses Stem Cell Research Strategy, *Cell Stem Cell* (2007) 2: 435-436.
[428] Nancy Witty, Strategic Planning: Progress and Potential, *Cell Stem Cell* (2007) 1: 383-386, at 383.

Stem cell researchers in Singapore have been involved in the scientific meetings of the ISSCR. On a number of occasions, members of the BAC have also been involved in the meetings as there were ethics components to them. It has been in part through such engagements that the views of the ISSCR are incorporated into the deliberations of the BAC. For the BAC Secretariat, being acquainted with a number of the scientists and policy-makers involved in the ISSCR added familiarity and perspective. Recognition by the ISSCR of the need to constantly recreate itself to enhance relevance and distinction contributes to their credibility among policymakers.[429]

Until 2015, three documents provide guidance for the conduct of all human embryonic stem cell research, including research involving cytoplasmic hybrids and chimeras. The first set of guidelines published in December 2006 set out the general regulatory framework for hESC research.[430] They exclude research on animal stem cells, human stem cells that are not known to possess totipotent or pluripotent potential, or the transfer of animal cells into humans at any stage of development. As such, the focus of the ISSCR was on experimental rather than therapeutic application of human pluripotent cells. Similar to the ESCRO committee, the ISSCR proposes a separate review mechanism for stem cell research, but in the form of a process referred to as Stem Cell Research Oversight (or SCRO).[431] The three categories of stem cell research for experiments that are permissible

---

[429] Take for instance the ISSCR's letter to the German government expression support for revisions to the 2002 Stem Cell Act. International Society for Stem Cell Research, Press Release: *Letter to German Government supporting changes to Stem Cell Act, 2002*, 7 March 2008. It also provided feedback to the NIH on its 2009 guidelines for stem cell research: International Society for Stem Cell Research, Press Release: *ISSCR Comments on Draft Guidelines for Embryonic Stem Cell Funding*, 22 May 2009.

[430] International Society for Stem Cell Research, *Guidelines for the Conduct of Human Embryonic Stem Cell Research*, 2006.

[431] *Ibid*, at 5, paragraph 8 (Recommendations for Oversight).

after standard review, permissible after additional and comprehensive review, and impermissible, reflect the ethical framework of the NAS.[432] However, the ISSCR Guidelines differs from the NAS Guidelines in that the incorporation of hES cells into nonhuman primate embryos or any embryonic stem cell into human embryos is not prohibited. It does specify caveats relating to the proportion of human stem cells transferred, the likely integration into critical tissues such as the germline and central nervous system, and the transfer of human cells into non-human primates.

A year later, the Ethics and Public Policy Committee of the ISSCR published a report that specifically addressed the subject of animal chimeras. It emphasised the importance of animal chimeras as research tools and to avoid 'unwanted stem cell exceptionalism'.[433] Operationally, monitoring and data collection should be based upon a sound assessment of the developmental trajectories that are likely to be affected, and the epigenetic context of regulation in which the mixed genes or cells are going to be deployed should be taken into account. Data collection should be related to known functional links, and evaluated in a scientifically legitimate manner. The ISSCR observes that no single test, such as the percentage presence of human derived cells in the brain, should be necessarily required, unless its functional link to pertinent physical or mental qualities is either demonstrated or is consistent with scientific knowledge or scientifically reasonable inferences concerning whether, in the context of other data, it will be a valid predictor of sentience.[434] Chimera neuroscientific research involving human stem cells or their direct derivatives hypothetically approximates some aspects of human brain functioning. It may thus require specialised cognitive

---

432 *Ibid* at 6-7, paragraph 10 (Categories of research).
433 International Society for Stem Cell Research, Ethical Standards for Human-to-Animal Chimera Experiments in Stem Cell Research, *Cell Stem Cell* (2007) 1: 159-163, at 161.
434 *Ibid*.

assessments or otherwise assessments that are conducted in neuro-scientific research.

In 2009, a report was published to consider if the creation of cytoplasmic hybrids is scientifically justified. This scientific and (to a lesser degree) ethical evaluation was undertaken in the light of some recent developments, notably those in the UK.[435] Contextualising SCNT (referred to as 'iSCNT', where the technique of SCNT is applied to the creation of cytoplasmic hybrids, in contrast to the more conventional hSCNT in therapeutic cloning) alongside iPSC technique in the broader technology of nuclear reprogramming research, the ISSCR recognises that the latter is a much simpler way of deriving cells with pluripotent qualities. However, there are important differences between the two techniques. First, the questions that these techniques seek to answer in basic biology are different. The epigenetic reprogramming entailed in iPSC is essentially gene-based whereas SCNT is concerned with oocyte-driven reprogramming on human somatic cell nuclei. Second, SCNT provides important information on human embryogenesis, from which physiological mechanisms and pathological aberrations can be better understood. It is at that time unclear if a viable embryo can be produced from gametes or embryonic stem cells derived from iPSC. Third, not enough is known about iPSC to "confidently abandon all other research pathways aimed at obtaining pluripotent cells."[436] As we have seen, this is a position that is consistent with the BAC's in its HA Consultation Paper. The ISSCR concludes that rather than rendering SCNT obsolete or redundant, the iPSC technique is complementary. It further agrees with the proposal of the AMS that comparison between pluripotent cell lines derived by hSCNT versus iSCNT should be allowed.[437]

---

[435] International Society for Stem Cell Research, Ethics Report on Interspecies Somatic Cell Nuclear Transfer Research, *Cell Stem Cell* (2009) 5: 27-30, at 27.
[436] *Ibid*, at 28.
[437] *Ibid*.

As for the ethical aspects of the research, the ISSCR did not view these to be significantly different from those attending to animal chimeras, even if the latter involved a mixture of genetically different cells rather than a mixture of genetic material within a cell. It did recognise that continued emphasis on the importance of SCNT may result in the exploitation of women for eggs. However, the research should not be precluded only on the basis of this risk if the development of stem cell-based therapies is of social or humanitarian importance. The 'common good' basis similarly is evident.[438] In 2016, the ISSCR issued a revised set of guidelines in response to new discoveries and techniques like mitochondrial replacement and gene editing.[439] The oversight mechanism proposed in its earlier guidelines remains unchanged and its wider implications will be discussed later in this work.

4.4 California Institute for Regenerative Medicine

In November 2004, the California *Stem Cell Research and Cures Act* (Proposition 71) was passed by a state-wide ballot. The legislation created the CIRM, endowed it with a research fund of $3 billion (to be expended over a decade) and constituted a Standards Working Group (SWG) to recommend scientific, medical and ethical regulations. In July 2005, the SWG recommended that the 2005 NAS Guidelines be adopted as interim regulations. These regulations became the subject of a year-long public consultation from July 2005 to July 2006, and were finalised in November 2006 after the revisions were reviewed and approved by the California Office of Administrative Law.[440]

---

[438] *Ibid*, at 29.
[439] International Society for Stem Cell Research, *Guidelines for Stem Cell Science and Clinical Translation*, 2016.
[440] Geoffrey P Lomax, Zach W Hall and Bernard Lo. Responsible Oversight of Human Stem Cell Research: The California Institute of Regenerative Medicine's Medical and Ethical Standards, *PLoS Medicine* (2007) 4, 5: 0803-0805.

The connection between the BAC and the CIRM was Professor Bernard Lo, who was the co-Chair of the SWG of the CIRM and an expert advisor to the BAC. He was also a Council member of the Institute of Medicine, under the auspices of which the NAS Guidelines have been published. When we met in August 2008, Professor Lo said that the guiding principle of the CIRM is to encourage institutions to develop best practices, to oversee the new and rapidly developing field and to ensure flexibility in the SCRO structure and function.[441] He added that a regulatory regime should be rigorous, but flexible, in order to be effective in providing some assurance to those who are opposed to some (but not all) forms of stem cell research. He identified the regulatory challenges of the CIRM to include specificity and appropriate implementation of guidelines.[442]

On the subject of human-animal mixing, Professor Lo said that bioethics in the US tends to start with an emotive response. The reliance of the President's Council on an intuitive feeling of repugnance in developing moral arguments is illustrative.[443] Such research is also seen to violate religious doctrine and undermine human dignity. He disagreed with the approach of the President's Council, and indicated the need to distinguish between religious beliefs that guide personal behaviour from values that guide public policy. The reasons underlying public policies must be understandable and persuasive. An instance when human dignity is seen to be violated is if an animal develops characteristics considered to be specifically human, such as neurological functions or production of human germ cells. There may also be such a concern when large portions of human genetic materials are transferred into an animal. The importance of distinguishing among the different types of

---

441 *CIRM Medical and Ethical Standards Regulations*, Title 17, California Code of Regulations, §100040, 25 August 2011 (Reformatted and Approved).
442 Interview with Professor Bernard Lo, 16 August 2008.
443 See William Saletan, The Thing Is: At the bioethics council, human nature denies human nature. *Slate*, 7 March 2005.

human-animal mixing, some of which has been extensively conducted already, includes:

(a) Introducing human genes into nonhuman animals, as in the case of transgenic animals, and

(b) Injecting human stem cells into nonhuman animals, which is undertaken to demonstrate pluripotentiality through the formation of teratomas in immune deficient mice.

Testing on animal models is also carried out before clinical trials in humans for proof of principle or as preclinical studies to establish safety and dosage.

As the NAS Guidelines have been substantially adopted by the CIRM, the introduction of hESC into animals at any stage of development will require SCRO review.[444] In particular, there must be acceptable scientific rationale and the probable differentiation and integration of human cells into animal tissue must be evaluated. In addition, the following research is currently not eligible for CIRM funding:[445]

(1) Breeding of nonhuman animal into which hESCs have been introduced;

(2) Introducing hESCs into nonhuman primate blastocysts; and

(3) Introducing hESCs into human blastocysts, as this could lead to confusion as to which DNA is controlling.

The CIRM has extended this prohibition to all pluripotent stem cells. Professor Bernard Lo explained that regulations must change to keep pace with scientific developments. In addition, he was of the view that attention would most likely shift to iPSC technology since pluripotent stem cell lines could be derived through it. The CIRM

---

[444] *CIRM Medical and Ethical Standards Regulations*, Title 17, California Code of Regulations, §100070(e), 25 August 2011.
[445] *Ibid*, §100030.

further requires that donors of materials for CIRM-funded research be informed that derived cells may be transplanted into animals.[446] This is to give effect to another core ethical principle of the CIRM, which is the requirement for informed consent from donors of biological materials to be obtained (with some exceptions).[447] The core principles or objectives of the CIRM were also mentioned when I met with Dr Geoffrey Lomax at his San Francisco office in May 2009. Dr Lomax was the senior officer who supports the work of the SWG, and was also the co-chair of the Interstate Alliance on Stem Cell Research. In a paper that he co-authored, the overall objectives of the CIRM regulations are set out as:

(a) Encourage research institutions and researchers to develop best practices for ethical conduct of human stem cell research,

(b) Avoid unnecessary regulatory burdens,

(c) Facilitate collaboration to accelerate scientific progress,

(d) Be consistent with existing laws, regulations and ethical guidelines, and

(e) Involve the public in developing regulations.[448]

Much of our discussion at the meeting and then over lunch was focused on public involvement.[449] Understandably, public support has been critical to the CIRM by virtue of its very existence. This may account for the sense of openness that the CIRM office exuded, undoubtedly enhanced by colourful electro-microscopic portraits of

---

[446] *Ibid*, §100100(b)(1)(E).
[447] The other two core ethical principles are: Review by independent committee (SCRO Committees in particular); and no payment beyond expenses to research oocyte donors (although payment may be made for oocytes donated for fertility treatment).
[448] Geoffrey P Lomax, Zach W Hall and Bernard Lo. Responsible Oversight of Human Stem Cell Research: The California Institute of Regenerative Medicine's Medical and Ethical Standards. In *PLoS Medicine* (2007) 4, 5: 0803-0805.
[449] Interview with Dr Geoffrey Lomax, Senior Officer, Standards Working Group, CIRM, 12 May 2009.

stem cells that seemed to reach out to you in their own language. Quite aptly, a sign placed next to the main reception desk read: 'Stem Cell Place'.

When I asked about the NAS Guidelines, he said that while it served as a model for the CIRM regulations, federal laws and guidelines – particularly the Common Rule and the NIH Guidelines – were also influential. Even then, the regulations must be tailored to suit local requirements. He viewed the harmonisation of standards on a nationwide (and even at an international) level to be important, although individual states will still be key drivers of stem cell policies in view of the difficulties in forging a broad consensus on the subject and in engaging with the public on a very broad scale. Prior to heading out for lunch, I was given a draft manuscript that he wrote.[450] The locally-tailored character of the Californian regulation reminded me of Professor Lo's comment that Proposition 71 is more specific in contrast to the UK HFE Amendment Bill. The latter does in fact encompass many broad social issues relating to reproduction and familial relations. Furthermore, public misapprehension of research involving human-animal mixing would likely be high in the US, and hence it would not be politically expedient to craft a broad legislation. An informant familiar with the situation in the UK said that the British government attempted to get through as many political objectives as possible, because the HFE Act of 1990 turned out to be too restrictive for research. While he did have some reservation about the breadth of the legislation, he noted that the British Parliament has been relatively liberal on the subject. Allowing the creation of a human embryo for research is a good example of its unique position in Europe.[451]

---

[450] Geoffrey P Lomax. Rejuvenated Federalism: State-Based Stem Cell Research Policy. In Benjamin J Capps and Alastair V Campbell (eds.), *Contested Cells: Global Perspectives on the Stem Cell Debate*. London: Imperial College Press, 2010, pp 359-375.

[451] Fieldnotes, 15 August 2008.

4.5 Academy of Medical Sciences

With the prospect that stem cell research could be curtailed when the time came for policy review of the regulatory framework established by the HFE Act, the AMS's report on interspecies embryos became the focal point in offering a counter trajectory. As we have also seen, the report has been important in a number of ways, including the provision of a vocabulary to better enable discussion on human stem cell research and inter-species embryos, and the specification of the four main types of human-animal combinations as hybrid, chimera, transgenic animal and cytoplasmic hybrid.[452] Here, we consider the key principles and governance framework proposed by the AMS for transgenic and chimeric animals that contain significant amounts of human genetic material.

Where human gametes and embryos are concerned, the AMS attempted to work within the regime established by the HFE Act. However, the more important discussion in the report related to the broader governance structure that extended beyond the established statutory regime to cover human-animal combinations in stem cell research more generally. It is in this respect that the ISSCR has been a dominant influence, especially in structuring governance as a categorical review process.[453] In particular, three categories of review were proposed. Like the ISSCR the AMS does not disapprove of the introduction of human pluripotent stem cells into a non-human primate or human embryo if there is sufficient justification for the research. It similarly sets out caveats relating to the proportion of human stem cells transferred, the likely integration into critical tissues such as the germ-line and central nervous system, and the transfer of human cells into non-human primates. If transgenic and

---

452 Academy of Medical Sciences. *Inter-species embryos*, London: Academy of Medical Sciences, June 2007, at 22. A table sets out the definitions of hybrids, chimeras, transgenic and cytoplasmic hybrids at three different stages of development: as cells and cell-lines, as embryo and as animals.
453 *Ibid,* at 35.

chimeric animals contain significant amounts of human genetic material, an appropriate conceptual and regulatory framework will have to be considered.

When I met with Dr Helen Munn in April 2008, the HFE Amendment Bill has successfully passed through the House of Lords and was being debated in the House of Commons. The HFE Amendment Bill was introduced in the House of Lords on 8 November 2007. The intent was to update (but otherwise retain) the "current model of regulation and the basic foundations of the existing law contained in the Human Fertilisation and Embryology Act 1990" in order to "help maintain the UK's position as a world leader in reproductive technologies and research".[454]

One of the main elements of the Bill is to increase the scope of legitimate embryo research activities, including 'interspecies embryo'. The Bill initially followed the terminology of the AMS report in its reference to 'interspecies embryos', but this was replaced by 'human admixed embryos'. Dr Munn, a young Oxford-trained scientist, was the Director of Medical Science Policy at the AMS, and also served as Secretariat to the report's Working Group. She said that this change was introduced by Lord MacKay so as to indicate that a cytoplasmic hybrid embryo is effectively 'human'. This classification is important because the HFEA does not regulate non-human embryo research. And as noted in the AMS 2007 report, *in vitro* animal embryo research did not appear to fall within any regulatory purview. Apart from this, (then) British Prime Minister Gordon Brown has lifted the 'Party Whip' to allow free vote on the issue after strong protest was received as some members of his party felt that they could not act against their conscience.[455] Dr Munn shared that those in the government who

---

[454] Elizabeth Shepherd, *Human Fertilisation and Embryology Bill [HL]*, HL Bill 6, 2007-2008. London: House of Lords Library Notes, 2007, at 1.

[455] Polly Tonybee, Religion doesn't rule in this clash of moral universes, *The Guardian*, 25 March 2008.

opposed the use of 'human admixed embryos' are also those who said 'no' to hESC research. On the whole, there was strong support for the HFE Amendment Bill as it is seen as the "flagship of knowledge economy in the UK".[456]

Earlier on, Professor Martin Bobrow told me that he personally did not expect the Bill's provisions for interspecific hybrids to be especially controversial in the UK, although there was a vocal minority in strong opposition.[457] Many of the legislative amendments proposed in the Bill related to sociological issues such as marital status and the welfare and rights of children. The provisions that related to human-animal combinations were included to ensure that these constructs would fall within the regulatory purview of the HFEA. He indicated that the term 'interspecies embryos' had been revised to 'human admixed embryos', which referred to human embryos with some non-human genetic material, as opposed to animal embryos with human material. The Bill was specifically concerned with human embryos and so would not include transgenic animals. As for animal chimeras, Professor Bobrow said that they would require more thought, especially in relation to the introduction of human cells (such as neural cells) into an animal (such as a monkey). In addition, it would be important not to confuse research involving human-animal combinations at an embryonic level with research using animal chimeras. Even in 2008, it was anticipated that the UK would have to deliberate on the latter in the near future, as there had been reports of significant amounts of human neural cells being introduced into non-human primates. Such research is contentious in the eyes of the public and there was no legal or practical control mechanisms apart from IRB review. Reflecting the concerns of researchers in general, Professor Bobrow similarly indicated that care should be taken not to interfere with certain well-established use of human-animal

---

456 Fieldnotes, 1 April 2008.
457 Fieldnotes, 19 January 2008.

combinations such as transgenic animals. Careful working through is required to determine where the problems lie, what the regulations are, who should be the controller and related issues.

The AMS shares a mission that is similar to the NAS. It was formed in 1998 to develop and support UK medical science and individual biomedical researchers into the future. As an independent academy of experts, it acts as a champion for exploration of knowledge, a guardian of intellectual rigor and excellence, and an advisor on national public policy issues. It is housed in the impressive No. 10 Carlton Terrace of the British Academy, with an interior that has largely survived the Second World War. The three-flight black marble staircase was modelled in French classical tradition, and the largest of the grand corniced ceilings in the Lecture Hall has an unfinished *trompe l'oeil* in the style of late Delacroix.[458] The area itself is home to many other learned societies and academic organisations including the Institute of Materials, Minerals and Mining, the Royal College of Pathologists, the Royal Academy of Engineers, and the Royal Society. Dr Munn said that the 2007 report was put together relatively quickly in view of the political developments on the subject. At that time, there was 'not much around' by way of relevant materials from the EU. But as is evident from the report, the guidelines of the NAS and the ISSCR as well as the regulations of the CIRM, were relied on by the AMS. Consultations were conducted with regulatory authorities like the HFEA and some assistance was sought from collaborative partners like the Wellcome Trust and the Science Media Centre. Reflecting back, Professor Bobrow said that the report has been important in directing scientific interests in a way that could help steer policy development.[459] Its substantive effect was perhaps most evident at the meeting with parliamentarians, where science and scientific interests appeared to speak with one voice.

---

[458] British Academy, *Carlton House Terrace*. London: British Academy, 2007, at 4.
[459] Interview with Professor Martin Bobrow, 2 August 2010.

4.6 Danish Council of Ethics

Shortly after the publication of the AMS 2007 report, the Danish Council of Ethics (DCE) and the Danish Ethical Council for Animals produced a report on research involving human-animal combinations entitled *Man or Mouse*.[460] The BAC did not have any direct connection with its Danish counterpart, but the report provided some (needless to say timely) insight into European thinking on the subject.[461] The two main issues considered in the report are, whether human-animal hybrid and chimera research should be prohibited altogether, and what considerations policy-makers should take note of if such research is not prohibited.

A majority of both councils did not consider ethical and moral concerns to be so convincing that hybrid and chimera research should be prohibited. Six ethical arguments, based on dignity of humans and animals, were identified as reasons for intuitive revulsion against human-animal admixtures, and each of these arguments were found to be inadequate.[462] Instead, an approach based on concrete assessment carried out on a case-by-case basis was preferred. In order to facilitate this approach, the councils were of the view that the current regulatory framework would have to be reviewed by policy-makers. In particular, the councils indicated that the current research legislation should be amended to empower

---

[460] Danish Council of Ethics (with the Danish Ethical Council for Animals). *Man or Mouse: Ethical aspects of chimera research*. Copenhagen: Danish Council of Ethics, 2007.

[461] Arguably, the approach is Scandinavian rather than continental European. However, the reasoning applied is European in the sense that it has been undertaken within a conceptual framework demarcated by European documents such as the *Convention for the Protection of Human Rights and Dignity of the Human Being with Regard to the Application of Biology and Medicine. Ibid*, at 27-28.

[462] Danish Council of Ethics (with the Danish Ethical Council for Animals). *Man or Mouse: Ethical aspects of chimera research*. Copenhagen: Danish Council of Ethics, 2007, at 97-99.

the relevant authority to regulate (and/or prohibit) experiments that relate to cognitive functions and reproduction.[463]

In the scientific review conducted up to 2006, various types of research involving a variety of human to animal and animal to animal combinations are discussed.[464] A number of examples involving the transplantation of animal cells (e.g. neurons from pig foetuses), tissues or organs from animals into humans are also described. It reports that there is no published example of true hybrids between humans and animals, transplantation of cell nuclei from animals to enucleated human ova, chimeras of human embryos or foetuses with non-human cells, insertion of human embryonic stem cells into blastocysts from animals and human embryos inserted into an animal womb. Similar to the approach of the BAC, current scientific work was used to frame the scope of ethical and legal discussions.

In a view similar to that of the AMS, the creation and use of transgenic animals have been earmarked for consideration in a separate report as such research is "a very extensive and wide-ranging sphere".[465] The councils also indicate the need to harmonise a number of different laws that would apply separately to the human or animal portion of an experiment. The DCE observes that Danish law currently draws a sharp division between 'human' and 'animal'. The difficulty posed by research involving chimeras and hybrids is that they are either unregulated or will have to be forced within one of these categories, which could result in much ambiguity. Professor Agger said that as a practical matter, it was unclear if cytoplasmic hybrids would fall within the regulatory purview of the Ministry of Justice (which regulated research involving animals) or the Ministry of Health (since human biological materials are entailed).[466] As we

---

463 *Ibid,* at 99-100.
464 *Ibid,* at 68-86 (Appendix).
465 *Ibid,* at 10.
466 Interview with Professor Peder Agger, Chairperson of the Danish Council of Ethics, 31 July 2010.

have seen, the UK was confronted with the same challenge. Also related to the difficulty of legal categorisation, it is unclear if the creation of a cytoplasmic hybrid embryo is regulated by law as it is equivalent to a 'human' embryo if assessed in terms of its genetic composition.[467] If so, it may be precluded by another legal provision that prohibits the creation of human-animal crossbreeds.[468] The applicability of this provision is ambiguous given that there is no scientific interest in developing a cytoplasmic hybrid embryo into a fully grown organism. A more fundamental difficulty lies in the prohibition against creating a 'human' embryo for research.[469] Still, this would depend on how a cytoplasmic hybrid embryo is to be classified. If – based on its genetic composition – the creation of a cytoplasmic hybrid embryo amounts to the creation of a human embryo even if not through the process of IVF, such research is prohibited.[470] The DCE did not consider this outcome to be satisfactory as a cytoplasmic hybrid embryo could not be understood as ethically equivalent to a human embryo created through IVF. In addition, preference is expressed for a single overall evaluative

---

[467] Section 25 of the Danish *Act on a Scientific-ethical Committee System and Handling of Biomedical Research Projects* (1992) is the key provision that governs embryo research, but it applies only to human embryos, not animal embryos. This begs the question as to whether a cytoplasmic hybrid created through the transplantation of a human somatic nucleus into an animal egg will result in a human embryo. Danish Council of Ethics (with the Danish Ethical Council for Animals). *Man or Mouse: Ethical aspects of chimera research*. Copenhagen: Danish Council of Ethics, 2007, at 27-28.

[468] *Ibid*, at 32-33. Section 28(3) of the Danish *Act on a Scientific-ethical Committee System and Handling of Biomedical Research Projects* (1992) prohibits: "Experiments whose purpose is to make possible the production of live human individuals who are crossbreeds with a gene stock incorporating elements from other species".

[469] *Ibid*, at 28-29. However, it has been observed elsewhere that the creation of human embryos for research is permissible if it is for the purpose of improving or providing instruction in ART. See: Tetsuya Ishii, Renee A Reijo Pera and Henry T Greely, Ethical and Legal Issues Arising in Research on Inducing Human Germ Cells from Pluripotent Stem Cells, *Cell Stem Cell* (2013) 13, 2: 145-148.

[470] *Ibid*, at 31.

framework that could apply to both human and animal research rather than two separate and distinct systems.[471] This arrangement, if taken up, will be a major contrast from the approach in the US, Singapore and to some degree the UK where, as we have seen, distinct institutions have been developed to govern exclusively human or animal research, not both. However, the research governance structure in Denmark is different in that its research ethics committees (equivalent to IRBs in the US and in Singapore) are not institution-based. Instead, they are grouped together by regions and are hierarchical in that researchers may appeal against a decision at the National Committee on Health Research Ethics.[472] There are some similarities with the UK system of ethics review, possibly modelled after the National Health Service.

I visited the Secretariat of the DCE in March 2008 and met with Ms Anne Lykkeskov. The office was housed in a traditional multi-storey terrace building with a classic elevator no taller than two meters and could admit a maximum of five persons. The office itself was impressively modern and the design *avant garde*. It so happened that on that day, Ms Lykkeskov would also be giving a lecture to a group of visiting Austrian graduate students. We spoke for about an hour and a half before the lecture began. The lecture itself was structured in a manner similar to lectures that I have given about the BAC – history of the organisation, past activities, current activities, future activities, and finally, a question and answer session. The DCE was established in 1987 as politicians did not feel adequate to regulate matters relating to the human body.[473] In 2005, its original mandate set out in legislation was expanded. Earlier on in our meeting, Ms Lykkeskov

---

[471] *Ibid*, at 100.
[472] Pursuant to Section 43 of the *Act on Research Ethics Review of Health Research Projects* (2013), the National Committee on Health Research Ethics has replaced the Central Research Ethics Committee, which was established under the *Act on a Biomedical Research Ethics Committee System and the Processing of Biomedical Research Projects* (2003).
[473] Fieldnotes, 14 March 2008.

told me that the main function of the DCE is not to direct policy but to inform politicians by setting out sensible arguments and approaches. Its link to the legislature is hence not as close as its counterparts in Sweden and Norway. In this respect, the DCE resembles the role of the BAC. Neither the Danish government nor the Singapore government is obliged to follow the recommendations proposed by its respective bioethics advisors. When I met the Chairperson of the DCE in 2010, Professor Peder Agger similarly indicated that the Council's role was to highlight the complex dilemmas in biomedical research, and it was for the Danish government to decide on the best course of action, if any was to be taken.[474]

As for the selection of topics for consideration, the DCE operates in a manner similar to the AMS in that it is for a council member (or academy fellow in the case of the AMS) to initiate. The topic of hybrids and chimeras is considered appropriate as there is strong public interest in the impact of science on the environment and human reproduction. Since the publication of its report, the Danish parliament (Christiansborg) has asked for hearings and workshops to be organised. I met Ms Lykkeskov's colleague, Ms Lise Wied Kirkegaard several months later in Paris and was given a copy of publicity for a public forum. It drew about two to three hundred participants, many of whom were civil servants, politicians and students.[475]

Ms Lykkeskov shared that, in preparing the report, the guidelines of the NAS and ISSCR were considered. However, the emphasis was on setting out arguments that were relevant to local conditions. As such, discussion on law and ethics was relatively extensive. When I asked about how the phenomenon of 'law' is perceived in Denmark, Ms Lykkeskov said that it is decisive and directive, and not really seen

---

[474] Interview with Professor Peder Agger, Chairperson of the Danish Council of Ethics, 31 July 2010.

[475] Interview with Ms Lise Wied Kirkegaard, Head of the Secretariat, Danish Council of Ethics, 31 July 2010.

Chimaera research – ethical and legal aspects

**Parliamentary Hall, Christiansborg,
Wednesday, 5 November 2008**

Organized by the Danish Council of Ethics,
the Danish Ethical Council for Animals and
the Nordic Committee on Bioethics
for the Parliamentary Committee on the Council of Ethics
and the Health Committee

THE PARLIAMENTARY COMMITTEES have requested the conference by way of follow-up to the report: *"Man or Mouse? Ethical Aspects of Chimaera Research"* from the Council of Ethics and the Ethical Council for Animals. In it, the ground is prepared for a debate on adjusting the legislation so as to take into account the latest research into chimaeras and hybrids—crossbreeds of animals and humans.

In recent decades researchers have developed chimaeras by moving cells—and entire organs—from one individual to another, particularly in connection with stem cell research. In some cases this involves mixing cells from animals and humans.

With the creation of human-animal crossbreeds, research is compelling us to question one of the conditions in life that we have thus far taken for granted. In our culture and legislation we see animals and people as two clearly distinct categories. People are largely protected by the law, while animals can be involved in risky medical experiments, killed, kept as pets or husbandry and eaten.

A CHIMAERA is a creature that has cells from two or more individuals in it. A chimaera, then, has cells with different genomes side by side in its organism.

A HYBRID is a crossbreed formed by uniting the gametes (egg and sperm cells) from different species—for instance, a mule is a hybrid between a horse and a donkey. Here all the cells in the individual have the same genetic make-up, a mixed genome with genetic material from both species.

However, the majority of the members on the two councils do not think that all experiments to create crossbreeds should be banned. Some clear lines do need to be drawn in the sand, however. The councils consider that the new research should give rise to a thorough review of current legislation on the basis of the ethical guidelines discussed in the report. Among other things, more detailed criteria should be provided as to what it means for an individual to be human.

The conference will discuss what types of research are potentially capable of altering identity-forming organs and thus becoming an ethical problem, as well as how to modify the legislation to avoid such problematic experimentation.

THE DANISH COUNCIL OF ETHICS   norden Nordic Committee on Bioethics   **The Danish Ethical Council for Animals**

Illustration 4.1. Publicity for Workshop on Chimera Research in Denmark

as part of everyday life. Her impression is that people are 'generally satisfied' with the current operation of law although some changes may be required in the light of scientific advancement. In a separate interview,[476] Ms Kirkegaard said that the Council of Europe's *Convention on Human Rights and Biomedicine* provided an important deliberative and analytical framework,[477] and there was as such much deliberation over its application to the subject of hybrids and chimeras. A lawyer by training, Ms Kirkegaard explained that this Convention is important as it has been ratified by Denmark. However, international treaties do not automatically become part of Danish law, as international law is considered a separate system of law under the dualistic principle of Danish legal tradition (arguably embodied in Article 19 of the Danish Constitution). In particular, there has been much discussion on whether the creation of cytoplasmic hybrids and chimeras could be interpreted as violating human dignity under the Convention, and the implications on the legality of these constructs under Danish law.

At the lecture to a group of Austrian students, Ms Lykkeskov explained that various types of human-animal combinations have been created for decades although the moral or ethical implications have not been fully engaged with. This may be attributable to the formal distinction drawn between 'humans' and 'animals' in law, and at some point, legal change may be required to address the blurring of this distinction. Some of the Austrian students did not think that a formal change in law can resolve the underlying moral and ethical challenges that arise from compromised human dignity. The notion of 'dignity' is used extensively in European documents but its precise meaning is unclear. The ethical focal points that the councils identify

---

[476] *Ibid.*

[477] Council of Europe. Convention for the Protection of Human Rights and Dignity of the Human Being with regard to the Application of Biology and Medicine: Convention on Human Rights and Biomedicine (Oviedo 4.IV, 1997).

as underpinning human dignity do not differ in practical substance from the focal points of the NAS, CIRM, ISSCR and AMS,
especially where they relate to human cognitive ability and human
reproduction.[478] The AMS suggests that human form may also be
an important way in which dignity is conceptualised.[479] In another
European-based discussion on the subject known as the Chimbrids
project, 'dignity' continued to be the key focal point.

4.7 European Union

We became aware of the Chimbrids project, a two-year project funded
by the EU under the Science and Society Priority 9 of the Sixth
Framework Programme of Research for Structuring the European
Research Area by Research on Ethics, through Professor Bartha
Knoppers. Professor Knoppers was one of the members of this inter-
disciplinary EU project team, set up to address questions that are
expected to emerge from new technologies such as SCNT. The project
deals only with human-animal chimeras and hybrids (not animal-
animal chimbrids) and aimed to analyse fundamental problems in
research that mixed human and animal materials in Europe and
abroad.

The overall approach of the Chimbrids project team does not differ
from those of policy bodies that we have considered in segregating
issues in terms of science, ethics and law. There are a number of
distinctive features in their published report (the 'EU Chimbrids
Report') however. Most evident is the focus on key international or
regional documents, rather than on expert guidelines such as those
issued by the ISSCR (with the exception of the Declaration of Helsinki).
Ethical and legal evaluation was mainly conducted within the

---

478 Danish Council of Ethics (with the Danish Ethical Council for Animals). *Man or Mouse: Ethical aspects of chimera research.* Copenhagen: Danish Council of Ethics, 2007, at 97-98.
479 Academy of Medical Sciences. *Inter-species embryos*, London: Academy of Medical Sciences, June 2007, at 29.

analytical framework constituted by the *Charter of Fundamental Rights of the European Union*, the Council of Europe's *Convention on Human Rights and Biomedicine* and United Nation's *Declarations on Human Cloning and Human Rights*. Apart from this, specific case studies are also considered in a cross-jurisdictional manner. Referred to as country reports, experts from Germany, the UK, France, Sweden, Spain, Austria, Switzerland, USA, Canada, Israel and Japan provided comments on ethical, regulatory and societal concerns arising from ten factual cases involving different research uses of human-animal combinations.[480] In addition, the report includes attempts to address more fundamental philosophical-anthropological questions (e.g. What does 'human nature' mean?).[481]

The outcome of an examination of scientific developments is a tabular matrix of the various types of human-to-animal and animal-to-human mixtures.[482] This matrix does not differ significantly from the one produced by the BAC in the early stages of its deliberation. This should not be at all surprising as information is essentially drawn from a common pool of scientific sources. In its ethical evaluation, the Chimbrids team continues to apply 'moral status' as its principal framework. The justification is drawn from a sense of inevitability as "it is impossible to genuinely avoid making decisions about the moral status of beings."[483] Under this approach, the features of sentience, rationality and autonomy, and species-membership have been identified as conferring human beings with moral status.[484] A similarly categorical approach was adopted in legal analysis. Moral

---

[480] Jochen Taupitz and Marion Weschka (eds.), *CHIMBRIDS – Chimeras and Hybrids in Comparative European and International Research*. Heidelberg: Springer, 2009, Annex B (at 829-1030).
[481] *Ibid*, at 17.
[482] *Ibid*, at 57-58.
[483] *Ibid*, at 62.
[484] *Ibid*.

status in ethics found equivalence in the notion of legal personhood – both arguably the legacies of the Enlightenment. Personhood is in turn the formal characteristic to which legal rights and obligetions articulated in key European Union documents draw reference and attachment.[485] Even then, none of these documents provide a clear answer to the philosophical-anthropological issues at hand, other than reproductive cloning as the only exception.

On the issue of whether a human embryo, however derived, is a person (or 'everyone') under Article 2 of the *European Convention on Human Rights*,[486] both the European Commission of Human Rights and the European Court of Human Rights have indicated that the answer would depend on member states. In *Evans v. The United Kingdom*,[487] the European Court of Human Rights was not prepared to grant any rights to human embryos further than what the relevant national legislation was prepared to confer. Earlier on, the European Commission of Human Rights has expressed a similar stance in *H. v. Norway*.[488] The contrasting national positions in Europe on this issue are well-know, with possibly the UK as among the most liberal, and Germany as among the most conservative, of the EU member states.[489] Similarly, the Council of Europe's *Convention on Human Rights and Biomedicine*,[490] as well as the *Additional Protocol on the Prohibition of*

---

[485] *Ibid,* at 88.

[486] Council of Europe, *Convention for the Protection of Human Rights and Fundamental Freedoms* as amended by Protocol 11, CETS No. 005, Rome 4.VI, 1950.

[487] European Court of Human Rights, Judgment of 7 March 2006, Application No. 6339/05, para. 46-47.

[488] European Commission of Human Rights, Decision of 19 May 1992 on the admissibility of the application, Application No. 17004/90, Decisions and Reports 73, pp 155-171, 168.

[489] Jochen Taupitz and Marion Weschka (eds.), *CHIMBRIDS – Chimeras and Hybrids in Comparative European and International Research.* Heidelberg: Springer, 2009, at 93.

[490] *Convention for the Protection of Human Rights and Dignity of the Human Being with Regard to the Application of Biology and Medicine – Convention on Human Rights and Biomedicine,* European Treaty Series – No. 164, Oviedo 4.IV.1997.

Cloning Human Beings,[491] does not define a 'human being' although it requires human dignity to be protected. Although 'dignity' is also not defined, Article 18(2) of the Convention prohibits the creation of a human embryo by fertilisation for any research purpose. Whether this prohibition extends to a cytoplasmic hybrid embryo will depend on the significance attributed to the presence of animal mitochondrial DNA, and ultimately on the way in which an 'embryo' is defined.[492] The Chimbrids team notes that in Spain, an embryo or pre-embryo requires – by definition – the fertilisation of an ovum. The biological construct of SCNT will not be an 'embryo' under this definition even though it will have all the features and potential of one.[493] Also relevant is Article 13 of the Convention, which prohibits any modification in the genome of any descendants unless undertaken for preventive, diagnostic or therapeutic purposes.[494] In addition, Article 1 of the Additional Protocol makes clear that reproductive cloning is a violation of human dignity and is thereby prohibited. As with the Additional Protocol, Article 3 of the EU's *Charter of Fundamental Rights* prohibits reproductive cloning as a violation of human dignity.[495] As for the status of a human embryo however derived, the Chimbrids team indicates this is for member states to decide since

---

[491] *Additional Protocol to the Convention for the Protection of Human Rights and Dignity of the Human Being with Regard to the Application of Biology and Medicine, on the Prohibition of Cloning Human Beings*, European Treaty Series – No. 168, Paris, 12.I.1998.

[492] Jochen Taupitz and Marion Weschka (eds.), *CHIMBRIDS – Chimeras and Hybrids in Comparative European and International Research*. Heidelberg: Springer, 2009, at 109.

[493] *Ibid*, at 107, footnote 199.

[494] However, the Explanatory Report to the Convention indicates this provision does not apply to medical research involving genetic modification but not for the purposes of procreation: see paragraph 91 of Explanatory Report.

[495] *Charter of Fundamental Rights of the European Union*, Official Journal of the European Communities 2000/C 364/01, of 18/12/2000.

Article 2 of the EU Charter corresponds to Article 2 of the *European Convention on Human Rights.*[496]

As we have seen, 'human dignity' is a notion central to European ethical and legal norms, and it is undoubtedly related to the ethical notion of 'moral status' as well as to legal personhood. Although not clearly defined, there are certain parameters entailed in the concept. We have seen that reproductive cloning and germline genetic modification (with limited exceptions) are two boundaries that should not be transgressed. Within the scope of activities that are permissible, we find a variety of policy orientations. The recommendations of the Chimbrids team are proposed from a more liberal standpoint, perhaps to maximise the policy options that are available to member states. However, chimbrids research should only be conducted following careful consideration of its scientific merit, human research ethics, animal ethics, legal aspects and societal and environmental implications.[497]

The specific recommendations set out in the EU Chimbrids Report do not detract from those of the other jurisdictions we have considered.[498] However, it is interesting to observe that while the Chimbrids team is similarly concerned with safeguarding human dignity, it seems to have adopted a position that is more liberal than that of the NAS in allowing the incorporation of animal pluripotent cells into a human blastocyst. On the issue of reproduction, the EU's position is similar to that of the NAS. Maintaining human dignity precludes the transfer of a human embryo into an animal and the transfer of an animal embryo into a woman.[499] Not surprisingly, a particularly striking feature of the recommendations in the Chimbrids

[496] Jochen Taupitz and Marion Weschka (eds.), *CHIMBRIDS – Chimeras and Hybrids in Comparative European and International Research*. Heidelberg: Springer, 2009, at 111.

[497] *Ibid,* at 456.

[498] *Ibid,* at 457.

[499] *Ibid,* Recommendations 18 and 19 respectively.

Report is that there are at least five specific recommendations relating to reproduction and germline genetic modification.[500] This emphasis may be attributable to requirements under the Council of Europe's *Convention on Human Rights and Biomedicine* that we have considered.

The opinion of the German Ethics Council (GEC) published after the EU Chimbrids Report maintains a robust reading of 'dignity' within the legislative framework of the German *Embryo Protection Act*.[501] On the basis of potential violation of human dignity, it endorsed the legal prohibition against fertilisation involving mixture of human and animal gametes, fusion of a human embryo with an animal embryo, and introduction of animal cells into a human embryo.[502] The council further recommends the prohibition of the insertion of animal material into human germline, or similar interventions that could undermine the dignity ascribed to the human species. The creation and use of cytoplasmic hybrids are considered to be ethically acceptable by a small majority of the council members mainly because no independently living organisms are expected to be produced.[503] Like the AMS, the German Ethics Council has proposed for the German animal welfare commission to consider the appropriateness of interventions that could drastically alter the appearance or capabilities (including cognitive ones) of an animal.[504] Outside of Europe, the Japanese Cabinet Office's Expert Panel on Bioethics also adopted a dignity-based approach and has made similar recommendations on the creation and use of human-animal combinations.[505]

---

[500] *Ibid*, Recommendations 13 to 17.

[501] German Ethics Council, *Human-animal mixtures in research: Opinion*. Berlin: German Ethics Council, 2011.

[502] *Ibid*, at 112-113, Recommendation 1.2.

[503] *Ibid*, at 114-115, Recommendation II; See also discussion on human dignity in relation to the *German Basic Law* and the *European Convention on Human Rights and Biomedicine, and the Additional Protocol concerning Biomedical Research*: at 52-59.

[504] *Ibid*, at 113, Recommendation I.3.

[505] Hiroshi Mizuno, Hidenori Akutsu, and Kazuto Kato, Ethical acceptability of research on human-animal chimeric embryos: summary of opinions by the

4.8 Synthesising an Approach

Prior to the public consultation on human-animal combinations in 2008, it was felt that the current system of review in Singapore could be relied upon with some 'adjustments'. Under this system, IRBs will bear much of the burden in deciding if research involving chimeras and hybrids should proceed. However, the negative reaction that chimeras and hybrids invoked, especially among certain religious groups and some policy-makers, sent a clear message to the BAC that any research involving human-animal combinations could only proceed on a regulated basis. Yet even if regulation was to be introduced, a number of respondents in the public consultation have queried the credibility of institutional self-regulation. Still others observed that the current research governance framework did not extend to researchers working outside of a healthcare setting. These reactions contributed to a shift in policy orientation from self-regulation to a more stringent and pervasive regulatory approach. To better secure public confidence, assurance as to the effectiveness of any regulation when introduced was also considered to be necessary. In both these respects, the policies, proposals and experiences of other jurisdictions were studied.[506] Throughout the process of policy formulation and discussion, the key documents that we have considered above have been important to the BAC's deliberations. These documents were exemplars of policy rationalities in the identification of ethical and regulatory issues, and in their resolution. Although these documents are context-bound, the rationalities, issues

---

Japanese Expert Panel on Bioethics, *Life Sciences, Society and Policy* (2015) 11: 15-21. See also: Hiroshi Mizuno, Recommended Ethical Safeguards on Fertilization of Human Germ Cells Derived from Pluripotent Stem Cells Solely for Research Purposes, *Stem Cell Reviews and Reports* (2016) 12: 377-384.

[506] Paragraph 4.1 of the BAC's report on human-animal combinations clearly indicates the importance of regulatory experiences in a number of key jurisdictions. Bioethics Advisory Committee, *Human-Animal Combinations in Stem Cell Research*. Singapore: Bioethics Advisory Committee, September 2010, at 20.

and goals have been generalisable and resonated with policy-makers in Singapore.

In the identification of ethical and regulatory issues, the documents of the NAS (along with ISSCR and AMS, as broadly sharing a particular ethical orientation), DCE and the EU Chimbrids project exhibited a degree of convergence. In essence, the integrity of two 'human' capacities was regarded as sufficiently fundamental to require regulatory safeguard. The first of these related to human sentience or consciousness, while the second was concerned with human reproduction. These concerns were similarly reflected in the feedback received by the BAC through its public consultation. To address these concerns, the BAC recommended that, for research involving chimeras, "particular attention should be paid to the need to avoid the creation of entities in which human sentience or consciousness might be expected to occur"[507] and that animals into which "any pluripotent stem cells have been introduced should not be allowed to breed".[508] In relation to cytoplasmic hybrids, the substantive categorisation of these biological constructs as effectively 'human' and thereby falling under the 14 day rule precludes concerns relating to human sentience or consciousness and reproduction from materialising.[509] For this, the BAC has in effect adopted the rationale of the AMS, even in the absence of any legislative framework like that of the HFE Act.

Unlike the NAS, but similar to the ISSCR, the BAC did not consider it necessary to impose a moratorium over research involving:

(i) The introduction of any embryonic stem cells (human or non-human) into human embryos, and

(ii) The introduction of human embryonic stem cells into non-human primate embryos.

---

[507] *Ibid*, at 3, Recommendation 3.
[508] *Ibid*, at 3, Recommendation 4.
[509] *Ibid*, at 3, Recommendation 2.

In relation to the first category, the ethical justification for this limitation was queried since there are potentially valid experiments that involve the making of human chimeras *in vitro*. For instance, they are useful in studying early gene activation. As for the second category, the introduction of a large amount of human cells into primates would be more contentious than creating human chimeras *in vitro*. This contention was felt not to be grounded in scientific logic, but on the perceived evolutionary proximity between humans and primates. It was also not entirely clear if primates were needed for such research at this time.

Unlike in earlier discussions on regulatory framework, a national or central stem cell ethics review body to review all human embryonic stem cell research in Singapore, including research involving cytoplasmic hybrids and human-animal chimeras, was proposed for the first time.[510] The BAC explained that this was necessary "in the public interest to provide clear and comprehensive legal guidance that explicitly addresses the subject of research involving human-animal combinations".[511] Apart from this, IRBs have indicated that they do not have the necessary expertise to review research relating to embryonic stem cells. Individual IRBs that currently provide oversight for stem cell research are not composed of people with the relevant expertise. It was envisaged that this national ethics review body will be composed of members with the relevant expertise. In addition, given Singapore's small size relative to larger countries like the US, centralisation of such a review mechanism makes better sense than to implement a dual system of review (as proposed by the NAS). It was also felt that standardisation through compliance with a set of national guidelines would minimise bureaucratic paperwork and ensure consistency in the ethics review process. Such a scheme would also be consistent with the ISSCR's recommendation for such an ethics body to be configured to suit the circumstance of each country.

---

[510] *Ibid*, at 3, Recommendation 1.
[511] *Ibid*, at 22, paragraph 4.10.

This national stem cell ethics review body should ensure that there is evidence that the cell lines are from a reliable source and have been derived ethically (with documentation of the use of an IRB-approved informed consent process, etc.) and that it complies with any additional review by an institutional animal ethics committee, an institutional biosafety committee and/or other institutionally mandated review.[512] As this area of research was considered to fall under the broad category of human embryonic stem cell research, the conscientious objection provision that was initially set out in the SC Report has been re-stated as a recommendation.[513]

4.9 Policy Construction of a Limited Anthropology

Although it was not the intent of the BAC to posit any definition of 'human being', the recommendations of the HA Report ironically had this effect, albeit a limited one. Drawing on discourses in science, ethics and law, and in un-orchestrated synchrony with other policy bodies, the HA Report similarly identifies certain 'focal points' as essential characteristics of a 'human being'. These could be generally set out as:

(a) Consciousness (as manifest in language, culture and religion) and sentience,

(b) Reproduction, and

(c) Human form, gestures and mannerism.

These 'focal points' objectify the 'human being', through identification of the qualifying features for species membership, and also through objectification of the 'other' in chimeras and hybrids. These biological constructs have been the subject of all the documents considered. They all share a similar context in human stem cell research, and

---

512 *Ibid*, at 22-23, paragraph 4.11.
513 *Ibid*, at 3.

rely on – as justificatory rationale – a notion of 'common good' (to be discussed below) grounded in the belief that human welfare would be greatly advanced if knowledge of nuclear reprogramming could be perfected and applied. In all the documents considered, reliance on the triad of science, ethics and law in policy construction seemed almost programmatic. To borrow the language of Carol Heimer, this could well be taken as the cognitive structure that has enabled a particular construction of the 'human being' to be advanced in public policy.[514]

This cognitive structure that the policy documents appear to share places considerable emphasis on the empirical grounding of ethics and law, essentially by interpreting chimeras and hybrids as first and foremost scientific materials. We know, as a matter of scientific knowledge, that a viable organism can be produced from mixing human and nonhuman materials, as well as the reasons for doing so. We also understand from the scientific community that biology cannot at the present time tell us what it is that makes us distinctively human – not in a material sense at least. From the human genome map, we learn that much of our genetic makeup is not extremely different from animals, lending some support to Darwinian postulation of evolutionary continuity. One could perhaps draw broad postulations on what 'humanness' amounts to on the basis of scientific knowledge alone, but this would be inconsistent with the character of science. Stem cell scientists work in the particular, and their preference is not to generalise. This has been my impression in attempting to get feedback from stem cell researchers and subsequently meeting with them. Dr Munn relates a similar experience in that scientists "like to

---

[514] Carol A Heimer, Conceiving Children: How Documents Support Case versus Biographical Analyses. In Annelise Riles (ed.), *Documents: Artefacts of Modern Knowledge*. Ann Arbor: University of Michigan Press, 2006, pp 95-126, at 121. In her study of documents in neonatal intensive care units, Heimer observes (at 121).

use a lot of caveats".[515] What they can tell us is that a human being is more than the sum of its material parts. Quite understandably, if chimeras and hybrids are biological 'tools' for researchers, their meaning will depend on usage.[516]

As we have seen, human stem cell research is the critical context for the policy documents that we have considered. It serves the dual function of enabling practical scientific definitions for chimera and hybrid to be formulated, and of securing legitimacy for research that will not yield immediate benefits. This may appear to be an obvious point, but it took some time for this association of object with context to sink in, perhaps due in part to the complexity of the artefacts and their distinct treatment in a separate report. Hence it was necessary for the HA Report to make clear in its title that the context remains human stem cell research. It is here that policy documents serve as a specific technology that enables comprehension through definition of context and focus.

Even working within specific settings or relatively more limited discourses, scientists are unable to agree on the likely impact or scientific merit of implanting human pluripotent cells into primates, for instance. As we have seen, the NAS, the NIH and the CIRM disallow the implantation of such cells into primate embryos. In contrast, the AMS, possibly the DCE, the EU Chimbrids team and the BAC do not consider this to be an issue provided that the 14 day or equivalent rule is applied. Arguably, this issue is likely to be more consequential in ethics than it is in science. On this point, Phillip Karpowicz and others do not think that introduction of human neural stem cells into a primate will confer it with human cognitive ability as neural cells proliferate at different rate depending on the host environment.[517]

---

515 Interview with Dr Helen Munn, 1 April 2008. Dr Munn points to page 7 of the AMS 2007 Report as illustration.

516 Phillip Karpowicz, Cynthia B Cohen and Derek van der Kooy, It is ethical to transplant human stem cells into nonhuman embryos, *Nature Medicine* (2004) 10, 4: 331-335, at 331.

517 *Ibid,* at 334.

David Degrazia argues that it is insufficient to limit our analysis of 'humanness' to the material aspects or to 'cognition' as a physiological and psychological trait. In order to safeguard dignity, it is necessary to inquire into what 'personhood' entails. The term 'person' does not mean 'human being' or even 'human being [with certain capacities]'.[518] 'Person' is not merely descriptive, and thereby limited to certain capacities, but also prescriptive or moral. He explains that:

> ['Personhood' is] associated with a cluster of more specific properties without being precisely analysable in terms of any specific subset: autonomy, rationality, self-awareness, linguistic competence, sociability, moral agency, and the capacity for intentional action. Not all of these properties are strictly necessary for being a person.[519]

On this basis, he argues that a 'person' is sufficiently constituted by "a being with the capacity for sufficiently complex forms of consciousness (each of the properties representing a form of consciousness)".[520] By this analysis, great apes are viewed as falling in a 'grey zone' between humans and animals,[521] and should have a moral status that is higher than rodents.[522]

The notion of 'personhood' has in fact developed over time. More than ten years ago, the same question was asked of human embryos. There was a single 'focal point' in the 14 day rule, in that an embryo (or 'pre-embryo') prior to having developed a 'primitive streak' is incapable of sentience. It is as such no more than a cluster of cells.

---

[518] David Degrazia, Human-Animal Chimeras: Human Dignity, Moral Status, and Species Prejudice, *Metaphilosophy* (2007) 38, 2-3: 309-329, at 319.
[519] *Ibid*, at 320.
[520] *Ibid*.
[521] *Ibid*, at 322.
[522] *Ibid*, at 326.

Some people consider the 14 day rule to be arbitrary and hence incapable of acquiring ethical stature for the lack of rational basis.[523] However, Mary Warnock explains how a biological basis has been attributed to the 14 day rule.[524] It has justification in that it is approximately at this stage of development that an IVF embryo would be implanted.[525] As such, the rationality of the 14 day rule is derived not from pure logic and theory, but an empirical basis and the practicality of technology. It is from this 'focal point' of when sentient life begins that the broader notion of 'personhood' is derived. At least one 'focal point' – that of consciousness – has a material source, and this is supplemented by other prescribed 'focal points'. In other words, chimeras and hybrids would not have had the meanings that they now do without the groundwork laid by the SC Report in 2002. Hence, the argument I am making here is that the policy epistemology of 'humanness' is incremental and contingent. It is characterised by 'focal points' that are in turn mapped onto broader scientific, ethical and/or legal discourses. In themselves, these 'focal points' are without meaning and could be regarded as arbitrary. But when linked to broader discourses and placed in context, they achieve a level of coherence that enables comprehension and justification. We see a parallel in the incremental manner in which scientific knowledge accrues. A stem cell researcher tells me that knowledge of nuclear reprogramming from SCNT did in fact enable the development of iPSC technology.[526]

---

523 Interview with philosopher and ethicist Professor Daniel Wilker, 10 May 2009.
524 Mary Warnock, *Nature and Mortality: recollections of a philosopher in public life*. London and New York: Continuum, 2003, at 95. She also points out (at 83) that "[m]ost people thought of the early embryo as a tiny homunculus, recognisably human."
525 Robert Winston, *A Child Against All Odds*. Reading: Bantam Books, 2007, at 42.
526 Interview with stem cell researcher Dr Pauline Tay, 18 August 2009.

These 'focal points' resemble what Bruno Latour labels as "circulating reference".[527] The concept of human-animal combinations could be in some ways seen as derived from similar notions that were circulated along the "reversible chain of transformations,"[528] which one could read as a reversible chain of documents. In this connection, the HA Report could be perceived as a link in this 'chain'. While the link possesses certain features that are distinctive to Singapore, it exhibits a cognitive structure, or "already-established centres of calculation", that would enable its identification and application outside of the local context. Even so, it would be imprudent to gloss over the fact that these 'focal points' are embedded within a particular cognitive structure and are developed within specific time and space to deal with particular challenges.

Whereas the NAS, AMS and BAC appeared to have relied on science as an analytical starting point, the DCE, the GEC and the EU Chimbrids project group were somewhat more predisposed to assuming a stronger ethical basis in the science-ethics-law cognitive triad. In Denmark, Germany and in the EU Chimbrids project, deliberations have largely been pertaining to the notion of 'dignity' as articulated in key European documents. In the case of Denmark, less reliance on institutional-based review may have affected the way in which the DCE thought about the appropriate set-up for ethics review. Like the NAS, the deliberations of the Chimbrids project team are more generic and broad. Its conclusions do not significantly detract from those of the NAS but there is substantial focus on human reproduction and germline genetic modification. These may in turn be traced back to the ways in which 'dignity' is construed. Drawing from ethical and social theories, Christian Smith argues that humans possess an

---

[527] Bruno Latour, *Pandora's hope: Essays on the reality of science studies*. Cambridge MA: Harvard University Press, 1999, pp 24-79 (Circulating Reference: Sampling the Soil in the Amazon Forest), at 24.

[528] *Ibid*, at 71.

inherent dignity by virtue of "the kinds of creatures they are ontologically".[529] He considers this to be real and objective in that it is not culturally relative or conferred upon by social contract or positive law. It is not an institutional fact or a social fact, but a 'brute fact' of ontological reality.[530]

In essence, Smith proposes that human persons are ontologically real and causally capacitated, but not autonomous or self-sufficient. Social construction depends on our capacities of personhood, and the former in turn help to define and sustain our durable identities, moral commitments and social communications.[531] He argues that humans are naturally highly capacitated and these capacities entail natural structures, directions and limits.[532] However, the knowledge that arises from these capacities (such as language, which he considers to be enabling rather than limiting) is always human and personal knowledge. It is subjective unless institutionalised or otherwise related to an ontological reality.[533] Smith observes that human dignity is real at an institutional level. However, he assumes that whether language or knowledge, they accurately map onto an ontological reality, and does not quite explain how this 'overlap' between social construction and 'reality' maps onto each other, and to what extent. In

---

[529] Christian Smith, *What is a Person? Rethinking Humanity, Social Life, and the Moral Good from the Person Up*. Chicago and London: University of Chicago Press, 2010, at 434. In analytical approach, he proposes a critical realist personalism as a third way between materialism, which he considers to ignore meanings, language, and interpretation, and strong form social constructionism, which conflate reality into meaning, language, and interpretation (at 198). Materiality is constituted and governed by natural laws of existence and function – what the hard sciences relate to (at 169).

[530] *Ibid*, at 444.

[531] *Ibid*, at 197.

[532] *Ibid*, at 173-179.

[533] On this point, Smith observes: "There is no Universal, Generic Knowledge out there for us to acquire. There is rather for humans only human knowledge – knowledge fitted for and appropriate to humans as particular beings. There appears to be other kinds of knowledge that are not human knowledge ... bats possess 'bat knowledge' of reality ..." *Ibid*, at 180.

relying on a cognitive structure composed of the science-ethics-law triad, the policy (and policy-related) bodies that we considered have drawn on all three institutions in the crystallisation of the 'focal points' that would objectify the 'human being'. The 'focal points' have in turn been associated with or otherwise subsumed within the broad notion of dignity, providing much needed vigour to both. On their own, these 'focal points' are matters-of-fact that lack moral force. In contrast, human dignity in some form or other has moral persuasion but is often devoid of substantive and practically useful content. Collectively, these policy documents on hybrids and chimeras have united 'focal points' to dignity in the context of human stem cell research and under a justificatory analytic of the 'common good'.[534] In addition, by way of recourse to science, ethics and law, the 'overlap' is essentially assumed, to the extent that all three institutions represent varying degrees of 'naturalness' or 'found-ness' in nature, the right and order. From a more pragmatic standpoint, the presence or absence of an overlap is perhaps not important given that a notion of dignity has been implicitly or explicitly subscribed to in all of the policy documents considered.

Still, the anthropology that has emerged in these policy documents is limited and fragmentary. In other words, we still do not quite know what is essentially 'human' from a non-anthropocentric point of view – if this vantage point can be assumed at all. As Annelise Riles has noted, policy documents are often less interested in expounding concepts or terminologies (such as 'women' in her study) than they are in ensuring institutional continuity.[535] Nevertheless, this

---

[534] The Warnock Report has itself resorted to claims of naturalness in conceptualising the family and parenthood. See Fenella Cannell, Concepts of Parenthood: the Warnock Report, the Gillick debate, and modern myths, *American Ethnologist* (1990) 17, 4: 667-686; and Peter Rivière, Unscrambling Parenthood, *Anthropology Today* (1985) 1, 4: 2-7.

[535] Annelise Riles, *The Network Inside Out*. Ann Arbor: University of Michigan Press, 2001, at 80-81. At page 80, she observes: "For example, if one takes the general subject of this conference 'women', certainly the word *women* appeared

minimum content has been sufficient in expunging hybrids and chimeras from the sanctity of human dignity, as the 'other'. In other words, a moralistic and naturalistic viewpoint that human beings belong to a higher moral order is sustained. Humans are self-aware, cultural, spiritual and capable of complex reasoning; not animals. The sacred is again clearly demarcated from the profane.[536] The cognitive structure thereby confers legitimacy through analogies that further entrench the perceived distinctions between humans and nonhuman animals. The reports that include substantive discussions (i.e. those of the NAS, AMS, DCE, EU Chimbrids project and BAC) all indicate that various forms of human-animal combinations have been useful to humanity for a long time. There is as such nothing unusual or detrimental about continuing to work with chimeras and hybrids under controlled conditions and for socially beneficial reasons. In *We Have Never Been Modern*, Bruno Latour observes that science has created a whole range of hybrids, or 'quasi-objects' which are neither merely natural things nor people or subjects.[537] But even though scientists have been creating these hybrid beings, people have denied this hybridity and preferred to demarcate 'nature' clearly from 'society'.[538] He thus surmised that: "We have never plunged into a homogeneous and planetary flow arriving either from the future or from the depths of time. Modernization has never occurred."[539] Yet Latour is aware that a difficult political issue would arise if we take up the challenge of constituting a 'Parliament of Things'. The present

---

frequently enough in the thousands of documents that circulated through the meeting. Yet in practice, it was hardly clear what this word 'meant' at all and how it might be delineated by the scope of other UN conferences on subjects such as development, human rights, population, children, or environment."

[536] Emile Durkheim (translated by Karen E Fields). *The Elementary Forms of Religious Life*. New York: The Free Press, 1995 [1912], at 34.

[537] Bruno Latour, *We Have Never Been Modern*. New York and London: Harvester Wheatsheaf, 1993 [1991], at 6.

[538] *Ibid*, at 10.

[539] *Ibid*, at 76.

scenario illustrates the institutional constraints in accommodating certain nonhuman animals as 'humans' or like-'human', let alone as a category that is neither 'human' nor 'animal' (i.e. 'thing').

4.10 Public Acceptability and the 'Common Good'

An informant told me over lunch that some years back, she decided not to pursue a career as a research scientist in spite of having had post-graduate training. In order to excel and ultimately become a Principal Investigator, you will have to "ask the right questions".[540] I pursued the point further, and learnt that a Principal Investigator must not only be able to carry out scientific experiments that answer issues of relevance to science, she must also ensure that they are of interest to funders. If we assume for simplicity that society follows ethics, then difficulties could arise when the questions that scientists are interested in do not conjoin with those of ethics. In a lecture at Raffles' Girls School – one of the most prestigious secondary schools in Singapore, a student asked what the scientific criteria for 'humanness' are.[541] It is I think a fair question as one might expect science to provide useful insights. It was also one of the questions that I had in mind when I first began research on the subject of human-animal combinations. This question was directed to Professor Davor Solter, one of the foremost stem cell researchers, who worked in Germany and the US before coming to Singapore. In response, he said that while biology may point to some important differences between human beings as a species from some other species, ultimately the question of 'humanness' is not one that scientists regard as meaningful to pursue. He queried: "When does a grain of rice become a pile of rice?" It could be an interesting question, but he considered it to be a waste of time for scientists to work on when an organism

---

[540] Fieldnotes, 17 July 2008.
[541] Fieldnotes, 3 October 2008.

becomes 'human'. He observed that if half of all the cells in a mouse is composed of human cells but looked and behaved like a mouse, it would not be regarded as 'human'. Even if an animal has a human organ, it would still not be regarded as an animal. At this point, I am reminded of my conversation with Professor Martin Bobrow at the start of my research. He shared a similar view in that the issue of 'what makes a human' is a philosophical question and cannot at this point be answered by biology. Hence, he said in a half-joking manner that a pragmatic test to go by could be formulated as:[542] "If it [the chimera or hybrid] walks past you in the street and you say it is 'human', it is 'human'. It is a little like a jury trial." As we will see in the next chapter, this also appears to be the position of NACLAR. In follow-up interviews that I conducted with stem cell scientists, their remarks are similar to those noted by Michael Gazzaniga:[543]

> A cell is a cell is a cell. It's a universal unit of processing that only scales in size between the bee and the human … There are differences in the types of neurons within a brain, and response properties of neurons within a brain. But across mammals – I think a neuron is a neuron.

It seems clear that if one attempts to search for a fundamental divide between humans and nonhuman animals, the answer will not (or not completely at least) be in biology. Jason Robert and Françoise Baylis agree that there is no sharp biological division between humans and animals. Any feeling of abomination or disgust towards the creation of interspecies organisms is a moral and social construct.[544] They argue that it is erroneous to think of species identities as fixed and that, by virtue of this putative fixity, there is a

---

[542] Fieldnotes, 25 September 2007.

[543] Michael S Gazzaniga. *Human: The science behind what makes your brain unique.* New York: HarperCollins Publishing, 2008, at 8.

[544] Jason Scott Robert and Françoise Baylis, Crossing Species Boundaries, *American Journal of Bioethics* (2003) 3, 3: 1-13, at 8.

scientific, political and moral imperative to protect and preserve the integrity of human beings and the human genome. However, they consider the most plausible objection to the creation of such creatures to rest on the notion of moral confusion, in that "countless social institutions, structures, and practices depend upon the moral distinction drawn between human and nonhuman."[545] Chimeras and hybrids could undermine moral and social order as it forces one "to confront the possibility that humanness is neither necessary nor sufficient for personhood."[546] As we shall consider further, there is a fundamental divide between humans as *persona* and animals as *res* is sustained by treating human-animal combinations as *res*. If Jacques Derrida is right that there is something ontological about shame in human consciousness that necessitates this aggression towards our 'other' in nonhuman animals,[547] it is certainly not the place for a policy paper to fundamentally reconfigure the existing moral and social order. In this sense, law and ethics have served as a means by which moral and social orders have been adjusted to accommodate a novel construct of science.

Professor Bobrow provided me with a helpful lead in his indication that while there is no standard definition of 'humanness', certain traits are associated with being 'human'. Human consciousness, reproduction and form have all been identified as demarcating features. For instance, the public would understandably be alarmed if a chimeric mouse started to walk around like a human being. The risk of this occurrence is low since the objective of stem cell research is not to confer human traits on non-human animals. To understand the creation of human-animal combinations in terms of its research end

---

[545] *Ibid,* at 10.
[546] *Ibid.*
[547] Laurence Simmons, Shame, Levinas's Dog, Derrida's Cat (and Some Fish). In Laurence Simmons and Philip Armstrong (eds.), *Knowing Animals.* Leiden: Brill, 2007, pp 27-42. Simmons uses Derrida's critique of specieism to show the ontological basis of shame in human consciousness.

goals suggests that it is possible to move forward with regulatory policies on chimeras and hybrids without having to determine what makes us 'human'. The end goals of stem cell research are clear and, as we have considered, supported by some level of public opinion. Concern over the moral status of an embryo has to some degree been answered in the artefact of the 'pre-embryo'. Legal pragmatism in particular, comes to mind. Justice Cardozo wrote some time back:[548]

> There had arisen a new situation which could not force itself without mutilation into any of the existing moulds. When we find a situation of this kind, the choice that will approve itself to this judge or that, will be determined largely by his conception of the end of the law, the function of legal liability; and this question of ends and functions is a question of philosophy.

A more recent manifestation of this pragmatism at law is evident in the decision of *In re A*.[549] The issue before the court was whether Jodie and Mary as conjoined twins should be separated since separation would inevitably cause Mary's death. If not separated, both Jodie and Mary would die. The parents were unable to consent to the operation as they sincerely believed – being devout Roman Catholics – that the twins were equal in value and it would be against the will of God to kill one in order to save the other. Drawing on medical evidence, the Court ruled that the twins could be separated because they have distinct individuality, and one has the capacity to live independently whereas the other did not. Relying instead on the doctrine of double-effect and on the legal defence of necessity, a pragmatic solution was arrived at, whilst sidestepping the controversial and indeterminate question of personhood.

---

548 Benjamin N Cardozo, *The Growth of Law*. New Haven: Yale University Press, 1924, at 101.
549 *In Re A (Children) (Conjoined Twins: Surgical Separation)* [2001] Fam 147, CA.

Purely intellectual pursuit to address first order questions such as when the moral identity of a person begins, is a luxury in policy work. Due to constraints of politics, resources and time, difficult policy issues require judgment based on public standards and morality.[550] Baroness Mary Warnock expresses this sentiment when she chaired the *Committee of Inquiry into Human Fertilisation and Embryology*. She was motivated to assume the role by her intellectual interest in the subject (which includes the relationship between law and morality), but ultimately concluded that two years was too short a time for serious intellectual engagement. For her, as it has been for me, time is itself an epistemological frame – albeit in the manner of a constraint – and more importantly, an assurance of currency and relevance.[551] Ethical reasoning has provided a basis by which stem cell research involving chimeras and hybrids could proceed. Regardless of whether one considers the ethical premises to be morally right, it was necessary for arguments raised in the BAC's documents to be acceptable. My experience in public policy work on stem cell research is consistent with the observation by Baroness Warnock, that what is considered to be morally right should be distinguished from what is acceptable.[552] The constraints that time and other factors imposed require a focus on what is acceptable as a matter of public policy. As she then explains, what is 'acceptable' often depends on what is believed to advance the common good of society.[553]

---

[550] Ronald Dworkin, *Law's Empire*. Cambridge MA: Harvard University Press, 1986, at 256. Dworkin argues that law as integrity requires a judge (i.e. Hercules J) to choose between eligible interpretations by asking which shows the community's structure of institutions and decisions – its public standards as a whole from the standpoint of public morality.

[551] Mary Warnock. *Nature and Mortality: recollections of a philosopher in public life*. London and New York: Continuum, 2003, at 104: "What's so sacred about June 26th?" This was the day which the committee has agreed to hand over the report, the press conference had been called and "everyone had adjusted their diaries".

[552] *Ibid*, at 98-99.

[553] *Ibid* at 100.

Annelise Riles makes a similar observation. In her study of the United Nations' Fourth World Conference on Women, Riles observes:[554] "If the chair's authority was always contentious, the authority of time went unquestioned." In order to achieve 'progress', 'gender' as a central subject matter was not finally addressed, but an acceptable document was produced.[555] Charles Yablon argues that court judgments are no different in that they present what is considered to be acceptable rather than what is true or right.[556] Crafting the BAC's documents was made easier by the fact that there is a notion of 'common good' under the broader discourse of stem cell research. Consequently, the emphasis was on explaining and justifying proposed courses of action that are likely to advance the 'common good', which in this case continues to be centred around the hope of regenerative medicine. As we shall discuss further, the metaphorical content of chimeras and hybrids is reconstituted in terms of certain ethical, scientific and social goals and specifications. The involutionary process was a means of rationalising and systematising a social phenomenon through the construction of hierarchical categories. Legal objectification has been a means of explaining and justifying a regulated approach, very much in the spirit of the SC Report. It has been relatively effective in meeting particular policy objectives, essentially by rendering visible and calculable certain concerns as regulatory risks. The drive to explain and justify also necessitated the search for allies. The rationale was that the more one's position is shared by others, the greater the sense of 'common good'.

---

554 Annelise Riles. [Deadlines]: Removing the Brackets on Politics in Bureaucratic and Anthropological Analysis. In Annelise Riles (ed.), *Documents: Artefacts of Modern Knowledge*. Ann Arbor: University of Michigan Press, 2006, pp 71-92, at 86.
555 *Ibid*, at 87.
556 Charles M Yablon, Are Judges Liars? A Wittgensteinian Critique of Law's Empire, *Canadian Journal of Law and Jurisprudence* (1990) 3: 123, at 124-125, and 135-138.

4.11 Global Scripts on Hybrids and Chimeras

In their study of the impact of international institutions on law-making in China, Indonesia and Korea over a period of 15 years, Terence Halliday and Bruce Carruthers argue that the globalisation of bankruptcy law has proceeded through recursive or iterative cycles at three levels: national, global and intermediate.[557] Recursive cycles could be relatively simple or highly complex:[558]

> The simplest patterns stay within cycles of a particular kind of law: an iteration from statutes to practice to amended statutes, or from court decisions to practice to further decisions, or from regulations to compliance to further regulations. More complex cycles can take several forms ... [where] earlier states in a cycle, or even earlier cycles, produce momentum that constrains the direction and impact of subsequent law-making and implementation.

Drawing on Lauren Edelman's theory of the endogeneity of law in national law-making as involving endogenous actors and mechanisms, they consider recursivity to be a better account of legal change as a dynamic and inclusive process, where new law arises less from law-making bodies and more from sites of practice, especially corporations.[559] This endogeneity of law is regarded as:

> a special instance of recursivity ... [in that it] ... incorporates full cycles of change from one kind of law (statutes) through creation of another kind of 'law' in practice through to its institutionalization via judicial rulings (case law). It has something of the invisibility of

---

[557] Terence C Halliday and Bruce G Carruthers, The Recursivity of Law: Global Norm Making and National Lawmaking in the Globalization of Corporate Insolvency Regimes, *American Journal of Sociology* (January 2007) 12, 4: 1135-1202. In this paper, the model of recursivity proposed is considered to be an approach to legal change that is "dynamic, evolutionary and nested": *Ibid*, at 1192.

[558] *Ibid*, at 1144.

[559] *Ibid*.

legalistic reform for it unfolds far from the interest-group hurly-burly of legislatures and more through the technical advances negotiated among human resource experts, lawyers, and judges.

In national law-making, endogenous change is attributed to the continuous interactions between actors and mechanisms in law-making and implementation,[560] which could otherwise be articulated as an interaction between formal law (statutes, cases and regulations) and law in practice (institutional behaviour). Experiences in national law-making, as Halliday and Carruthers observe, frequently influence global norm making through exogenous actors (such as international financial institutions, governance organisations and professional associations) and exogenous processes (which includes economic coercion, persuasion and modelling).[561]

As illustration of the constitutive power of legal concepts, Halliday and Carruthers point to global scripts that instantiate norms for adoption.[562] Elsewhere, they observe that, as different script producers were involved, several varieties of formalisation could exist.[563] The various scripts could in turn be categorised into two main types: those that were descriptive or prescriptive codes (as represented by the IMF, World Bank, Asian Development Bank, and UNCITRAL (United Nations Commission on International Trade Law) documents), and those that were developed and used by international financial

---

560 Four mechanisms that drive recursive cycles are identified as the *indeterminacy of law*, *contradictions*, *diagnostic struggles* and *actor mismatch*. *Ibid*, at 1149-1153.
561 *Ibid*, at 1148.
562 Norms are defined, for heuristic purposes, as "formalized codifications of behavioural prescriptions that are accepted by subjects as legitimate and authoritative." Terence C Halliday, Recursivity of Global Normmaking: A Sociolegal Agenda, *Annual Review of Law and Social Science* (2009) 5: 263-289, at 268.
563 Bruce G Carruthers and Terence C Halliday, Negotiating Globalization: Global Scripts and Intermediation in the Construction of Asian Insolvency Regimes. *Law & Social Inquiry* (2006) 31, 3: 521-584, at 536.

institutions and consultants as diagnostic tools.[564] These scripts emerged, following the Asian Financial Crisis in 1997. Consolidation followed when the UN articulated a single consensual norm in 2004, so that by 2005, all countries in the region were expected to conform to this legitimated standard.[565] In her study of human rights abuses in Burkina Faso and Kenya, Sally Falk Moore has similarly alluded to the presence of a 'global script' in the form of universal standards of morality in international human rights instruments that enables local struggles to be mapped against. Hence she observes that:

> Worldwide connections are being created out of the episodes of local struggles. And those connections involve a common, diffuse, value-laden symbolic content, as well as implying that practice consequences may emerge for individuals, institutions, and organizations.[566]

However, it is unclear if there is uniform agreement over whether 'global scripts' are intrinsic or otherwise necessary to processes of globalisation, especially where the law is a contributory force. For instance, the existence of a similar 'global script' is more ambiguous in Sally Engle Merry's study of the adoption of human rights interventions for gender violence. It is not entirely clear if there is an essential human rights content that could be appropriated, localised, transformed or otherwise imposed. For Merry, all script – if there is one – is neither 'local' nor 'global' (but possibly 'glocal').[567]

---

564 *Ibid*, at 570-571. Variations in forms of global scripts related largely to the level of discretion that nation-states had in different analytical possibilities: *Ibid*, at 540.

565 *Ibid*, at 539. Between 1998 and 2005, Carruthers and Halliday observe four main phases (at 569-571): (1) multiple actors and no formal script; (2) multiple actors and multiple formal scripts; (3) competing scripts and actors leading to hybrid forms; and (4) multiple actors and a single script.

566 Sally Falk Moore, Political Struggles in Legal Arenas: Some African Instances. In Max Kirsch (ed.), *Inclusion and Exclusion in the Global Arena*. New York: Routledge, 2006, pp 269-286, at 284.

567 Sally Engle Merry, New Legal Realism and the Ethnography of Transnational Law, *Law & Social Inquiry* (2006) 31, 4: 975-995, at 986.

Marina Kurkchiyan's study of the failure to set up UK-styled media self-regulatory bodies in two Russian cities, Rostov-on-Don and Nizhniy Novgorod, appears to support Merry's position. Referring to Douglas North's notion of institutions as 'rules of the game', institutional transplant could be regarded as a means by which new rules (both formal and informal) are set for local players.[568] The attempt to introduce an ethical means of regulation failed when, as Kurkchiyan finds, the core concept (in the transplantation exercise) of moral or ethical restraint was immediately understood as (or perhaps replaced by) legal restraint.[569] Consequently, all media disputes were managed legalistically, in direct contrast to the original intent of a less formalistic approach in the Anglo-American system of alternative dispute resolution. Kurkchiyan explains that as "both the idea of industrial self-regulation and of mediation as a means of dispute resolution, more generally, were not part of the local know-how", these notions and related practices "had to be explained, understood, interpreted, and implemented from scratch".[570] The outcome of her research suggests that, in thinking about what got transplanted, the emergent set of thinking and practices were neither 'local' (in the sense of conventional Russian institutional practices) nor 'global' (in the UK-styled self-regulatory practices), but perhaps a hybrid of the two, at best. Otherwise, it is questionable if transplantation arose at all, if there has been no significant change in the dominant mentality in conventional Russian practices, albeit with some modifications.

At least initially, the documents of the NAS appears to have created a 'script' that is akin to a form of globalised localism. In the years between 2005 and 2010, we observe a similar recursivity described by Halliday and Carruthers in initial creation of the guidelines of the NAS, their endorsement by the ISSCR (albeit with some exceptions),

---

568 Marina Kurkchiyan, Russian Legal Culture: An Analysis of Adaptive Response to an Institutional Transplant, *Law & Social Inquiry* (2009) 34, 2: 337-364, at 340.
569 *Ibid*, at 359.
570 *Ibid*, at 348.

and subsequent revisions made by both the NAS and ISSCR. Jenson and Santos define this process as one whereby certain local conditions succeed in traversing borders and so acquire the status of the 'global', either by constituting or otherwise by defining the dominant features of global consciousness on the subject. This status further enables it to designate rival conditions as local.[571] A similar, though possibly less recursive, process has been observed in Europe, mainly centred on the *Convention of Human Rights and Biomedicine*. However, we also do observe what Sally Engle Merry describes as indigenisation, or localised globalism, which entails the selective adaptation of a global ideal to local conditions.[572] The approaches of the BAC, and to some degree, the AMS, bear features of indigenisation to varying degrees.

Due to similar factors, it was found in another study that, together with greater mortality burden as an epidemiological condition, medical globalisation resulted in greater global institutional hetero-geneity across 58 countries.[573] The co-development of western allopathic medicine and traditional-alternative medicine did not support the homogeneity thesis in globalisation literature, which quite understandably assumed substitution of the latter by the former given the dominance of the world polity of medicine by western-allopathic medical organisations. Much to the contrary, greater heterogeneity is perhaps to be anticipated with the expansion of the world polity of medicine to include other international agendas such as human rights and development. From the standpoint of the HA Report at least, there were two 'global' scripts: one that could be

---

571 Jane Jenson and Boaventura de Sousa Santos. Introduction: Case Studies and Common Trends in Globalizations, in *Globalizing Institutions: Case Studies in Regulation and Innovation*, Jane Jenson and Boaventura de Sousa Santos (eds.). Aldershot: Ashgate, 2000, pp 9-26.

572 Sally Engle Merry. *Human Rights and Gender Violence: Translating International Law into Local Justice*. Chicago: University of Chicago Press, 2005.

573 Jae-Mahn Shim, Gerard Bodeker and Gemma Burford. Institutional heterogeneity in globalization: Co-development of western-allopathic medicine and traditional-alternative medicine, *International Sociology* (2011) 26, 6: 769-788, at 781-782.

traced to the NAS, and another to continental European sources. Developments in the UK were not quite of 'global' proportion, but important for reasons we will consider in the next chapter. The point to be noted is that the diversity of 'globalisation' experiences, including various theorised forms of institutional dynamics such as translation, isomorphism, decoupling and hybridisation,[574] may well account for the diversity of what could be regarded as 'global scripts'. Yet, for various policy reasons that have been noted earlier, a consolidated reading of these scripts as a 'global' or 'international' script, was adopted for the HA Report. This was possible as the 'focal points' advanced by these scripts shared the same place-holding notion of the 'common good' and were basically complementary.

4.12 Bioethical Accounts Scripted Upwards

Globalisation has been in a significant way an account of relationships. In 1974, Immanuel Wallerstein provided a macrosocial account of globalisation as division of labour among different geographical regions and countries.[575] In essence, Wallerstein proposes a tri-modal structure involving three regions: a core region of high-wage, capital intensive and skilled labour, a peripheral region focused on raw material production and intensive in unskilled labour, and a semi-periphery region with mixed forms of labour and capital intensity. In this world-system paradigm, Wallerstein attempts to describe how countries and regions compete to impose dominant cultures, which could be broadly understood as a system of shared meanings and symbols. His account has been criticised over time on a number

---

574 Gili S Drori, John W Meyer, Francisco O Ramirez, and Evan Schofer. *Science in the Modern World Polity: Institutionalization and Globalization.* Stanford, CA: Stanford University Press, 2003. See also Jan Niederveen Pieterse. *Globalization and Culture: Global Melange.* Lanham: Rowman and Littlefield, 2004.

575 Immanuel Wallerstein. *The Modern World-System I: Capitalist Agriculture and the Origins of the European World-Economy in the Sixteenth Century.* New York: Academic Press, 1974.

of bases, including a lack of descriptive rigour due in part to its generality. In my view, William Robinson correctly observes that the notion of globalisation depends very much on what we understand as being circulated in global systems.[576] In analysing global scripting on hybrids and chimeras, what captivated me was the circulation of policy documents and the 'focal points' that they encapsulated, not quite the transnational capitalist class that Robinson points to.[577] Again, 'focal points' seem appropriate as the process of policy development was focused on (primarily 'local') coordination, but not in a planned or orchestrated way. In addition, there did not appear to be an explicit agenda of network building or network power,[578] although earlier attempts to create international norms on human embryonic stem cell research did. The global scripting process, in the initial stages at least, appeared to be more happenstance, where the circulation of normative frames and norms, as well as sense-making endeavours, was made manifest in the exchange of policy documents.

It is further important to recognise the role of institutions (and their documents) as 'script carriers'. In a study on the attitudes towards, and the practice of, female genital cutting in five African countries, it was found that institutions that carry 'modern' scripts all

---

[576] William I Robinson. Globalization and the sociology of Immanuel Wallerstein: A critical appraisal. *International Sociology* (2011) 26, 6: 723-745.

[577] *Ibid*, at 741.

[578] David Singh Grewal similarly draws on Thomas Schelling's notion of 'focal points' in analysing network power. However, the networks that he addresses appear to me to be constituted by relatively fixed or structured relationships. Zeev Maos presents a similar (although significantly more quantitative) analysis of network relations. I did not find rigid or structured relations among the institutions that I have studied. The representatives from these institutions whom I interviewed similarly did not consider their various institutions to be part of a 'network'. Neither the NAS nor the CIRM, which shared close working relationships on a number of projects, considered themselves to be associated in this way. David Singh Grewal, *Network Power: The Social Dynamics of Globalization*. New Haven and London: Yale University Press, 2008; and Zeev Maoz, *Networks of Nations: The Evolution, Structure, and Impact of International Networks*, 1816-2001. New York: Cambridge University Press, 2011.

reduce the probability that women will favour the continuation of 'circumcision' of their daughters.[579] Adopting a neo-institutionalist approach, 'modern' institutions such as education, college, mass media and employment, have been identified as 'script carriers'; they provide institutional logics that could be drawn upon for constructing individual identities and understandings about the world.[580] Modernisation is thereby seen as a process of reshaping an individual's entire cultural universe, and not just perspectives in 'modern' environments. Adding to this, a materialist element was also noted as a contributing factor. Professionalised international governmental organisations and international non-governmental organisations with relatively large amounts of resources have played a prominent role in the neo-institutionalist account of how changes have occurred through globalisation.

Documents are artefacts of (post?)modern knowledge in that they are relational, not so much in and of themselves, but as an essentialised component of their originating institutions – the 'script-carriers'. At one level, they mediate relationships within institutions. In sending the HA Consultation Paper and receiving feedback in return, the BAC establishes a relationship with its consultation party. The act of giving a document creates an information potentiality that motivates contact. The very construct of ethical or legal rules has the effect of enjoining the public, the state and researchers in a three-way relationship. Sarah Franklin and Celia Roberts liken this to a social contract. They argue that the 'Warnock strategy' entails a certain 'give-and-take' such that in exchange for permitting a limited amount of embryo research, the state would assure the public of strict regulation that is subject to the very highest standards of public

---

579 Elizabeth Heger Boyle, Barbara J McMorris and Mayra Gomez. Local Conformity to International Norms. *International Sociology* (2002) 17, 1: 5-33.

580 *Ibid*, at 6-7 and 25-26. Neoinstitutionalism and modernism are regarded as differing from each other in the former's emphasis on international systems and scripts, whereas the latter focuses on individual-nature relationship.

accountability. It was in this context that Mary Warnock posed a question about feeling, judgement and belonging to which she offered a solution of tolerance, compromise and regulation.[581] In creating a sense of a whole that is greater than the sum of its parts, a kind of 'social contract' emerges that marks the 'British way forward' with techniques such as PGD and IVF, as well as with human cloning, stem cell technology and biobanking. Franklin and Roberts allegorises this as a firm hand that disciplines the troops, so that if discipline and order can be maintained, much faster progress will be made – to everyone's benefit.[582] The 'common good' is thus actualised and lived. In addition, these documents put forward various forms of orderings and co-ordinations. We can broadly group them as institutional-based review (NAS, NIH, CIRM), centralised regulation (DCE, EU Chimbrids project, GEC), and mixed approaches (AMS, ISSCR, BAC). Such social configurations lower uncertainty as to how scientists are expected to behave and how the public would (and should) react. They confine the conduct of scientists to what is permissible and assure the public that scientists will conform to these prescriptions. What was unpredictable is now within expectation.

In considering and adopting some of the 'focal points' in the NAS Guidelines, the BAC and the NAS became 'related' by commonality. In contrast to this analysis, the notion of 'circulating references' suggests that there is some form of collective effort at developing 'focal points'. While this may be the case in certain situations, I have not found any conscious effort toward collaboration as such. One institution borrows from another to a degree, but the concerns that each institution sets out to address is uniquely its own and often peculiar to its time and context. But as we have seen, this does not mean that there is no commonality. The indebtedness is often paid towards the

---

[581] Sarah Franklin and Celia Roberts. *Born and Made: An Ethnography of Preimplantation Genetic Diagnosis.* Princeton, NJ: Princeton University Press, 2006, at 197.
[582] *Ibid,* at 198.

advancement of commonalities and arguable *is* the cause of social relations. It is one reason why the BAC is concerned with developments that occur outside of its territory, and *vice versa*. In addition, documents are a basis of (or trigger for) institutional learning. They are also means by which various knowledge systems 'come together' in the production of a 'collective consciousness' of sorts, or perhaps a discourse among discourses – a very generic 'global script'. In legal analysis, it is akin to the association of cases through the derivation of their respective *ratio decidendi*.

The documentary bases upon which these 'focal points' subsist should not be overlooked. The documents of the institutions that we have considered all embody the essence of their respective institutional sponsors and thereby have meaning quite apart from the broader socio-political climate. They are, in a sense, samples of Weber's basic model of society; that is an equilibrium between different institutional sectors taken on a global scale.[583] In their portrayal of what constitutes human and non-human, these documents enable us to learn about ourselves from the societies they represent, in the way that perhaps Durkheim's idea of *anomie* in his book on suicide does.[584] But the HA Report, like the documents of the NAS, CIRM, ISSCR, AMS, DCE, GEC and the EU Chimbrids project, each retain their own distinct character and form. It is their 'focal points' that serve as 'social technologies' that enable re-imagining and the generation of other social facts.[585]

The 'focal points' are means by which a level of shared consciousness, or an intersubjective space, is accessed. As we have seen, documents are communicative in the substantive information that

---

[583] Mary Douglas. *How Institutions Think*. Syracuse: Syracuse University Press, 1986, at 93.

[584] *Ibid*, at 97.

[585] Stephen J Collier and Aihwa Ong. Global Assemblages and Anthropological Problems. In Aihwa Ong and Stephen J Collier, *Global Assemblages: Technology, Politics, and Ethics as Anthropological Problems*. Singapore: Blackwell Publishing, 2005, pp 3-21, at 7.

they embody, particularly in terms of the 'focal point' issues by which they are framed. In addition, they are instruments by which discursive and normative categories, as well as practices, are de-constructed, created or sustained. Social facts are scripted into documents and are directed at generating different forms of action. In addition, documents allow an attentive reader to get a sense of how a society or community understands itself.[586] Collectively, documents contribute to a 'global script' through the intermediation of 'focal points'. The reflexivity of scripts – whether local, global or glocal – is not confined to commentary on social institutions but they are set up to be interpreted. Scripts offer unique insight into their own operations as acts of cultural instauration, and are capable of revealing something about the inner processes of instauration.[587]

---

[586] Karin Barber. *The Anthropology of Texts, Persons and Publics: Oral and written culture in Africa and beyond.* Cambridge: Cambridge University Press, 2007, at 4.
[587] *Ibid*, at 5.

5

Chimeras and Hybrids as Regulatory Placeholders

5.1 Constituting Chimeras and Hybrids

I learnt of Dr Irving Weissman's proposed creation of a mouse with a human brain when assisting in research that would culminate in the SC Report. That was in 2001. But as the proposal – however interesting – was not an issue of immediate interest or relevance at that time, the matter was put aside only to be taken up again some years later. By 2007, the institutional framework developed for hESC research conferred on his work a sense of place and a sensibility of purpose. Weissman proposed to create a mouse with a brain composed of human-derived neurons within a structure of mouse glial cells. This could be done in a number of ways; one of which was through transplanting human brain stem cells into an inbred strain of an immunologically deficient (called severe combined immune deficiency or 'SCID') foetal mouse just before the degeneration of its own brain cells. The objective of the research was to study human neurons *in vivo* in a laboratory animal.[588] An earlier experiment involving the introduction of human brain stem cells into a fully

---

[588] Henry T Greely, Mildred K Cho, Linda F Hogle and Debra M Satz, Thinking About the Human Neuron Mouse. *The American Journal of Bioethics* (2007) 7, 5: 27-40, at 31.

functioning brain of a mouse showed the former behaving like murine brain cells. So if a mouse could be created to possess only human brain cells but functioning within a murine brain structure, the outcome might allow something to be said about whether there is anything 'human' about the brain cells, and more generally, about characteristics that are essentially 'human'. Although the experiment was approved by Stanford University's IRB, the research was not carried out due possibly to the (scientific) difficulty in determining if the firing of human-derived neurons in a mouse could be said to be the same as their counterparts in a human being.[589] Still, this episode is important for a number of reasons. First, it is an indication of a scientific rationality and trajectory. Second, it marks the beginning of formal (or institutional) deliberation on chimeras and hybrids. Third, it triggers critical reflection on what we know about these constructs and how much more is to be known. It further raises questions on what should be regarded as 'human' characteristics. As we shall see, these questions will require (albeit tentative) regulatory responses if the research is to have meaning beyond the realm of science.

Chimeras and hybrids of the HA Report are creatures of human design and exist only in the sanitised confines of the laboratory. With very limited exceptions, they do not differ significantly in form from their counterparts in the natural environment. In the usual course of life, ordinary people are unlikely to come into contact with these wondrous creatures. But chimeras and hybrids also exist in human imagination, in myths and, to some degree, in day-to-day language under the more generic expression of 'monsters'. They are metaphors made vivid in Michael Crichton's *Next*.[590] We see them even in discussions of contemporary affairs. Niall Ferguson's 'Chimerica' depicts the negative consequence of combining Chinese surplus and American deficit as having contributed to the most severe credit

---

[589] *Ibid.*
[590] Michael Crichton. *Next*. New York: HarperCollins Publishers, 2006.

crisis since the Great Depression.[591] As metaphors in biomedical sciences however, the negative connotations present an almost implacable obstacle to any meaningful discussion. More daunting was the complexity and breadth of the subject matter. As a lawyer, my initially reaction was an unsettling excitement. Legal training in matching social phenomena to legal paradigms did not at first seem relevant. The purpose was not to constitute chimeras and hybrids as legal 'subjects' in a strict sense – not immediately at least. Furthermore, the law has in almost all cases clearly distinguished between humans and nonhuman animals. The chimeras and hybrids that we are to deal with have components of both. Even if these constructs did fit into an existing legal category, what are the rules that should apply? And to whom? My colleagues and I also expected the public to be interested, grave and possibly adverse. Perhaps in anticipation of this, the approach adopted has been systematic and cautious. Consequently, the consultation paper on the subject was less directive than previous consultation papers, and no recommendations or guidelines were proposed for consideration. Shortly after the commencement of public consultation, a faculty member of a law school in Singapore commented that lawyers are not generally accustomed to such open-endedness in consultation documents. In what sounds to me like Lon Fuller,[592] he added that there would be little that the Law Reform Committee of the Singapore Academy of Law (of which he was a member) could provide by way of feedback given the absence of legal rules on the subject.

Ironically, it was the ethical and legal techniques of categorisation, systematisation, distantiation and objectification that gave form to chimeras and hybrids. The 'focal points' that we considered in the

---

591 Niall Ferguson. *The Ascent of Money: A Financial History of the World*. New York: Penguin Books, 2008, at 333-341.

592 Lon L Fuller. *The Morality of Law*. New Haven: Yale University Press, 1969. Fuller indicates (at 47) that an 'internal morality of law' is that there must be rules. These rules need not be in the nature of legislation and would include those promulgated by administrative agencies (at 168-173).

previous chapter operated as ethical and legal analytics and techniques that laid the foundation for instauration in a number of ways. First, they discredited existing models *of* chimeras and hybrids. Second, they co-constructed a model *for* these biological constructs through a process of categorisation. This construction was based on science and ethics but through a process akin to legal adjudication. My field experience suggests a direct contribution of juridical knowledge and technique in the making of chimeras and hybrids in the BAC's documents. But why create these categories? One reason is that the instauration (or substitution) of 'old' or more conventional meanings embedded in the metaphors for new ones enables discussion, especially in public forums. Another reason just as important is that ethical and legal categories create regulatory objects. By definition, regulatory objects can be controlled through means of ethical values and 'law'. This in turn gives meaning to regulatory risk and further enables a response to certain modes of arguments, such as a concern with descent down the 'slippery slope'. Hence the third reason ethics and law have been important in the policy process relating to chimeras and hybrids is that it is not only anticipatory; it realises what Annelise Riles refers to as 'as if' legal fictions or placeholders.[593] This way, it pre-empted public reaction and thereby stabilised what could have been a volatile discursive terrain. The deployment of ethical and legal knowledge in sustaining certain distinctions, such as the great chasm that has been built between humans and nonhuman animals is illustrative. But there are also limitations to categorisation through objectification and instauration. In a policy environment, a danger lies in the treatment of these 'objects' as truisms.

Drawing on Annelise Riles's analysis of legal techniques in a variety of forms, this chapter provides an account of the application of ethical and legal techniques within bureaucratic and public environments.

---

[593] Annelise Riles. Collateral Expertise: Legal Knowledge in the Global Financial Markets. *Current Anthropology* (2010) 51, 6: 795-818, at 802-803, and 815. See also Annelise Riles. *Collateral Knowledge: Legal Reasoning in the Global Financial Markets*. Chicago and London: University of Chicago Press, 2011, at 172-175.

Broadly speaking, these techniques are regulatory and entail styles of argumentation and systematic reasoning. We focus in particular on the use of these techniques in constructing metaphors as conceptual models, which is another major theme of this Chapter. It is argued that the metaphorical construction of 'hybrids' and 'chimeras' as models of 'Seeing As-if' enables regulatory control. Referring to the works of Lakoff and Johnston on metaphors, James Underhill identifies fundamental claims in metaphors as influencing the way people formulate ideas and express them (e.g. 'time is money'), form systematic constructs (e.g. refusing to 'waste' one's time in a 'profitless venture'), highlight and hide (e.g. 'Argument is War' conceals the fact that it can also be constructive), contradict one another (especially since conceptual metaphors can be mutually exclusive), grounded in experience that corresponds with one's experience of reality (e.g. 'Ideas are Food'), create similarity (e.g. 'The Stock Market is up today' where 'More is Up'), and widen cardinal trope to embrace other forms of comparison (e.g. 'pretty as a rose').[594] While the 'hybrids' and 'chimeras' in the BAC's documents may be more limited in discursive substance and temporality relative to the metaphors that Underhill considers, they have been effectively deployed as placeholders. In the context of this study, the metaphorical effectiveness of 'hybrids' and 'chimeras' as regulatory devices has been dependent on their capability to be applied as placeholders. The construction of these placeholders has not been limited to Singapore, but involved – as we have discussed in the previous chapter – iterative interactions across several jurisdictions. I also want to return to the concept of instauration, which has a primary meaning of being 'restorative', but has a secondary meaning in juxtaposition rather than succession. As bioethical creations, 'hybrids' and 'chimeras' instaurate the chasm between human and

---

[594] James W Underhill. *Creating Worldviews: Metaphor, Ideology and Language.* Edinburgh: Edinburg University Press, 2011, at 25-29.

nonhuman entities. But they also embody a transgression, or a state of *qui n'avait pu être* (what was not able to be).

5.2 Defining Human-Animal Combinations in Singapore

Almost immediately following the publication by the BAC of its recommendations on egg donation for stem cell research on 7 November 2007,[595] a consultation paper (HA Consultation Paper) on the creation of cytoplasmic hybrid embryos and chimeric animals (under the broader rubric of human-animal combination) was released to the public on 8 January 2008.[596] The overall format of the HA Consultation Paper did not differ substantially from earlier consultation papers prepared by the BAC in that there was relatively clear segmentation of discussion relating to the scientific, ethical and legal implications of the subjects. But unlike its predecessors, the HA Consultation Paper did not propose any recommendation for consideration. The overall tone of the Consultation Paper was task oriented, and hence pragmatic. In devising a definition for chimeras and hybrids, it did not attempt to explain the essence of 'humanity'. Instead, the focus fell on the types of human-animal combinations that were already used in research or in facilitating medical therapy and those that researchers have a prospective interest in developing. The action-orientation of policy documents required the outlay of information to be made in a way that can direct meaningful responses to policy challenges. As an interest was in exploring the possibility of using animal eggs for SCNT, the creation of a cytoplasmic hybrid embryo was further elaborated on in the draft consultation paper. It was schematically represented as:[597]

---

595 Bioethics Advisory Committee, *Donation of Human Eggs for Research*. Singapore: Bioethics Advisory Committee, 3 November 2008.

596 Bioethics Advisory Committee, *Human-Animal Combinations for Biomedical Research: A Consultation Paper*, Singapore: Bioethics Advisory Committee, 8 January 2008.

597 Fieldnotes, 27 July 2007: Draft Consultation Paper, at 4.

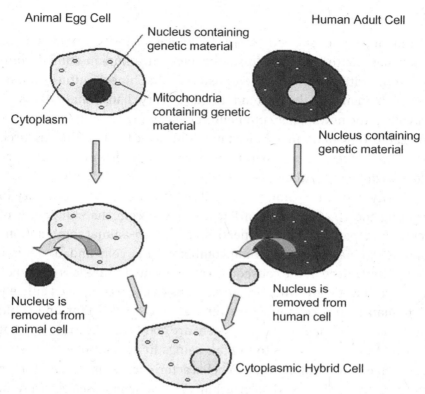

Nucleus from human adult cell is inserted into animal egg cell. The resultant cell called a cytoplasmic hybrid cell has human genetic material from the human cell and animal genetic material from the mitochondria of the animal cell. If activated, cell division would occur and each resulting cell would contain genetic material from both animal and human sources.

Figure 5.1. Creating a Cytoplasmic Hybrid Embryo

In fact, prior to the release of the HA Consultation Paper, human-animal combination was already a moot topic in the public domain. For instance, a commentary specifically on the subject was published in the mainstream local Chinese newspaper on 1 July 2007.[598] The

---

[598] Fieldnotes, 21 August 2008.

commentary was entitled '人面兽身', which suggests a tendency for a lay person to associate research involving human-animal combinations with the creation of monsters.[599] In Chinese culture, unions between man and beast tend to have very bad connotations.[600] However, the newspaper commentator – a biology graduate student – indicated that most people he knew did not object to the research after the objectives and nature of these scientific constructs were clearly explained to them.

Clarity in defining 'human-animal combinations' was necessary in drafting the HA Consultation Paper. Purely from the standpoint of scientific capability, a broad spectrum of human-animal combinations can be produced through some combination of cells and/or genetic materials. However, the consequences of the mixing are less clear. For instance, it is not known if a mouse that has a brain composed entirely of human neural cells would exhibit characteristics that one could recognise as 'human'. Even then, there are good reasons to expect that a primate (being 'closer' to human beings in evolutionary terms) is more likely to exhibit 'human' characteristics if its brain (being structurally similar to that of a human) was composed entirely of human neurons than would a mouse. In addition, the developmental stage of the research entity (be it an embryo or a fully developed organism) is relevant as this may have an effect on the extent of integration between host tissues and the introduced cells or genetic materials. Hence, despite the uncertainties, useful analytical measures have been identified as including the extensiveness of the human-animal mix, the type of organism concerned, and the developmental stage of this organism. A general taxonomy comprising three main types of human-animal combination, being chimeras, hybrids and

---

[599] 陈华彪, 人面兽身, 联合早报 [Chen H B. Human Face Beast Body, Combined Morning Paper], 1 July 2007.
[600] Interview with sociologist and BAC member, Professor Eddie Kuo, 28 April 2009.

transgenic organisms, [601] was devised after a relatively detailed review of scientific, ethical, legal and policy literatures on the subject. Table 5.1 sets out the possibilities categorically.[602]

Table 5.1. Types of Human-Animal Combination

	Definition Embryo	Definition Developed Entity	Examples of Uses in Research
Human Chimera (With Some Animal Cellular Material)	An embryo created by introducing one or more animal cells, usually stem cells, into a human embryo at an early stage of development. Any particular cell from the resulting embryo could be traced back either to the human or animal source.	An entity brought to term from a preponderantly human chimeric embryo. Animal cells would be present in many or all of its tissues. This entity may also be created by introducing animal cells into a person or into a human embryo at a later stage of development. Such an entity would have animal cells present only in a few tissues.	No known proposals to create such chimeric embryos or entities for research purposes (other than for clinical transplant research).

(Continued)

---

[601] In the HA Consultation Paper, a chimera is defined as an "organism whose body contains cells from another organism of the same or a different species", whereas a hybrid is an "organism whose cells contain genetic material from organisms of different species." A transgenic animal is an "animal that has a genome containing genes from another species". See Bioethics Advisory Committee, *Human-Animal Combinations for Biomedical Research: A Consultation Paper.* Singapore: Bioethics Advisory Committee, 8 January 2008, pp. 40–42.

[602] Important sources of information for this table include documents of the US National Academy of Sciences and the UK Academy of Medical Sciences. See The National Academy of Sciences, USA, *Guidelines for Human Embryonic Stem Cell Research*, 2005 (amended 2007 and 2008); and The Academy of Medical Sciences, *Inter-species embryos: A report by the Academy of Medical Sciences.* London: Academy of Medical Sciences, June 2007.

Table 5.1.   (*Continued*)

	Definition Embryo	Definition Developed Entity	Examples of Uses in Research
Animal Chimera (With Some Human Cellular Material)	An embryo created by introducing one or more human cells, usually stem cells, into an animal embryo at an early stage of development. Any particular cell from the resulting embryo could be traced back either to the human or animal source.	An entity brought to term from a preponderantly animal chimeric embryo. Human cells would be present in many or all of its tissues. This entity may also be created by introducing human cells into an animal or into an animal embryo at a later stage of development. Such an entity would have human cells present only in a few tissues.	• Growing human organs in animals for the purpose of transplantation into humans. • For testing the pluripotence of stem cells, for example, via the transplantation of such cells into immuno-deficient mice. • To evaluate the potential usefulness and safety of transplanting human stem cells for clinical treatment, by testing such stem cells in animals. • For creating disease-specific research models such as the HIV infected SCID-Hu mouse.
Human-Animal Cytoplasmic Hybrid or Cybrid (With a Human Nuclear Genome)	An embryo created by replacing the nucleus of an animal egg with the nucleus of an adult human somatic cell.	An entity brought to term from a human-animal cytoplasmic hybrid embryo with a human nuclear genome.	The embryo may be used for studying the processes involved in nuclear reprogramming, which may lead to deriving patient-specific stem cell lines. May also potentially be used to derive disease-specific stem cell lines for the purpose of research on specific diseases. No known proposals to bring a human-animal cytoplasmic hybrid embryo to term for research purposes.
Animal-Human Cytoplasmic Hybrid (With an Animal Nuclear Genome)	An embryo created by replacing the nucleus of a human egg with the nucleus of an adult animal somatic cell.	An entity brought to term from a human-animal cytoplasmic hybrid embryo with an animal nuclear genome.	No known proposals to create animal-human cytoplasmic hybrid embryos or entities for research.

Table 5.1. (*Continued*)

	Definition Embryo	Definition Developed Entity	Examples of Uses in Research
True Human-Animal Hybrid	An embryo created by fertilising an animal egg with a human sperm or vice versa. Any particular cell from the resulting embryo contains almost equal genetic contributions from both human and animal source.	An entity developed from a human-animal true hybrid embryo.	Not used in research, although the human-animal true hybrid embryo has been used to assess or diagnosis sub-fertility.
Transgenic Human (With Some Animal Genetic Material)	A human embryo with animal genes inserted.	A human being developed from a human embryo that has integrated animal genes.	No known proposals to create such transgenic human embryos or human beings.
Transgenic Animal (With Some Human Genetic Material)	An animal embryo with human genes inserted.	An animal developed from an animal embryo that has integrated human genes.	Transgenic animals with human genetic material are widely used as disease-specific research models and many examples exist. One such example is the Oncomouse.

However, the scope of the HA Consultation Paper is much narrower in order to aid comprehension and facilitate discussion. In narrowing down the possibilities, all categories of human-animal combinations that either did not draw any scientific interest or were ethically less controversial were excluded. Transgenic animals have not been included in the HA Consultation Paper, as those routinely used in research tend to carry a very small number of human genes and hence are not considered to be ethically controversial. However, transgenic animals could be a matter for future deliberation if whole human chromosomes are incorporated into non-human animals. As for transgenic humans, there is no known scientific interest in such experimentation. Being a matter of public policy, it would not be necessary to consider all the types of human-animal combination that can be created, even if there might have been academic reasons to do so. Even in the broader deliberation of other policy bodies such as the AMS, the contingency of free roaming human-animal creatures was precluded as the subject matter was mainly confined to embryos.

Apart from narrowing the scope through the categorical exclusion of certain human-animal combinations, a processual limitation has also been adopted in that only 'human-to-animal' combinations would fall within its purview. A chimera or hybrid could arise through the incorporation of animal materials into human ('animal-to-human' or 'human' chimera), or through the incorporation of human materials into animals ('human-to-animal', or 'animal' chimera or hybrid). Focus would only be on the latter process as the former was either ethically unambiguous at that time or already captured within an existing regulatory framework. For instance, the creation of an animal cytoplasmic hybrid (by introducing an animal nucleus into an enucleated human egg) would be unethical as the scarcity of human eggs implied that eggs should not be 'wasted' unless there is overwhelming scientific imperative. As for any research on human embryos, specific approval from the MOH is required. Hence, any attempt to create a human embryo with non-human material could only be done with the approval of the Ministry. Similarly, the incorporation of animal materials into human at any point from the foetal stage of development would be regulated as research involving human subjects. With the successive narrowing of focus and the exclusion of theoretical possibilities from current consideration, the broad scope of 'human-animal combinations' was cropped down to 'human-to-animal' chimeras (or animal chimera) and cytoplasmic hybrids.

The much narrower scope is apparent in the table on the types of human-animal combination set out in the HA Consultation Paper (see Table 5.2).[603] Although 'transgenic animals' are included in the table, they have not been considered in the HA Consultation Paper, but serve only to emphasise that they have not been considered to "raise any new ethical difficulties."[604]

Table 5.2. Creation and Use of Chimeras and Cytoplasmic Hybrids

	How It Is Created	**Examples of Use in Research**
Animal Chimeras	By introducing human cells, usually stem cells, into an animal or an early animal embryo or an animal foetus.	• Testing the developmental potential of human stem cells or their derivatives. • Evaluating the potential usefulness and safety of transplanting human stem cells for clinical treatment. • In vivo drug testing giving an approximation to human responses. • Studying the possibility of growing human tissues and organs in animals for the purpose of transplantation into humans.
Cytoplasmic Hybrid Embryos	By the transfer of the nucleus of a human somatic cell into an animal egg from which the nucleus has been removed (see Figure 2 [of HA Consultation Paper]).	• A source of pluripotent stem cells for research. • Studying the processes involved in nuclear reprogramming. • A source of disease-specific stem cells for the study of specific disease processes and methods of treatment.
Transgenic Animals	By introducing human genes into an animal embryo.	Routinely used in research to understand the cause of diseases, to develop more effective treatment for these diseases, to test the safety of new products and vaccines, and to study the possibility of producing organs for transplantation that will not be rejected.

---

603 Bioethics Advisory Committee, Singapore, Human-Animal Combinations for Biomedical Research: A Consultation Paper, 8 January 2008, at 15.
604 *Ibid*, at 13, paragraph 14.

Given the narrower focus, the HA Consultation Paper could have been re-titled 'chimeras and hybrids'. However, a generic expression like 'human-animal combinations' was considered to be more neutral than an explicit reference to 'chimeras' and 'hybrids'.[605] In addition, if the draft consultation paper was to be renamed 'chimeras and hybrids', it could be confused with the recently concluded public consultation of the HFEA. Hence in spite of the narrower focus of the draft consultation paper, the title of 'human-animal combination' was used. A further possibility was for the term 'inter-species cell transplantation' to be used in place of 'chimera', since the latter was regarded as emotionally charged and carried negative connotations.[606] However, such a terminological substitution might be perceived as an attempt to sidestep ethical controversy by using a different label for something generally understood as referring to chimeras. Given that the term 'chimera' has already been used in a variety of literature to refer to the mixing of human and animal biological materials at a cellular level, the terminology was used.

5.3 Ethical Evaluation in the HA Consultation Paper

The ethical discussion was similarly focused on narrowing the scope of the discussion to those that relate to the types of hybrids and chimeras of interest at that time. In particular, it was directed at refuting what Leon Kass – Chairman of President George W Bush's Council of Bioethics from 2002 to 2005 – regarded as the 'Wisdom of Repugnance'. Kass argues that we shudder at the prospect of human cloning not because of the novelty of the technology, but because "we intuit and feel, immediately and without argument, the violation of things that we rightfully hold dear."[607] If cloning causes one to shudder, the prospect of human-animal chimeras and hybrids will

---

605 Fieldnotes, 21 August 2007.
606 Fieldnotes, 14 November 2007.
607 Leon R Kass. The Wisdom of Repugnance, *New Republic* (2 June 1997) 216, 22: 17-26.

quite possibly create convulsions. Some scholars provide convincing reasons not to dismiss feelings lightly, even if they were merely initial reactions. For example, following Martin Heidegger and Maurice Merleau-Ponty, Kim MacLauren argues that emotions are not located in some 'solipsistic consciousness' but in our embodied engagement with the world and with others.[608] In addressing this reaction, a moralistic attitude was not adopted as this would come across as fundamentally dismissive of emotional expressions.[609] The problem with reactions of disgust, repugnance or like feelings is that they are a poor guide to collective action and public policy. Their seemingly subjective character further impedes an appropriate legal response given the impersonal nature of law. Such feelings could well be related to political and ideological views of the world, but both feelings and views change over time.[610] There also did not appear to be any effective policy means to address purely emotional concerns. On this rationale, the BAC considered emotional neutrality in ethical discussion to be a balanced manner in setting out and addressing commonly articulated or anticipated concerns and fears.[611] Substantive issues have been introduced and counter-arguments presented in order for the discussion to be rounded on the whole. Still, in a meeting with religious group leaders on 13 August 2008, it was observed

---

608 Kim MacLaren. Emotional Metamorphoses: The Role of Others in Becoming a Subject, in *Embodiment and Agency*. In Sue Campbell, Letitia Meynell and Susan Sherwin (eds.). University Park PA: The Pennsylvania State University, 2009, pp 25-45, at 26.

609 MacLauren indicates that emotional responses are often assumed to be simply irrational ways of configuring reality, and that a person already knows better, or already has access to the 'rational' response. *Ibid*, at 43.

610 Dan Jones, Moral psychology: the depths of disgust, *Nature* (14 June 2007) 447, 7146: 768-771. Jones writes (at 771): "... data from psychology and neuroscience should make us think twice about drawing on revulsion as a basis for our personal moral judgements. History seems to bear this out. Women (especially menstruating ones), the mentally and physically disabled, and inter-racial sex have all been viewed with disgust, and are still viewed as such by some ... If disgust wasn't a good moral indicator then, why should it be now?"

611 Fieldnotes, 21 August 2007.

by some that the ethical discussion in the HA Consultation Paper came across as 'consequentialist' in general orientation. This perception may be attributable to the categorical (and taxonomic) approach that sought to balance current and potential uses against anticipated risks. This was also a critique, by some bioethicists, of Henry Greely's allegedly utilitarian approach.[612] It is questionable if public policy could comprehensively capture all ethical concerns.[613] As the HA Consultation Paper sought to update the SC Report, the principles of justness and sustainability continue to guide the BAC's deliberation.[614]

The application of these principles is evident in the ethical identification of interests. An issue arose as to whether a discussion of 'Imago Dei' (Image of God) from an expert paper should be incorporated into the HA Consultation Paper. The concern was that this would be too targeted at a particular community (i.e. those of the Christian faith).[615] There is no similar concept of 'Imago Dei' in the Islamic faith, and although there are deities with human-animal forms

---

[612] Françoise Baylis and Jason Scott Robert. Part-Human Chimeras: Worrying the Facts, Probing the Ethics, *American Journal of Bioethics* (2007) 7, 5: 41-45. Baylis and Robert state (at 44): "... the general utilitarian framework relied upon by Greely and colleagues in their analysis of the ethics of creating human neuron mice ... is not, in our view, sufficiently rich as to capture the range of ethical concerns. The ethical concerns with this research are not just about weighing putative harms and benefits ... chimeric research raises deep philosophical questions about what it means to be human and these questions cannot be addressed by appeal to utility maximizing strategies."

[613] Interview with Associate Professor John Elliott, former member of the BAC and a member of the Secretariat, 27 August 2009.

[614] The BAC indicates that its recommendations are intended to lead to results that are 'just' and 'sustainable'. The former favours research with tremendous potential therapeutic benefits to mankind while the latter requires research to have little biological or genetic impact on future generations. See Bioethics Advisory Committee, *Ethical, Legal and Social Issues in Human Stem Cell Research, Reproductive and Therapeutic Cloning*. Singapore: Bioethics Advisory Committee, 21 June 2002, at 35, paragraph 47.

[615] Nuyen A T, Stem Cell Research and Interspecies Fusion: Some Philosophical Issues, 2007, at 3. Available at http://www.bioethics-singapore.org.

in Buddhism and Taoism, this did not necessarily imply that Buddhists and Taoists would be more receptive to research involving human-animal combinations since the mixing of human and animal features tend to have negative connotations in Chinese culture. This concern did not find ready or expedient solution, but the discussion on 'Imago Dei' was not specifically raised in the HA Consultation Paper. It was nevertheless implicit in the ethical discussion on objecting to the research due to repugnance or 'playing God'.[616] The fact that 'God' has been set out in upper case suggests the Abrahamic conception of a monotheistic deity.

As the intent was to keep discussion in the HA Consultation Paper open-ended, effective regulation was more difficult to present as it could be seen as pre-empting the discussion if specific regulatory approaches were proposed.[617] The significance attributed to regulatory control was nevertheless clear.[618] Instead of recommending specific regulatory approaches, regulatory principles were discussed.[619] The BAC indicated that research involving human-animal combinations should – as a baseline standard – remain governed within an existing ethical framework. Under the framework proposed by the ISSCR, four factors to be taken into account in the creation of human-non-human primate neural tissue chimeras via the implantation of human neural stem cells into an animal are stated essentially as scientifically-grounded ethical considerations. These factors, adopted by the BAC as ethical premises, are:[620]

---

[616] Bioethics Advisory Committee, *Human-Animal Combinations for Biomedical Research: A Consultation Paper*. Singapore: Bioethics Advisory Committee, 8 January 2008, at 20-22.

[617] Fieldnotes, 14 November 2007.

[618] *Ibid*.

[619] Bioethics Advisory Committee, *Human-Animal Combinations for Biomedical Research: A Consultation Paper*. Singapore: Bioethics Advisory Committee, 8 January 2008, at 27, paragraph 56.

[620] *Ibid*, at 23, paragraph 43.

(1) Proportion or ratio of human to animal cells in the animal's brain;

(2) Site of integration of the human neural cells;

(3) Recipient species; and

(4) Brain size of the animal involved.

Ethical constraints are also not clearly distinguished from regulatory measures in the HA Consultation Paper for reasons considered earlier on. Not surprisingly, the Executive Summary of the HA Consultation Paper emphasised that ethical constraints should be effective *as* regulatory safeguards in the event that research involving human-animal combinations is allowed. It was also made clear what would not be permitted, such as allowing human-animal combinations to develop to term or for them to be implanted into a womb. The possibility of setting out regulatory parameters to enable the measured advancement of science was used against the 'slippery slope' concern, which will be elaborated on below.[621]

In the next two sections, we consider responses from stem cell researchers in Singapore and members of a national advisory body on the use of laboratory animals. My hope at the beginning of this project was that science could perhaps provide some insights on whether or not human beings could be set apart as a particular kind of entity. Conventional ethical and legal theories are essentially anthropocentric, in that one's moral status is derived from one's biological relationship to the human species (i.e. *homo sapiens*). Some have considered anthropocentrism to unfairly discriminate against nonhuman species, and have attempted to advance more inclusive approaches to determine moral status. For instance, a capacity-based approach has been put forward, so that a creature's moral status will be determined by considering what it is capable of doing.[622] However,

---

[621] *Ibid*, at 29, paragraphs 60-63.
[622] Monika Piotrowska, Transferring Morality to Human-Nonhuman Chimeras, *American Journal of Bioethics* (2014) 14, 2: 4-12.

such a limited criterion seems to reinforce anthropocentrism on the one hand, or otherwise provide little guidance if moral status is to be determined based on the origin of the transferred cells if the capacity concerned is difficult to detect. Ultimately, the publication of the HA Report and the enactment of the Human Biomedical Research Act served to reinforce traditional speciesist divide, but the controversial that emerged did illustrate the domestication of wildly imaginative metaphors like chimeras and hybrids within the confines of bioethics.

5.4 Reactions from the Scientific Community

The SC Report specifies the categories of stem cell research that are permitted under varying degrees of regulatory purview. One such categories relates to the creation of human embryos specifically for research, which can only be justified under relatively stringent conditions, including the absence of an acceptable alternative.[623] The requirement of 'no acceptable alternative exists' is ambiguous as it would depend on who decides on what is acceptable. It could now be given a very restrictive reading by IRBs, in view of iPSC technology that has recently gained prominence. It is also ambiguous as to whether the three conditions set out for the creation of an embryo for research are applicable only to embryos created by SCNT or more generally to the creation of embryos through the combination of gametes. The creation of embryos for research by SCNT could be interpreted as being subject to a more stringent requirement than creation of embryos by other means, such as IVF.

It used to be thought that a main source of pluripotent stem cells would be embryos. And if such pluripotent stem cells were to be patient-specific, then SCNT was considered to be an important technique that would enable the derivation. As we have discussed in

---

[623] Bioethics Advisory Committee, *Ethical, Legal and Social Issues in Human Stem Cell Research, Reproductive and Therapeutic Cloning*. Singapore: Bioethics Advisory Committee, 21 June 2002, at vii (Recommendation 5).

Chapter 2, human pluripotent stem cells could be derived without using embryos.[624] In essence, adult dermal fibroblasts (skin cells) were re-programmed (induced) to function like pluripotent stem cells through the use of viral factors. This represented an important proof of principle that pluripotent stem cells can be generated from somatic cells by the combination of a small number of factors. Such cells were referred to as iPSC.

This development immediately raised a question as to whether SCNT had been rendered obsolete. It was at that time still unclear if the technology could be used to derive human iPSCs from other types of human tissue. Even if this could be done, the level of pluripotence of iPSCs may not be as effective or efficient as stem cells derived through SCNT. Despite these uncertainties, the planned public consultation on human-animal combinations was conducted as planned. It was explained in the HA Consultation Paper that allowing research to progress on all fronts would be in the public interest.[625]

Separately, a survey of stem cell researchers in Singapore was conducted to obtain more information on possible impact of iPSC technology, as well as the relevance and level of interest in research involving human-animal combinations. A questionnaire comprising six questions was sent to 68 stem cell scientists. These scientists were identified from a researchers' database maintained by A*STAR and the Stem Cell Club's List of Group Leaders. They were contacted through email and the questionnaire was attached together with some reference materials. A total of 30 responses were received (or 44%), which is considered to be a good response rate. Of these, only four of the thirty researchers who responded used human-animal

---

624 Takahashi K, *et al.*, Induction of Pluripotent Stem Cells from Adult Human Fibroblasts by Defined Factors, *Cell*, 131, 5 (2007): 1-12. See also Yu J *et al.* Induced Pluripotent Stem Cell Lines Derived from Human Somatic Cells, *Science* 318, 5858 (21 Dec 2007): 1917-1920.

625 Bioethics Advisory Committee, Singapore, *Human-Animal Combinations for Biomedical Research: A Consultation Paper*. Singapore: Bioethics Advisory Committee, 8 January 2008, at 11, paragraph 8.

combinations in their research. However, the respondents were mostly in support of the use of human-animal combinations in research. Two main points were highlighted in almost all the responses, regardless of whether they were for or against the use of human-animal combinations: the first was the need for clear and effective regulation, and the second was the importance attributed to informing and engaging the public on the subject.

Some respondents were not supportive of research involving cytoplasmic hybrids and argued that greater investment should be channelled into iPSC technology. However, there is also an understanding in scientific ventures that it is important not to close an alternative until it is known with certainty that the favoured method actually works.[626] If iPSC technology should prove to be the better method, then nuclear transfer technology would be redundant, given that it is ethically contentious and inefficient in deriving embryonic stem cells. In retrospect, this policy orientation has been vindicated as recent research suggests that iPSC cells have characteristics that are different from SCNT cells. Feedback from stem cell researchers also suggested that the requirement of 'no acceptable alternative exists' was considered to be ambiguous as it would depend on who decides on what is acceptable. In addition, it might be given a very restrictive reading by IRBs, particularly in view of iPSC technology. It is also questionable as to whether the hierarchy of sources for human embryonic stem cells[627] remains relevant (i.e. a concept that surplus embryo should be used before an embryo may be created for research). One view is that there are insufficient left-over embryos from IVF treatment for research. Most of these embryos are not donated for research, and this problem is not specific to Singapore. Thus the statement that: "As long as there are sufficient

---

[626] Fieldnotes, 16 January 2008, M2.

[627] Bioethics Advisory Committee, Singapore, *Ethical, Legal and Social Issues in Human Stem Cell Research, Reproductive and Therapeutic Cloning*, 21 June 2002, at vii, reading Recommendations 4 and 5 of the Stem Cell Report together.

and appropriately donated surplus embryos from fertility treatments available for use in research ..."[628] could be inaccurate in the light of current experience. An advisor to the BAC observed that it is not only a question of numbers.[629] Potential uses of stem cells include allowing researchers to study and understand the processes in developmental biology, to test new drugs, and to generate cells and tissues for therapy.

Apart from the issues already highlighted in the survey, feedback from researchers during the public consultation raised a concern over 'red-tape'. This concern over the burdening of research involving human-animal combinations already commonplace in the scientific world prompted the meeting with senior stem cell researchers in May 2009. In that meeting, researchers were of the view that standard types of human-animal combinations should not require extensive ethics review. As such, it would be necessary to demarcate clearly between chimeras that are routinely created, such as those created as a result of a standard scientific procedure like teratoma testing, from less conventional research like SCNT. For 'non-conventional' human-animal combinations such as cytoplasmic hybrids, the researchers agreed that more detailed ethical scrutiny may be required. For instance, a researcher may want to take progenitor cells from a patient with leukaemia and put these into a mouse. While it is highly unlikely that human DNA will enter into the germline of the mouse, this possibility could not be completely ruled out. Like stem cells, progenitor cells have the capacity to differentiate into specific cell types. Hence such research was considered to be a borderline case and might require full ethics review, although it should be noted that such a mouse will not be allowed to breed, and will be confined to a laboratory environment. The use of pluripotent cells in neurological research should also require ethical review. It was noted that the

---

[628] *Ibid*, paragraph 30, at 28.
[629] Interview with Professor Martin Bobrow, 19 January 2008.

first human trial has been started by Geron and the implications of such neurological research will have to be carefully considered.[630] The researchers further recommended that the BAC highlight issues for an IACUC to decide, as it knows of the exact extent of research that could be done on laboratory animals. A researcher noted that "the IACUC counts all mice".[631] Hence more interaction between the IACUC and IRB could avoid duplicative review. However, another researcher said that, from his experience as a member of an IACUC, all research involving human cells will have to be reviewed by an IRB.[632] As such, it will be difficult to exclude either the IACUC or the IRB from reviewing a research proposal involving human-animal combinations.

Notwithstanding iPSC technology, there is a continuing need for ethical guidance on embryo research. Despite strong research interest in iPSC technology, ethical concerns with embryonic stem cell research would not be extinguished as 'engineered' oocyte and sperm created through iPSC could be used to create an embryo, thereby giving rise to a whole range of related issues. However, the level of research interest in creating an embryo through such means was unclear. A researcher was of the view that there would be research interest in the near future (in about 2 to 5 years' time) in creating embryos through iPSC technology given the increasing popularity of stem cell therapy.[633] It was further observed that iPSCs could be imported into Singapore for the purpose of deriving stem cell lines from embryos thereby created as this did not fall within any regulatory control.

The BAC's plurality of approaches was also supported as researchers generally recognised that SCNT remains a useful technology. Reprogramming research should be allowed so long as

---

630 Geron, Geron Initiates Clinical Trial of Human Embryonic Stem Cell-Based Therapy, Press Release, 11 October 2010.
631 Fieldnotes, 26 May 2009, HH.
632 Fieldnotes, 26 May 2009, PR.
633 Fieldnotes, 26 May 2009, MK.

the technology is not applied for reproduction, but the shortage of human oocytes will continue to be a major problem. In relation to the regulatory environment, the researchers did not consider the current regulations to be prohibitive of research involving human-animal combinations, although they were concerned that some aspects of the research may become over-regulated. The proposal to establish a central or national ethics review body for stem cell research was supported by the researchers. The efficacy of ethics review was felt to vary with different reviewing officers since their familiarity with the subject matter and the standards entailed differ. In addition, different IRBs have different 'house rules' and many IRBs are constituted of medically trained professionals who might not fully appreciate the research requirements of scientists.

My sense from the meeting (and also from subsequent individual interviews) has been that the researchers took a very practical and personal view of the issues as they did not want to speak on behalf of their community (which could be broadly associated with the Stem Cell Society). Hence they did not venture any opinion on what their peers were or were not interested to do. Although the BAC's decision to ask the researchers where the boundaries should be drawn is a sensible one, these were not the types of questions that researchers wanted to answer. The term 'human-animal combination' was somewhat confusing to them because they did not regard a chimeric mouse created as a means of testing pluripotency to fall within the definition – as conceived by them. Such a biological construct was to them a 'standard practice' in the field and should not be burdened with strict ethical scrutiny. From experience with such research, they appeared uniformly concerned about over-regulation. To some degree, this concern was justified. All stem cell research would have to undergo IRB review under the guidelines issued by the BAC. With the benefit of experience, ethical review of certain types of embryonic stem cell research may be relaxed. There was some confusion over terminology when a researcher said he objected to research involving 'human-animal combinations'. In the context of the discussion, he was likely to be referring to cytoplasmic hybrid, rather than a chimeric mouse for testing pluripotency - which he himself had a hand in creating. Once the matter of chimeric mouse as 'standard practice' was carved out of the rubric of 'human-animal combinations', the researchers did not disagreed with the proposed introduction of regulatory control, be it in terms of a proposed centralised regulatory mechanism, or in targeting specific areas for regulatory attention, such as research with neurological (hence sentience) and repro-ductive or germline implications. Their comments on the continuing relevance of ethical guidance and review for embryo research, notwithstanding the advent of iPSC technology, have been especially helpful in affirming the proposed approach.

5.5 Between Humans and Animals

Cytoplasmic hybrid embryos constitute a relatively small and perhaps even niche area of research involving human-animal combinations. As discussed above, transgenic animals and chimeric animals or chimeras created through the introduction of human cells such as stem cells, into animals at various stages of development or the grafting of human neural cells into primate brains, constitute the largest group of human-animal combinations. Until the HBRA comes into force in Singapore, the only regulation relating to such research was primarily concerned with animal welfare. Given this focus, a query arose as to whether there was a need for some sort of interface between the regulation of human subject research and the regulation of animal research. Like the BAC, NACLAR was established in 2003 to develop national guidelines for the care and use of animals for scientific research. The Agri-Food & Veterinary Authority of Singapore (AVA), which NACLAR advises, is the implementer of the guidelines. On October 2004, it issued a set of guidelines that addresses all aspects of the care and use of animals for scientific purposes.[634] The principles of replacement, reduction and refinement have been stated as encapsulating the guidelines. In 'replacement', researchers are encouraged to consider alternatives to animal models, and thereby 'reduce' the number of animals used. Where animals are used, projects and techniques should be 'refined' to minimise impact on animals. The NACLAR guidelines require all research facilities that house and use animals for scientific purposes to establish an IACUC, which is responsible for the oversight and evaluation of animal care and use programmes of the institution. In order to qualify for licensing from the AVA, it is a requirement for these research facilities to comply with the guidelines.

I met with members of NACLAR in a meeting organised by the BAC, and also in individual interviews to discuss the HA Consultation Paper and public feedback relating to animal welfare and care. An issue that was discussed related to the nature of a cytoplasmic hybrid embryo, and whether it should be regarded as predominantly human for regulatory purposes. Under the (then proposed) UK amending legislation on the subject,[635] a human 'admixed embryo' will fall within the regulatory purview of the HFEA regardless of the extent of admixture if the proposed legislation is to be a classificatory guide. In Singapore, human-animal combinations were considered to fall outside the guidelines unless they have an impact on animal welfare. If a cytoplasmic hybrid 'embryo' is considered 'human' for regulatory purposes, then it would fall outside of the NACLAR guidelines. In addition, the NACLAR guidelines apply only to subjects that are legally defined as 'animals' and do not apply to 'embryos'. NACLAR members further indicated that the guidelines would not ordinarily apply when animal material is used unless an animal is involved. If human material is introduced into an animal, the NACLAR guidelines would apply as animal welfare is an issue. If human material is introduced

---

634 National Advisory Committee on Laboratory Animal Research, *Guidelines on the Care and Use of Animal for Scientific Purposes in Singapore*. Singapore: National Advisory Committee on Laboratory Animal Research, 2004.

635 UK Human Fertilisation and Embryology Bill, HL Bill 6, 2007-2008.

into an animal embryo or foetus, and then allowed to develop into a live animal, the NACLAR guidelines would also apply. It follows that the welfare of an animal, as donor of embryos, is similarly covered by the NACLAR guidelines. However, as a cytoplasmic hybrid embryo will not be implanted, animal welfare is unlikely to be a concern.

In the absence of sound scientific rationale for mixing human and non-human gametes, it was queried if the creation of true hybrids through means such as this should be prohibited by law. If such a research avenue should not to be proscribed, it was then queried if there should be any requirements for ethics review that will be different from the existing requirements for ethics review, in respect of experiments using or creating humanised animals (i.e. chimeras or transgenic animals). The concern among some researchers in Singapore that this arrangement might lead to greater bureaucratisation of the ethics review process was again raised.

Members of NACLAR agreed that the creation of true hybrids by mixing human and non-human gametes for reproductive purposes should be prohibited by law. But NACLAR also agreed that while the creation of an animal that is partly humanised with a view to obtaining new knowledge about therapeutic possibilities should not be pro-hibited, approvals from both an IRB and an IACUC must be sought.[636] Humanised animals such as SCID-Hu mice are commonly created, and the NACLAR guidelines sought to secure the welfare of the animal through measures such as requiring tests to ensure that the animal did not become infected with human pathogens. Insofar as the creation and use of humanised animals were already addressed by the NACLAR guidelines, a new set of guidelines was considered to be unnecessary. As such, concern over greater bureaucratisation of the ethics review process was not considered to be well grounded. NACLAR members further indicated that it

---

[636] Danish Council of Ethics (with the Danish Ethical Council for Animals). *Man or Mouse: Ethical aspects of chimera research*. Copenhagen: Danish Council of Ethics, 2007, at 39.

has adopted the de-centralised approach of Australia, Canada, New Zealand and the US, preferring self-regulation by institutions handling laboratory animals to the UK practice of licensing at different levels. Even if a centralised ethics review system should be put in place, it was felt that the existing framework for animal ethics review through the IACUC should be retained, as animal ethics will continue to be the responsibility of the institutions concerned.[637]

Whether a distinction should be drawn among different types of animal recipients (such as mouse as opposed to primates) was also considered. A related issue was whether the introduction of a substantial amount of human material into an animal should be of regulatory concern. The general sense was that different types of animal recipients should be distinguished, largely on the basis of evolutionary biology. In addition, the introduction of a substantial amount of human material (such as human neurons) into an animal could be of regulatory concern. The extent to which a chimeric embryo is allowed to grow is still unclear, and such an embryo is usually terminated before birth. It was observed that the number of experiments involving the introduction of human embryonic stem cells into animals to test for pluripotency and to determine experimental conditions required for cell differentiation is likely to increase. For this reason, scientists will require clear guidelines on permissible research, such as the extent to which human neurons may be introduced into an animal.

There was ambiguity over what should be done if an animal with human sentience should emerge. Some members of NACLAR felt the threshold for the care of this animal may have to be increased. Even then, the baseline of care for the animal would still apply. If it is to be euthanised, this should be carried out in accordance with internationally accepted standards. As to how 'sentient' a chimeric animal is allowed to be, this would be an issue for the IRB, rather than an IACUC, to decide. However, there should not be a need to develop

---

[637] Fieldnotes, 15 April 2008, BO.

a formalised set of procedures directed at a chimeric animal with human sentience as this outcome should be avoided at the point of initial review. In the event that a sentient creature emerges without any known cause, then there should be a mechanism to address this particular contingency. In other words, this 'adverse outcome' should be handled on a case-by-case basis, rather than by general regulation. It may be considered unethical for such an animal to be euthanised like any other laboratory animal. Interestingly, it was observed by some that even in such a case, it is still an animal and that there are countries that allow human beings to be euthanised.[638] But a NACLAR member observed that the legal situation is far from clear, as an animal with human sentience would fall within a legal lacuna. It would arguably not be an 'animal' contemplated under the *Animals and Birds Act*,[639] and would thereby be outside of the regulatory purview of the AVA. It would be for the BAC ('or some higher level') to decide whether such a contingency should be anticipated in regulation, or it should be managed if and when this materialises.[640] It was felt that the latter option is preferable since Singapore has a more tightly regulated environment than a country like the US, where regulations would cover only certain animals unless the research is federally funded. With better control in Singapore, it was observed that regulatory oversight should not be overly prescriptive. For instance, it would be difficult to distinguish 'humans' from 'animals' by way of guidelines without being unduly prescriptive. Self-regulation was regarded as the best way to avoid stifling research. For the time being, death as an endpoint is strongly discouraged under the NACLAR guidelines, which states: "Death as an end-point must be avoided if at all possible. If death as end-point must be used, the Investigator must ensure that the animal's distress or pain is minimised and use

---

[638] *Ibid.*
[639] *Animals and Birds Act* (Cap. 7), 2002 Revised Edition.
[640] Fieldnotes, 15 April 2008, EC.

appropriate sedation, analgesia, or anaesthesia to relieve the animal's distress or pain."[641] Hence, while the creation of human-animal combinations is not opposed, researchers are strongly encouraged to seek alternatives to painful procedures, and to develop endpoints and criteria for premature termination as in Europe and America.

The necessity of including transgenic animals in the prospective HA Report was also raised. It was noted that transgenic animals have not been considered in the HA Consultation Paper although they have been identified by the AMS and the DCE for future consideration.[642] A transgenic primate might, for instance, raise more ethical concerns than a chimeric primate. For this reason, the oversight mechanism for transgenic animals would likely be different from a mechanism for chimeric animals, and a separate regime should be developed.

Feedback received on this issue has highlighted the need to ensure that chimeric animals:

(a) Do not breed,

(b) Are confined within a laboratory environment (and so do not enter the food chain), and

(c) Suitably comprehensive tests for pathogens should be carried out on cell lines and tissue used in human-animal combinations, as established cell line producers such as ATCC[643] may not run sufficiently complete tests for pathogens.

In essence, there was an indication that additional laboratory requirements might have to be introduced. However, the existing

---

[641] National Advisory Committee on Laboratory Animal Research, *Guidelines on the Care and Use of Animal for Scientific Purposes in Singapore*. Singapore: National Advisory Committee on Laboratory Animal Research, 2004, para 2.2.4 (h).

[642] The Academy of Medical Sciences, UK, *Inter-species embryos: A report by the Academy of Medical Sciences.* London: Academy of Medical Sciences, June 2007, at 40, and Danish Council of Ethics and the Danish Ethical Council for Animals, *Man or Mouse? Ethical aspects of chimera research.* Copenhagen: Danish Council of Ethics, 2007, at 10.

[643] ATCC (or American Type Cell Culture) cell lines are commercial cell lines generally recognised to have satisfied ethical requirements in their derivation.

guidelines should adequately address animal ethics concerns, including the contingency of a research animal (chimeric or not) escaping from a laboratory environment. The security of the research facility is one component of the site inspection carried out by the AVA. In addition, laboratories have protocols to deal with such a contingency. It was emphasised that at various points that the regulatory environment in Singapore should not be unduly restrictive. Human-animal chimeras that are already commonly created and used should not be burdened by additional regulatory control.

Human-animal combinations bring to mind Jacque Derrida's critique of the institution of speciesism in his neologism of *l'animot*. He argues that:

> [A]mong non-humans and separate from non-humans there is an immense multiplicity of other living things that cannot in any way be homogenised, except by means of violence and wilful ignorance, within the category of what is called the animal or animality in general ... The confusion of all non-human living creatures within the general and common category of the animal is not simply a sin against rigorous thinking, vigilance, lucidity, or empirical authority; it is also a crime.[644]

Certain 'constructs' of interspecies combination such as a human being with a pig's heart valve have been controversial, but they did not otherwise pose a serious threat to the moral and social boundaries that distinguish 'humans' from 'animals'. However, human embryonic stem cell technology has enabled a level of cellular integration between human and non-human animals that was not previously thought possible. For instance, human embryonic stem cells may be introduced into an animal embryo in order to study the development of particular diseases or in the creation of disease models. Once introduced, the dispersion of human cells within the animal embryo

---

[644] Jacques Derrida (trans. David Wills). The Animal That Therefore I Am (More to Follow), *Critical Inquiry* (2002) 28: 369-418, at 416.

will be difficult, if not impossible, to control. More critical is that the level of integration between human and non-human embryonic cells is expected to be profound, giving rise to a real concern that a creature with human features could be created if the embryo is drawn from an animal that is close to humans in evolutionary terms (such as primates). In other words, interspecies combinations generate a deconstructive force so strong that 'humans' again come face to face with its 'Other' in 'animals'. This is the great paradox that we witnessed in Darwinian deconstructionism in *On the Origin of Species* that contributed to a fundamental shift within the law from naturalism to positivism. As legal historian Michael Stolleis points out, the natural law (and naturalism in law) has itself arisen from a shift away from the 'Law of God' in the religious crisis of sixteenth and seventeenth century Europe.[645] With the ascent of natural science, and "the notion of the 'state as machine' functioning according to the rules of the natural sciences[,] ... jurists so optimistically sought their metaphors and analogies" in that field.[646]

As we have seen, STS scholars provide convincing arguments that in getting behind scientific objectification, we find a natural-cultural mix that in turn points to far more fluid ways in which relationships among sentient beings and non-sentient objects could be organised. Legal objectification through laws that both secure animal welfare and enable the utilisation of animals to meet certain human needs share some commonalities with scientific objectification. The challenge posed by human-animal combinations to the often assumed clarity of the distinction between humans and non-human animals represents the natural-cultural mix that objectification conceals. When the categorical breach first surfaced in science, the question of 'humanness' was transposed to ethics. Science has in that sense

---

[645] Michael Stolleis, The Legitimation of Law through God, Tradition, Will, Nature and Constitution. In Larraine Daston and Michael Stolleis (eds.), *Natural Law and Laws of Nature in Early Modern Europe: Jurisprudence, Theology, Moral and Natural Philosophy*. Cornwall: Ashgate Publishing, 2008.

[646] *Ibid*, at 52-53.

insulated itself from the paradox by labelling this an 'ethical' rather than 'scientific' issue. It is not because scientists are 'disinterested', but science is itself incapable of providing a response from within its own knowledge field. Within ethics (as we shall see), a rationalising process through categorisation and systematisation has been initiated to shield 'humanity' from its 'Other' by reinvigorating a compromised 'naturalism'. Arguably, there has been some level of success in demarcating the 'sacred' from the 'profane'. In the process, ethics – like religion – has to transcend both the 'Self' and its 'Other' in the form of a Third. There are two problems here. First, the transcendence to a standpoint of the Third is also to transcend reason. Hence in so doing, ethics itself encounters its paradox. But while it may share some likeness of being with religion, ethics is not religion. This presents the second difficulty in that ethics is confronted by its own impotence. At the most practical level, ethics has limited recourse to the exercise of legitimate power. Ethics needs science in overcoming the first difficulty. The ethical category of 'humanness' is projected back onto scientific material so that the 'rationality' is regained. Ethics also needs law, and the unifying basis for both has been in the 'common good'. Some perceive this union as consequentialist or utilitarian, based largely on a balance of perceived cost and benefit. But it is from this practical association that ethics switches back-and-forth with law, thereby allowing both to escape from the shocking encounter with its paradox.[647] As a stem cell researcher observed, the IACUC he worked with "... treated mice like they are humans",[648] and another said that his (institution's) IACUC "counted all mice".[649] Singling out experimental animals for exceptional protection serves to instaurate the hierarchical structure that

---

[647] In a different context, Annelise Riles has evaluated a similar shifting in and out of the law as movements between normative and reflexive knowledge. See: Annelise Riles, Representing In-Between: Law, Anthropology and the Rhetoric of Interdisciplinarity. *University of Illinois Law Review* (1994): 597-653, at 643-644.
[648] Interview with Professor Davor Solter, 22 February 2010.
[649] Fieldnotes, 26 May 2009, HH.

places human beings above other nonhuman species. If a similar response is considered to be necessary for human-animal combinations, then the concerns that the researchers and NACLAR members share over the prospect of excessive bureaucracy might not have been entirely unfounded.

Whether the BAC or NACLAR, policy bodies in Singapore and elsewhere appeared to have perpetuated the common perception of essentially two populations: of 'humans' and its 'Other'. This is similarly the case in substituting older metaphors *of* chimeras and hybrids with new metaphoric models *for* these biological constructs. The 'crime' that Derrida speaks of is perhaps mitigated by the fact that less violence is inflicted in the erasure of the difference among species, and individuals of a species, within institutions that relate to 'humans' and 'animals' in biomedicine. Still, it is necessary to sustain a distinction between humans and non-human animals in order for current practices in science, ethics and law to make sense. In the law, sustaining the distinction between *persona* and *res* is a critical premise by which a certain moral and social order is maintained. But as we have seen, the Great Apes continue to haunt us; persisting within the great chasm that distinguishes 'humans' from its 'Other'. Whereas some countries are prepared to allow some differentiation within the large category of 'animals' by distinguishing primates in particular, other countries like Singapore are not prepared to do so.

5.6 Categorisation and Classification

Drawing up categories has been a useful approach to understanding chimeras and hybrids, and for me, in presenting them as legal 'objects'. Reflecting on the brief conversation that I had along a corridor at the NUS Bukit Timah campus a little while back, legal categorisation arises principally through legislation and adjudication. Clear rules set out the investitive conditions, which in turn create categories that define legal subjects and objects. Eric Mitnick explains:[650]

> For the common law system of reference to precedents is based
> upon the principle of formal justice that like cases must be treated
> alike. Courts will thus determine any new claim of legislative right
> both with reference to explicit legislative criteria and by reasoning
> analogically from prior cases. The result, once again, will be a
> class of persons related by law one to another by virtue of some
> common characteristic(s). Indeed, even in the absence of legisla-
> tion, adjudicative generality works to similar effect, though the
> investitive conditions tend necessarily to develop in the opposite
> direction ... a right fashioned exclusively in adjudication begins with
> a particular claimant pressing a particular claim and then only
> gradually broadens into a rule of law.

As we have seen, the manner in which the BAC went about the
analysis was to set out in taxonomies the types of chimeras and
hybrids that occur naturally, those that have been created by
scientists, and those that could be created. For instance, a pregnant
woman is by definition a human-human 'chimera'. Being 'natural',
this benign 'chimera' does not provoke any feeling of disgust in
contemporary society. Hence 'natural' as opposed to 'unnatural' was
a premise on which categorisation was based, which also related to
current and potential uses. Henry Greely's approach is similar in that
he attempts to assess how taxonomy of chimeras might illuminate
ethical issues that categorisation creates.[651] He relied on four dimensions based on biological constituents, relationship between the
organisms, how mixing is done and when it took place, and arrived at
the conclusion that the ethical issues depend on the 'humanity',
'naturalness' and proposed uses of the chimeric organism.

---

[650] Eric J Mitnick. *Rights, Groups and Self-Invention: Group-differentiated Rights in
Liberal Theory.* Cornwall: Ashgate Publishing, 2006, at 58.
[651] Henry T. Greely, Defining Chimeras...and Chimeric Concerns. *American Journal of
Bioethics* (2003) 3, 3: 17-20.

For the purposes of public consultation, a neutral definition of 'chimeras' and 'hybrids' in the Chinese language was thought to be necessary since the subject matter was already being discussed in that language forum. The expression '嵌合体' is commonly used in scientific and ethical discussions in both China and Taiwan, and is also the expression used in the newspaper commentary. In addition, this expression has been applied in a number of English-Chinese dictionaries. In Japanese, Kanji (old script Chinese) characters have not been used to depict 'chimera' although they are used for the more generic reference to 'cell' (细胞). Instead, the term 'chimera' is set out in katakana as 'キメラ', which suggests the importation of a foreign terminology (and its corresponding meaning) into the Japanese lexicon. For instance, this term has been used by Japan's Ministry of Education, Culture, Sports, Science and Technology (文部科学省).[652]

Chimeras and hybrids are metaphors that enable the transmission of these concepts from myths and imagination to present day reality. Even though a chimeric mouse, let alone a cytoplasmic hybrid embryo, does not look anything like Homer's Medusa or the characters in the Chinese classic *Journey to the West* (西游记), the ontologically creative function of metaphors enable a cognitive equivalence to be drawn between the two metaphoric objects.[653] Hence in the public

---

[652] See for instance, 文部科学省. 生命倫理及び安全対策に係る留意事項 [Ministry of Education, Culture, Sports, Science and Technology, Japan. Notice on Bioethics and Safety Considerations]. See also 文部科学省. 人クローン胚の研究目的の作成・利用のあり方に関する検討経緯等について [Ministry of Education, Culture, Sports, Science and Technology, Japan. Background discussion on the purposes and uses of human cloned embryos]. The reference to chimeric embryo in Japanese (キメラ) appears to be a more generic reference to human-animal combinations (嵌合胚胎) in Chinese.

[653] Relying on the seminal work of Max Black, Terrell Carver and Jernej Pikalo indicate that metaphors are creative-productive function that shape thinking on discourses and contexts. They also act as discursive nodal points. See Terrell Carver and Jernej Pikalo. Editors' introduction. In *Political Language and Metaphor: Interpreting and changing the world*, Terrell Carver and Jernej Pikalo (eds.). London and New York: Routledge, 2008, pp 1-12, at 3-4. See also: Max Black. *Models and Metaphors: Studies in Language and Philosophy*. Ithaca and London: Cornell University Press, 1962.

imagination, the creation of chimeras or hybrids by scientists is no different from the creation of monsters (for instance, see Illustration 5.1 on images of chimeric creatures presented in a press report on the BAC's HA Consultation Paper). In fact, graphical illustrations were made by a member of the Secretariat during a discussion on how best to introduce a 'chimera' and 'cytoplasmic hybrid' (by considering how they could be created) to the public:

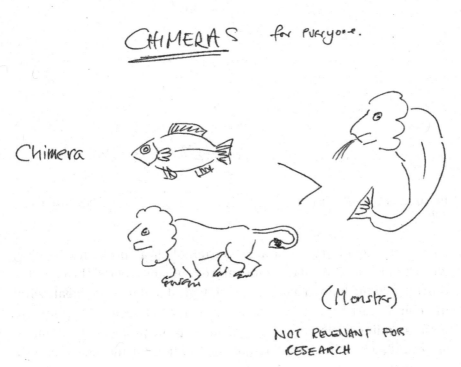

Illustration 5.1.   Sketch of a Chimera. (Used with kind permission of Professor John Elliott.)

Concerns over the pervasive metaphorical contents of chimeras and hybrids, a research group sponsored by the European Union considered the invention of a new term for these biological

CYTOPLASMIC HYBRID

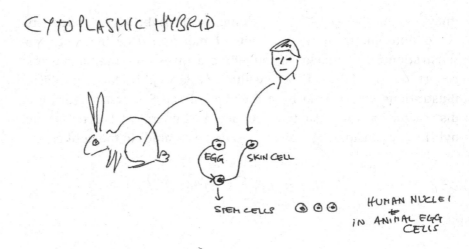

Illustration 5.2. Sketch of a Hybrid. (Used with kind permission of Professor John Elliott.)

constructs necessary to address terminological problems. [654] The word 'Chimbrid' is used to denote any organisms created through the mixing of living human and animal biological material and dealt with in their report. [655] It is hence a term distinct from the common understanding of chimeras and hybrids that the project team regards as grounded in culture and mythology, and thereby inconsistent with science.[656]

---

[654] Jochen Taupitz and Marion Weschka (eds.), CHIMBRIDS – Chimeras and Hybrids in Comparative European and International Research. Heidelberg: Springer, 2009, at 5.

[655] The Chimbrids team did observe that the scientific community was not unified on the distinctions between human and non-human chimeras: *Ibid*, at 16.

[656] *Ibid*, at 13.

Veronique Mottier's observation that metaphors inform and structure thinking as 'mini-narratives' acting against a backdrop of tacit knowledge is pertinent.[657] These 'mini-narratives' have the capacity to form identities through discursive mechanisms of boundary drawing, boundary maintenance, ordering and othering. A number of well-known Chinese didactical folklores with imaginary entities (that include foxes and ghosts) have these multi-fold, and evidently moralising, functions.[658] In our present situation, the familiar mythical metaphors constitute the identities of the biological constructs. They posed the most direct and immediate challenge as models of some prior and typically unarticulated understanding of the phenomena – perhaps related in some way to the 'yuk' feeling that some have raised in opposition to the creation of human-animal combinations in research. Dvora Yanow defines 'models *of* prior conceptualisation' as metaphors, or forms of 'seeing-as'. These metaphors "embody and reflect context-specific prior understanding of their subject matter, drawing – usually implicitly, through tacit knowledge – on metaphoric meaning in its source origins."[659] More insightful is her recognition that metaphors are also 'models *for*', in that "they embody seeds for subsequent, future action that follows from the underlying logic of the prior understanding on which they draw".[660] In order to counter the existing metaphors or models *of*

---

657 Veronique Mottier. Metaphors, mini-narratives and Foucauldian discourse theory. In Terrell Carver and Jernej Pikalo (eds.), *Political Language and Metaphor: Interpreting and changing the world*. London and New York: Routledge, 2008, pp 182-194, at 191-192.

658 Leo Tak-hung Chan. *The Discourse on Foxes and Ghosts: Ji Yun and Eighteenth-Century Literati Storytelling*. Hong Kong: Chinese University Press, 1998. See for instance, at 246-247.

659 Dvora Yanow. Cognition meets action: Metaphors as models of and models for. In Terrell Carver and Jernej Pikalo (eds.), *Political Language and Metaphor: Interpreting and changing the world*. London and New York: Routledge, 2008, pp 225-238, at 227 (emphasis in original).

660 *Ibid.*

chimeras and hybrids, it would be necessary to discredit them. Once discredited, these ideas would then have to be disembedded from the familiar mythical context and re-constituted within a new context that will enable the new to be understood in terms of the old. It may be inferred from the tabular display (Table 5.2) of human-animal combinations that the new context is grounded in the rationalities of ethics and science combined, and applied toward the maximisation of the common good (in that, the end goal is some therapeutic benefit). In contrast, the old context is projected as speculative, irrational and superstitious.

During the public consultation, the attempt to displace more commonplace notions of chimeras and hybrids was on the whole successful. It subsequently emerged during the public consultation that neither the English language nor Chinese language newspapers deployed the more common terminology 'chimera', but instead preferred a terminology that captured the essence of the biological construct. The English language papers used the term 'human-animal combinations' that was proposed by the BAC and attempted to present the discussion in relatively objective light. This was similarly the case for the mainstream Chinese language newspaper (联合早报) in Singapore.[661] Another two Chinese language newspaper attempted to sensationalise the subject with controversial cartoon pictures of creatures such as a pig with a human head, but the content of these articles was a reasonable presentation of the issues.[662] News reports from China, Taiwan and Hong Kong, as well as the news coverage by

---

661 谢燕燕, 生物道德资询委员会征询公众: 你是否接受人兽嵌合体, 联合早报 [Xie YY, Bioethics Advisory Committee Consults the Public: Can you accept human-animal combinations, Combined Morning Paper], 9 January 2008.

662 许翔宇, 人兽混合体? 生物道德资询委员会征询公众意见, 联合晚报 [Xu XY, Human-Animal Combinations? Bioethics Advisory Committee Seeks Public Opinion, Combined Night Paper], 8 January 2008. See also 郭秀芳与李腾宝, 人兽怪研究, 引发各种问题: 带人细胞的肉, 你敢吃吗?, 新民晚报 [Guo XF and Li TB, Human-Animal Strange Research, Raises All Kinds of Issues: Meat with Human Cells, do you dare eat?, New People's Night Paper], 8 January 2008.

the main Chinese language newspaper in Singapore referred to human-animal combinations as '人兽混合体'. There is some ambiguity in relation to the term '嵌合体', which has been defined to mean chimeras, but has also been used to refer to human-animal combinations in general. In relation to the HA Consultation Paper, the Chinese press used the term '嵌合体' to refer to human-animal combinations generally. The two main categories of human-animal combinations considered by the BAC have been translated by the Chinese press as '杂合体' for hybrids and '客迈拉' for chimeras. Cytoplasmic hybrid (or cybrid) embryo, which is a sub-category of hybrids, was defined as '胞质杂配胚胎'. This is consistent with the terminology used in China, notably by the Chinese Medical Doctor Association.[663] It follows that cytoplasmic hybrids are defined as '胞质杂合体'. In some reports, a more generic term '人兽混合胚胎' is used to describe cytoplasmic hybrids as human-animal interspecies embryos. Hence a function of the HA Consultation Paper was to displace the 'old' and conventional metaphoric notions of chimeras and hybrids with ethically and scientifically 'appropriate' ones.

The approach adopted by the BAC may also be described as an analytical (or displacement) technique that sets out in taxonomies the types of chimeras and hybrids that occur naturally, those that have been created by scientists, and those that could be created.[664] Being somewhat 'natural', a recipient of blood transfusion and a mule would technically be a 'chimera' and 'hybrid' respectively, without provoking any feeling of disgust in contemporary society. Categorisation based on 'natural' as opposed to 'unnatural' and further related to current and potential uses reflect (as we have discussed) Henry Greely's

---

[663] 中国医师协会, 人兽混合胚胎问世 [Chinese Medical Doctor Association, Birth of Human-Animal Hybrid Embryo], 3 April 2008. See also: 你能否接受人兽嵌合体? [Can you accept human-animal combinations?], 1 September 2008.

[664] Bioethics Advisory Committee, Singapore, *Human-Animal Combinations for Biomedical Research: A Consultation Paper*. Singapore: Bioethics Advisory Committee, 8 January 2008, at 6. The BAC distinguished between fictitious chimeras (e.g. centaur) from biological ones (e.g. pregnant woman).

approach, as well as his observation that the ethical issues depend on the 'humanity', 'naturalness' and proposed uses of the chimeric organism.

5.7 Reaction of the Singaporean Public

Public consultation in Singapore on the subject of human-animal combinations concluded on 10 March 2008. Similar to previous public consultations of the BAC, written submissions were received from scientists, lay members of the public, and from institutions. In addition, 58 entries were made on the REACH Discussion Forum[665] from at least 43 individuals.[666] Most comments on REACH are made anonymously (or pseudonymously).

Written submissions received from a majority of the respondents indicated some level of support for some or all forms of human-animal combinations. The main reasons or requirements (as the case may be) given for supporting or in order to allow research involving the creation and use of human-animal combinations are:

(1) No mixing of human and animal genetic materials;

(2) There are legal and/or ethical regulatory systems in place;

(3) Broader consultative process required;

(4) Alternative technology (such as induced pluripotent stem cell technology) should be explored;

(5) Clear informed consent and other procedures required;

(6) Research should be clearly beneficial; and

(7) Avoid over-regulation.

---

665 REACH (Reaching Everyone for Active Citizenry @ Home) is set by the Feedback Unit in 2006 to engage and reach out to as many Singaporean and permanent residents as possible to develop and promote an active citizenry through citizen participation and involvement.

666 Repeated entries on REACH Discussion Forum were excluded as far as practicable to avoid double-counting.

The main reasons for opposing the research by a minority of respondents are:

(1) Moral Outrage or Repugnance;

(2) Misunderstanding of what is intended;

(3) Concerns about objectivity or effectiveness of regulation;

(4) Challenging the effectiveness or value of the research, or highlighting its risk;

(5) Arguments based on human dignity and against instrumental use of human beings;

(6) Concern with maintaining the distinction between humans and animals;

(7) Objections based on the moral status of the embryo;

(8) 'Playing God', hubris and allowing scientific pragmatism to replace ethics;

(9) Violation of the laws of Nature; and

(10) 'Slippery slope' concerns.

Some respondents have segregated the different types of human-animal combination whereas four other respondents have treated such combinations as effectively cytoplasmic hybrids or combinations created at the cellular level and are thereby subject to the 14 day rule. Others have addressed human-animal combinations categorically. It has also been indicated that there may be a need to relate ethical and legal discussions to particular types of human-animal combination. In addition, several respondents have called for broader representation (especially non-governmental bodies and bodies that regulate the use of animals) in the governance of the creation and use of human-animal combinations.

Consistent with the feedback from stem cell researchers, not all scientists are supportive of the creation and use of cytoplasmic hybrids due to concern over feasibility and lack of justification.

Induced pluripotent stem cell technology has been welcomed by a number of respondents as a viable alternative although most respondents agree with the BAC's proposal for a multi-fronted approach.

Other members of the public are likely to be opposed to human-animal combinations if they are of the view that such combinations will not be confined to a laboratory environment or if they have religious concerns. Almost all religious bodies that have provided written responses are either opposed to or have indicated very limited support for human-animal combinations. Interestingly, the Islamic Religious Council of Singapore, an Islamic Religious organisation and a professional body with some religious affiliation to Islam have indicated support for the research provided that effective regulatory safeguards are in place. However, there is some concern over the possibility of over-regulation and the lack of explicit stem cell legislation.

Of the 43 individuals who provided feedback on the REACH Discussion Forum, a majority (18) have expressed some support for research using human-animal combinations. However, a large number of individuals (12) did not express any view, whereas the number of individuals who are neutral or did not express a clear view on the issue (seven respondents) is close to the number of individuals opposed to the research (six respondents). In addition, six comments were received via REACH on the Consultation Paper. Of these, five expressed opposition to the research.

On the whole, there was no clear indication of support or opposition for the research. A similar outcome was observed of the British public's reaction to research involving cytoplasmic hybrids. Nevertheless, the outcome of the public consultation was important to the BAC for a number of reasons. First, the absence of strong public reaction was an indication of public receptivity to the research. This may perhaps be attributed to the absence of a dominant group or discourse in the consultation. Second, there was no serious omission in the ethical identification of issues or interests. Strongest reaction for and against the research were for reasons that were within expectation. A level of agreement over ethical rules that can be applied is important for the purposes of legal objectification, as we shall consider. Third, emphasis on sound and effective regulation enabled a practical and measured response to a number of uncertainties and concerns.

5.8 Contributory Developments in the UK

The emphasis on regulation by the lay public and experts alike may at first seem surprising, but perhaps less so when viewed in context. There was considerably sensationalised reporting in the media on regulatory development in the UK on cytoplasmic hybrid embryos from the time before and extending right through the public consultation of the BAC. As a matter of public policy, developments in the UK have been highly influential in Singapore. Hence the UK's experience with this particular type of human-animal combination was instructive as to how such research could be understood as a policy concern. In the UK, human-animal combinations in research became a public issue when an expert advisory group recommended that the creation of cytoplasmic hybrid embryos should be prohibited.[667] However, the House of Lords Select Committee on stem cell research did not agree, and suggested that, on the contrary, research using a cytoplasmic hybrid embryo might be more acceptable to people given that human eggs would not be required.[668] The House of Commons Science and Technology Select Committee agreed, and proposed new legislation in 2005 to define the nature of

---

667 Department of Health, UK, *Stem Cell Research: Medical Progress with Responsibility*. London: Department of Health, June 2000. See Recommendation 6, at 47.
668 House of Lords Select Committee, UK, *Stem Cell Research*, 2002. See paragraph 8.18.

inter-species embryos and to make their creation legal for research purposes, subject to the 14 day rule.[669] In August that year, the Science Media Centre organised a background briefing on chimeras. At this briefing, the possibility of using cytoplasmic hybrid embryos in research was discussed, and concerns over regulatory loopholes were also raised. This was identified as the first step in what became a concerted attempt to keep public and politicians, via the media, fully informed.[670]

By December 2006, however, a government white paper proposed prohibiting the creation of hybrid and chimeric embryos.[671] This development followed from applications by researchers from King's College, London, and Newcastle University for permission to create cytoplasmic hybrid embryos for research. The possible imposition of legal limitation to embryonic stem cell research prompted the HFEA to conduct a full consultation to gauge public opinion,[672] and the pooling together of the efforts of the AMS, the Wellcome Trust, the Royal Society, the Medical Research Council, the Association of Medical Research Charities and many individual patient charities to amplify the message of possible benefits that could be gained by allowing the research. A consultation paper entitled 'Hybrids and Chimeras' was issued by the HFEA to solicit feedback over a period of

---

[669] House of Commons Science and Technology Select Committee, *Reproductive Technologies and the Law*, 2005, paragraph 66.

[670] Geoff Watts (ed.). *Hype Hope and hybrids: Science, policy and media perspectives of the Human Fertilisation and Embryology Bill*, London: The Academy of Medical Sciences, Medical Research Council, Science Media Centre and Wellcome Trust, 2009, at 11.

[671] Department of Health, UK, Review of the Human Fertilisation and Embryology Act: Proposals for revised legislation (including establishment of the Regulatory Authority for Tissue and Embryos). London: Department of Health, December 2006.

[672] Human Fertilisation and Embryology Authority, UK, *Hybrids and Chimeras: A report on the findings of the consultation*. London: Human Fertilisation and Embryology Authority, October 2007.

three months, from 26 April to 20 July 2007.[673] Those who responded to the poll or to public consultation had strong views one way or the other. The full consultation conducted by the HFEA revealed that while up to 67% of the respondents initially opposed creating hybrids in general, the opposition fell to 30% and support rose to 50% when it was explained that the research could help scientists understand diseases such as Parkinson's and Alzheimer's disease.[674] From the various polls and public consultations conducted, it was observed that on the whole, there was not a clear majority of the British public either opposed to or supporting the research.[675] However, the polls did suggest majority public support for the creation of hybrid embryos when the likelihood of treatments for named diseases was indicated. Where there were no claims of important potential medical advance (such as in the creation of 'true' hybrids), a majority was opposed.

It was during this time that the AMS published its 2007 report on the subject of inter-species embryos,[676] to clarify the terminology and the scientific issues in the debate. The report was put together relatively quickly in view of the political developments on the subject.[677] Consultations were conducted with regulatory authorities like the HFEA. The substantive report begins with an explanation of the value of human-animal combinations in the context of hESC research and SCNT. It emphasises that this research is directed at learning how to control stem cell differentiation and development, nuclear reprogramming and generating specialised tissues in culture

---

673 Human Fertilisation and Embryology Authority, UK, Press Statement, 26 April 2007.

674 David A Jones, What does the British public think about human-animal hybrid embryos? *Journal of Medical Ethics* 35, 3 (2009): 168-170, at 169.

675 *Ibid.*

676 The Academy of Medical Sciences, UK, *Inter-species embryos: A report by the Academy of Medical Sciences.* London: Academy of Medical Sciences, June 2007.

677 Interview with Dr Helen Munn, Executive Director (then Director, Medical Science Policy), Academy of Medical Sciences, 1 April 2008.

or animal models.[678] Human-animal combinations could help overcome the shortage of human oocytes for such research.[679]

Strong arguments are presented for extending the current legislation on human embryo research to inter-species embryos. Under such a framework of regulatory control, the AMS indicates that there would be no substantive ethical or moral reasons not to proceed with the research on cytoplasmic hybrid, human transgenic or human chimeric embryos.[680] It further argues that *in vitro* laboratory research involving cytoplasmic hybrids or other inter-species embryos would not raise any significant safety risks over and above regular cell culture, provided that good laboratory practice is rigorously followed. However, if cell lines derived from such embryos should ever be contemplated for therapeutic use, it would be prudent to scan the mitochondria and cytoplasmic RNA of the species to be used for pathogens.[681]

The AMS 2007 report was a galvanising force, and contributed to a briefing for Ministers of Parliament jointly undertaken by the AMS, the Medical Research Council, the Royal Society and the Wellcome Trust at the House of Commons on 6 May 2008. The concerted effort of scientific bodies and medical charities in the UK culminated in the successful passage of comprehensive legislation on the subject through Parliament. The HFE Act 2008 was passed in October 2008 and received the royal assent in November 2008.[682] It supersedes the 1990 version of the legislation. Of relevance to the BAC is Part 1 of the legislation, which ensures that all research on human embryos that occur outside the body, and research on human admixed embryos, where animal DNA is not predominant, are subject to strict regulation.

---

[678] The Academy of Medical Sciences, UK, *Inter-species embryos: A report by the Academy of Medical Sciences.* London: Academy of Medical Sciences, June 2007, at 7-14.

[679] *Ibid*, at 16-17.

[680] *Ibid*, at 30-31.

[681] *Ibid*, at 38.

[682] Human Fertilisation and Embryology Act, UK, 2008. See also Explanatory Notes to the legislation.

The Act, which is administered by the HFEA, was implemented in stages, with the legislative provisions that relate to research on embryos being effective from October 2009.

In the Act, the term 'embryo' means a live human embryo and includes "an egg that is in the process of fertilisation or is undergoing any other process capable of resulting in an embryo",[683] and a 'human admixed' embryo is specifically defined.[684]

Reference to human cells or animal cells means either cells from a human or human embryo, or cells from an animal or animal embryo, as the case may be. Thus human admixed embryos, which are created from a combination of human and animal genetic material, would include:

(1) Human cytoplasmic hybrid embryos;

(2) True human-animal hybrid embryos;

(3) Transgenic human embryos;

(4) Human-animal chimeric embryos; and

(5) Any other embryo that has human and animal nuclear or mitochondrial DNA, but in which the animal DNA is not predominant.

The creation and use of human-admixed embryos covered under the legislation is allowed under license if they are purely for laboratory research, and such research should not extend beyond 14 days of embryonic development. These embryos are to be destroyed after the 14 day limit is reached.[685] The Act also stipulates that a license cannot authorise placing a human admixed embryo in a woman[686] or in an animal.[687] In addition, the Act does not cover the creation or use of animal chimeric foetuses or animals, or (as

---

[683] *Ibid*, Section 1(2).
[684] *Ibid*, Section 4A (6).
[685] *Ibid*. Sections 4A (2) and 4A (3).
[686] *Ibid*. Section 4A (1) (a).
[687] *Ibid*. Section 4A (4).

indicated above) the creation or use of human admixed embryos in which animal DNA is predominant.

As discussed earlier, the AMS published a more comprehensive report on research involving inter-species mixtures in 2011. Here, the AMS noted three areas in which the creation of animal-human models through genetic engineering or stem cell methods might be particularly sensitive or approach current social, ethical or regulatory boundaries. These areas of public interest and concern identified through public dialogue are research involving the brain, research involving the reproductive system, and research involving aspects of human appearance or behavioural traits.[688] The AMS observed that, on the whole, a majority of participants in the public dialogue were supportive of research using animals containing human materials, provided that such research is conducted to improve human health or to combat disease. A majority of the participants also expressed greater concern for *in vivo* experiments than *in vitro* experiments, such as the creation of human-animal hybrid cells.

5.9 Report on Human-Animal Combinations

With the conclusion of the public consultation and with positive regulatory developments in the UK, a draft set of recommendations were prepared by the HECR Working Group. The substance of these recommendations was heavily influenced by the framework laid out by the NAS and the ISSCR (discussed in the previous chapter), legislative change and related developments in the UK, and local feedback. The recommendations were focused for a time on addressing the creation and use of pluripotent cells in general, but it reverted to specific focus on human-animal combinations after

---

[688] Academy of Medical Sciences, *Animals containing human material.* London: The Academy of Medical Sciences, July 2011, at 31. The Working Group for this report was chaired by Professor Martin Bobrow.

discussion continued at the level of the BAC.[689] This approach was felt to be expedient for three main reasons. First, the scientific community was concerned that an overly prescriptive treatment of all conceivable types of human-animal combinations could burden research. By limiting recommendations to the most controversial of human-animal combinations, there would be a clear signal to all concerned that a majority of the research involving such constructs is not considered to be ethically contentious. Second, feedback from the National Council of Churches in Singapore (NCCS) and the Catholic Medical Guild (CMG) made clear an expectation that the BAC was to respond to their specific ethical positions and contentions.[690] This message was reiterated when the BAC met with religious group leaders. Representatives of the NCCS and the CMG considered the BAC's ethical arguments to be lacking in comprehensiveness.[691] In response to this critique, a point-for-point rebuttal of ethical arguments raised by the NCCS and CMG was prepared, although it may queried if the debate was directed at the same concerns. Ultimately, a much more streamlined version of the ethical discussion was published in the HA Report.[692] The need to add focus to the ethical

---

[689] Bioethics Advisory Committee, *Human-Animal Combinations in Stem Cell Research*. Singapore: Bioethics Advisory Committee, September 2010. The BAC explicitly sets out (at paragraph 1.7, at 5-6) the two types of human-animal combinations that are considered in the HA Report as animal chimeras (in which human pluripotent cells have been introduced at various stages of the animal's development) and cytoplasmic hybrid embryos. It further states (at paragraph 1.8, at 6) that the HA Report "does not extend to consideration of ... other more speculative combinations."

[690] The NCCS indicates in its feedback to the BAC that: "[w]hile the consultation paper is very lucid and tightly argued, at the same time it suffers the disadvantage of being too general. Because there are many different types of chimera research, it is not only profitable but it is indeed necessary to evaluate the ethics of each. Only when this is done will a clearer and fairer picture emerge." *Ibid*, at C9-2.

[691] Fieldnotes, 13 August 2008. On the position of the NCCS, see also: Roland Chia, *Hybrids, Cybrids and Chimeras: The Ethics of Interspecies Research*. Singapore: National Council of Churches of Singapore, 2012.

[692] Bioethics Advisory Committee, *Human-Animal Combinations in Stem Cell Research*. Singapore: Bioethics Advisory Committee, September 2010, pp 16-19. In

discussion was another reason for limiting the scope of the HA Report to particular human-animal combinations. Third, a narrower scope was considered to more effectively direct public and regulatory attention to the 'pertinent issues'. Even then, the HA Report was only published towards the end of 2010, even though the recommendations were finalised and presented to the government at the end of 2009.[693] This delay was intended to provide regulators with more 'reaction time', especially since a recommendation of the BAC was for a single national body to be established to review and monitor all stem cell research involving human pluripotent stem cells or human-animal combinations conducted in Singapore.[694] The regulation of stem cell research *per se* was unlikely to have been the cause of the delay since a similar recommendation was in fact advanced earlier. The SC Report recommended that there should be a statutory body to license, control and monitor all stem cell research conducted in Singapore, together with a comprehensive legislative framework and guidelines.[695] However, a more direct form of control has not been instituted, perhaps owing to preference for a 'phased' or incremental regulatory approach, and to the fact that stem cell research did not have the volume or scale that justified intense regulatory attention. Hence, the more likely reason was the ambiguity as to which government agency should shoulder the regulatory burden, since different agencies were responsible for overseeing basic research as opposed to clinical trials, and human as opposed to animal

---

particular, the ethical contention of 'Playing God' has been explicitly addressed in the report (at 18), whereas this was only alluded to in the HA Consultation Paper.

[693] Fieldnotes, 20 November 2009.

[694] Bioethics Advisory Committee, *Human-Animal Combinations in Stem Cell Research.* Singapore: Bioethics Advisory Committee, September 2010, at 3.

[695] Bioethics Advisory Committee, *Ethical, Legal and Social Issues in Human Stem Cell Research, Reproductive and Therapeutic Cloning.* Singapore: Bioethics Advisory Committee, June 2002, Recommendation 8, at viii.

research.[696] In other words, there was a problem with regulatory categories. Another reason was to allow more time to observe developments in the UK following legislative changes introduced at the end of 2008.

Consequently, the HA Report is relatively concise, comprising only five recommendations, although bearing the generic title of 'human-animal combinations'. Of these, one recommendation is directed at cytoplasmic hybrid embryos, and another two relate to (human-to-animal) chimeras (which, as we have earlier noted, exclude animal-to-human chimeras). Together, these recommendations make clear the types of research that are permitted.

In order to include human-animal combinations within the rubric of the ethics framework, the regulated methods of deriving new stem cell lines have been enlarged to include newer methods such as parthenogenesis, reproductive semi-cloning, altered nuclear transfer, and inter-species SCNT. In addition, research involving the creation of chimeric animals through the introduction of human embryonic stem cells into non-human animals at any stage of embryonic, foetal, or postnatal development have also been brought within the framework. Consistent with the positions of key policy bodies, the BAC makes clear that animals into which any kind of pluripotent cells are introduced should not be allowed to breed.[697] For animals into which whole human embryonic stem cells had been introduced, a concern was that if such animals were allowed to breed, human gametes could be produced by chance, so that a substantial amount of human materials would be present in the next generation. While it is unlikely that such animals will reveal human features, the possibility remains.

---

[696] An observation to this effect was made in the HA Report: "Currently, no governmental body in Singapore has explicit statutory power to regulate human stem cell research involving human-animal combinations." Bioethics Advisory Committee, *Human-Animal Combinations in Stem Cell Research*. Singapore: Bioethics Advisory Committee, September 2010, paragraph 4.9, at 22.

[697] *Ibid*, Recommendation 4, at 3.

However, such a risk will not arise for transgenic animals, where only a very small quantity of human genes is incorporated.[698]

5.10 Chimeras and Hybrids as Regulatory Objects

In her contribution to the legal section of the European Union's Chimbrids project, Elisabeth Rynning observes that a difficulty in regulating chimeras and hybrids is the lack of knowledge regarding the potential future value and the risks involved. Consequently, "the necessary balancing of interests to a certain extent will amount to a balancing of two unknowns, making it virtually impossible to reach any well-founded conclusions on proportionality."[699] In managing this uncertainty, categorisation has the effect of lowering the informational deficiency by streamlining a social phenomenon on the basis of certain desired information qualities. Social and cognitive psychologists tell us that this is how we – as human beings – generally store and process information.[700] The generation of categories through rationalisation and systematisation in legal and regulatory processes does not detract significantly from our basic cognitive orientation. Reductionism in categorisation is evident in what Bruno Latour describes as involution in terms of a model of qualification as opposed to fictionalisation.[701] Latour argues that:

---

698 The BAC suggests that research involving certain types of transgenic animals (such as transgenic non-human primates) can be ethically contentions. Such animals could be the subject of another report to be produced by the BAC. *Ibid*, paragraph 1.8, at 6.

699 Elizabeth Rynning. Legal tools and strategies for the regulation of chimbrids, In J Taupitz and M Weschka (eds.), *CHIMBRIDS – Chimeras and Hybrids in Comparative European and International Research*. Heidelberg: Springer, 2009, pp 79-87, at 85.

700 Judith A Howard, Social Psychology of Identities, *Annual Review of Sociology* (2000) 26: 367-393.

701 Bruno Latour, Scientific Objects and Legal Objectivity. In Alain Pottage and Martha Mundy (eds.), *Law, Anthropology, and the Constitution of the Social: Making Persons and Things*. Cambridge: Cambridge University Press, 2004, pp 73-114, at 104.

[W]hereas in science everything is done to ensure that the impact of new information upon a body of established knowledge is as devastating as possible, in law things are arranged in such a way as to ensure that the particular facts are just the external occasion for a change which alters only the law itself, and not the particular facts, about which one can learn nothing further, beyond the name of the claimant.[702]

In this connection, Alain Pottage observes that an inquiry into the facts in the case of law "is confined to the question whether the facts are such as to trigger the application of the rule ... this is a mode of involution rather than just a mode of classification because qualification is less about cognition than it is about steering institutional action."[703]

The tabularised survey of a range of human-animal combinations based on certain scientific, ethical and social criteria (in Table 5.2) is an attempt at acquiring an understanding of the subject at hand for the purposes of steering institutional action. With understanding, it becomes possible to appreciate the regulatory risk[704] entailed as knowledge enables control. Hence categorisation through typifying human-animal combinations is also an exercise in the enumeration of risks entailed. Reification through objectification was also thereby achieved through the substitution of scientific, ethical and social content in a categorical manner for mythical ones in the metaphors of 'chimeras' and 'hybrids'. As earlier considered, the displacement technique may give description to the BAC's approach in the HA

---

[702] *Ibid*, at 105.

[703] Alain Pottage, Introduction: The Fabrication of Persons and Things. In Alain Pottage and Martha Mundy (eds.), *Law, Anthropology, and the Constitution of the Social: Making Persons and Things*. Cambridge: Cambridge University Press, 2004, pp 1-39, at 21-22.

[704] Regulatory risk relates to the risk of not achieving the regulatory objectives or the risk of generating other regulatory issues that are unanticipated when regulation was introduced. See: Cass Sunstein, Health-Health Tradeoffs. In Cass Sunstein (ed.), *Risk and Reason*. Cambridge: Cambridge University Press, 2002, pp 133-152.

Consultation Paper. Models *for* 'chimeras' and 'hybrids' were constructed to replace models *of* these constructs. The elimination
of categories that followed, from the many combinations down
to human-to-animal chimeras and cytoplasmic hybrid embryos
effectively reduces the uncertainty in and regulatory risks of the
subject matter, and this facilitates control, as well as action.

The involution that one observes in the BAC's deployment of
scientific and ethical (or regulatory) categories to objectify a particular metaphorical content for (or viewpoint of) hybrids and
chimeras is not dissimilar to the way in which factual 'objectivity' is
generated through science. Objectification enables reification, so that
hybrids and chimeras are no longer images of endless adverse
outcomes, but are objects that could be brought under some form of
institutional control. In this sense, reification renders calculability
and enables institutional action. In addition, a sense of 'found-ness'
through the erasure of context and association with perceptions of
'natural-ness' confer legitimacy on this otherwise limited content or
viewpoint. The largely positive public reaction to the BAC's recommendations suggests that the BAC has been relatively successful in
re-constituting conventional metaphors of hybrids and chimeras as
freestanding legal objects of chimeras and hybrids that could fall
under the power of regulatory control. We proceed to consider
further how this sense of institutional control could arise.

5.11 Metaphors that Arrest the Slide Downwards

Philosopher and BAC member, Professor Anh Tuan Nuyen, commenced his segment of the public lecture on 16 August 2008 with a
travesty of the 'slippery slope' argument.[705] He narrated a scene with

---

705 The public forum entitled 'Mixing human and animal tissues: Is such research
     ethical?' comprised three speakers: a stem cell scientist (Professor Lawrence
     Stanton), a philosopher (Professor Anh Tuan Nuyen) and a medical ethicist
     (Professor Bernard Lo). In a newspaper article that publicised this event, it was

two men chatting in a pub. One man told the other that he intends to emigrate. When asked for the reason, he said that same-sex marriage was initially illegal in the country. The government recently decided to repeal the prohibitive legislation. He surmised that given these developments, he should leave the country before he is forced to change his sexual orientation in the future.[706] From this vantage point, the flaw in reasoning is apparent. Yet, the metaphorical argument of 'slippery slope' has been raised in each and every public consultation conducted by the BAC. Feedback from the public consultation also indicates the persuasiveness of this argument in the mind of the public. And this phenomenon is by no means confined to Singapore. Dag Stenvoll provides illustrations of the extensive deployment of this argument in the Norwegian parliamentary debates on sexuality, abortion and new reproductive technologies from the 1950s through the 1990s. His analysis of the 'slippery slope' mechanics is instructive:[707]

> The slippery slope image works metaphorically in at least two ways. First, it sets up the physical world of solid objects as an analogy to political matters, implying that politics is like the physical world: if you 'move' something in the world of politics, like making

---

observed that: "Opponents fear that tinkering with the human genome puts science on the slippery slope to creating animal-human hybrids". The BAC's position was then indicated as: "But unlike Hollywood science, researchers are not looking to create half-man half-animal monstrosities ..." See Tania Tan, Forum on ethics of mixing human, animal genes, *The Straits Times*, 14 August 2008.

706 Certain homosexual conducts are technically illegal in Singapore and could constitute a criminal offence. At around the time of the public lecture, there has been ongoing debate as to whether this Edwardian legacy should be repealed. In order to pacify a vocal conservative minority, the government has adopted a pragmatic position of retaining the legislation, but providing an assurance that this legislation will not be enforced.

707 Dag Stenvoll. Slippery slopes in political discourse. In Terrell Carver and Jernej Pikalo (eds.), *Political Language and Metaphor: Interpreting and changing the world*. London and New York: Routledge, 2008, pp 28-40, at 29. Stenvoll observes (at 37) that metaphors are significant in politics because they have constitutive functions in that they contribute to the scene that set of a sequence that inevitably ends in tragedy.

or changing a particular law or policy, other things will inevitably follow ... Second, the slippery slope does in itself entail a particular image of movement: from a good or relatively good place to a relatively worse or natural world of determinism and laws of physics. It imposes a kind of unidirectional, unstoppable movement which, when used metaphorically about politics, binds phenomena together in a specific way ... The metaphorical expression of a slippery slope also involves a dual displacement of focus: regarding time perspective, from the present to the future, and regarding problematisation, from the instant to the danger case.

When applied in ethical debates, the determinism in Stenvoll's 'POLITICS IS PHYSICS' is no less forceful as 'ETHICS IS PHYSICS'. It became a subject for critique in the editorial of an issue of the *Journal of Medical Ethics*.[708] Whether a scientific possibility is seen as 'a slope going down' towards some detriment or an escalator going up towards some benefit is ultimately a prediction. This misleading metaphoric stealth of hand led to the BAC's decision to avoid using the phrase 'slippery slope'. Focus should instead be directed at the avoidance of adverse outcomes through means such as regulation, and on remedies should such outcomes materialise.

Of pertinence is the ethnographic finding of Sarah Franklin and Celia Roberts on the uptake of embryo research and new reproductive technologies in the UK. Contrary to the view of PGD as a socially destabilising technology in offering 'too much choice', their study suggests a much more careful and thoughtful engagement with the difficulties presented by PGD.[709] In the light of this, the BAC considers

---

[708] Søren Holm and T Takala. High hopes and automatic escalators: a critique of some new arguments in bioethics, *Journal of Medical Ethics* (2007) 33, 1: 1-4.
[709] *Ibid.*

effective regulation to be a means by which the determinism entailed in the 'slippery slope' argument could be countered.[710]

In the BAC's HA Report, the metaphors of 'hybrid' and 'chimera' could be broadly regarded as 'world-perceiving', in that they present conceptual frameworks of understanding that influence our perception of the world.[711] As we have seen, the minimum content of these metaphors are directed at displacing particular cultural mind-sets that range from the fear of bringing to life mythical creatures to religious concerns over transgressing 'natural' boundaries.[712] Their production is directed as reifying particular scientific and ethical notions in a way that not only enables institutional action (particularly regulatory control), but also the consumption or exploitation of particular biological constructs in scientific work. For instance, the creation and use of a cytoplasmic hybrid embryo would not have found support in prevailing cultural (and especially those of the Judeo-Christian traditions) beliefs. This is broadly speaking the context to the metaphors of 'hybrid' and 'chimera' in the HA Report. We have also seen the range of formats that the BAC has deployed, which include analytical tables, schematic diagrams, artistic portrait (even if limited to the level of the Secretariat) and comparative tables. Putting these constructed metaphorical models through public

---

[710] Bioethics Advisory Committee, Singapore, *Human-Animal Combinations for Biomedical Research: A Consultation Paper*. Singapore: Bioethics Advisory Committee, 8 January 2008, paragraph 60 at 29.

[711] Aside from 'world-perceiving', James Underhill indicates that metaphors could also be 'world-conceiving' (which we will further discuss in the next Chapter), and could relate to a cultural mind-set, personal world or otherwise a perspective. James W Underhill, *Creating Worldviews: Metaphors, Ideology and Language*. Edinburgh: Edinburgh University Press, 2011, at 7.

[712] Calum Mackellar and David Jones provide a broad overview of the different religious and ideological beliefs in relation to HACs. By their assessment, these beliefs are essentially premised on conventional distinctions that attempt to set *homo sapiens* apart from other living organisms. See: Calum Mackellar and David Albert Jones, *Chimera's Children: Ethical, philosophical and religious perspectives on human-nonhuman experimentation*. London and New York: Continuum, 2012, at 133-148.

consultation secures for them a degree of legitimacy, so that they become not only models of 'seeing-as', but also models of social (and ideological) mediation and consensus.[713] The BAC attempted to communicate this in the HA Report when it indicated that the faith of the Singaporean public in the regulatory approach was consistent with relatively concurrent developments in leading jurisdictions.[714] However, to say that 'hybrid' and 'chimera' are metaphors is an incomplete account, especially since the term 'metaphor' suggests a relatively well settled lexical content or meaning. In the next section, it is argued that Annelise Riles's analytic of a placeholder provides a more rigorous account.

5.12 Metaphors as Placeholders

Annelise Riles argues that collateral put up as security by a party to a financial swap transaction could be understood as a 'placeholder', which is "a device for governing the near future".[715] As a legal technique, it serves as "a tool for producing working truths, for the moment".[716] As for its substantive character, it could be understood as a kind of legal fiction, much like the notion that a corporation is a

---

713 Particularly where scientific models are concerned, they are means of theory construction, exploration, representation, measurement and learning, through a process that could be understood as incremental and pragmatically consensual. See: Margaret Morrison and Mary S Morgan, Models as mediating instruments. In Mary S Morgan and Margaret Morrison (eds.), *Models as Mediators: Perspectives on Natural and Social Science.* Cambridge: Cambridge University Press, 1999, pp 10-37.

714 Bioethics Advisory Committee, Singapore, *Human-Animal Combinations in Stem Cell Research.* Singapore: Bioethics Advisory Committee, September 2010, at 20-22.

715 Annelise Riles. *Collateral Knowledge: Legal Reasoning in the Global Financial Markets.* Chicago and London: University of Chicago Press, 2011, at 180. In the context of her research, a placeholder is understood as (at 169) "in the meantime, that is, for the near future, the parties simply agree to act as if the holder of the collateral (the pledgee) already has clear and complete rights over the collateral (as if the parties are no longer trapped in the messy 'meantime')."

716 *Ibid.*

person. It is an 'As If', or a consciously false statement that is irrefutable. Riles provides this explanation:[717]

> When I say that legal fictions are technicalities or techniques of private law, therefore, I mean that they are *nonrepresentational* ... Thus the legal fiction is not really so much an epistemological claim as it is a special kind of pause, for the moment. In mathematics, a placeholder is a "symbol, frequently an empty box, used in teaching to denote a missing quantity or operator in an expression." One creates a placeholder in order provisionally to overlook it. In other words, it is a technique for working with and in the meantime. As such it has no particular content or meaning, except that it defines and manages the near future – the time for which this particular commitment holds true. But it is also a political device, a kind of collective commitment: The original meaning of the term was overtly political ...

Elsewhere, Riles explains that unlike other kinds of legal fiction, a 'placeholder' emphasises an often overlooked temporal dimension (or "for the time being-ness"):[718]

> It is not that things are unsettled, not that we need to direct our attention to further inquiry (probabilities); it is just that they are settled only *for the time being*. It will be up to future actors to decide what the state of affairs is at that time.

---

[717] *Ibid*, at 173–174 (Emphasis in original). In a different forum, Riles indicates: "One creates a placeholder in order to overlook it for the moment. In other words, it is a technique for working with and in the meantime. As such, it has no particular content or meaning, except that it defines and manages the near future, the time for which this particular commitment holds true. But it is also a political device, a kind of collective commitment ... the placeholder's central feature is that it forecloses the question of the moment for the near future, but by resolving it, but by papering over it ... by creating a dummy solution subject to future reevaluation. The placeholder is the precise opposite, then, of pragmatist ways of thinking about the ambiguity or open-endedness of the present as an open zone of endless possibility and unpredictability." See Annelise Riles. Collateral Expertise: Legal Knowledge in the Global Financial Markets. *Current Anthropology* (2010) 51, 6: 795-818, at 803.

[718] *Ibid*, at 815 (Emphasis in original).

Temporality encapsulated in the notion of 'placeholder' is critical to appreciate fully the significance of metaphors in a policy environment. It is incomplete to think of 'chimera' and 'hybrid' only as models for 'seeing as'. When the endeavour was initiated to give meaning to such biological constructs by transposing the question of identities from the scientific to ethical domain, the models of scientific 'Seeing As' became models for 'Seeing As If'. In a sense, the transformation also reflects a movement from *is* to *ought*; from scientific facticity to a normative one. The 'papering over' was by way of a temporal truism that adds to the multiplicity of meanings over material constructs. Put differently, it was a temporal and purpose-specific semiotic superstructure (a *lingua franca* perhaps?) layered over a variedly composed material-semiotic substrate.[719] Many researchers and policy-makers continue to see this endeavour as one part durable (material) and one part temporal (semiotic). In the meeting with scientists, we find that many of them appeared to have their own classificatory scheme. Again, this is not a phenomenon that is confined to Singapore. Shortly after I started my fieldwork, Professor Martin Bobrow (who was in Singapore for a meeting) shared over dinner that scientists in the UK have adopted different definitions of chimeras and hybrids, making it necessary for the AMS and allied organisations to push for standardised meanings.[720] As we have seen, the situation was no less different in Singapore. At the BAC's meeting with scientists, chimeras routinely created in the course of research was not a problematic that fell within the definition of human-animal combinations. Prior to the meeting, many of them considered human-animal combinations to relate only to cytoplasmic hybrid embryos. As we have noted earlier, the NCCS indicated that the BAC did not go far enough in analysing the ethical implication of the full spectrum of chimeras and hybrids that

---

719 Annelise Riles's observation that placeholders are a material, sociotechnical phenomenon, not simply a concept, is relevant here. See: Annelise Riles. *Collateral Knowledge: Legal Reasoning in the Global Financial Markets.* Chicago and London: University of Chicago Press, 2011, at 175.

720 Fieldnotes, 25 September 2007.

could be created. This is a fair observation because the 'placeholders' could render other accounts of human-animal combinations 'invisible' by simply not giving recognition to them.

As placeholders, 'hybrids' and 'chimeras' thereby served (in the words of Riles) as political devices that foreclose the many un-answered questions of the moment for the near future by creating a dummy solution subject to future re-evaluation. Being devices for 'Seeing As-If', it is not the intent of the BAC to resolve more philosophical issues relating to the essence of human beings and animals through these re-constituted metaphors. A 'hybrid' in the HA Report is narrowly construed as referring to cytoplasmic hybrid, and in research, it is treated *as-if* it is a human embryo, so that the research must not extend "beyond 14 days or the appearance of the primitive streak, whichever is earlier, nor be implanted into any human or animal uterus."[721] In this way, the thorny issue of when human life begins is side-stepped, and taken to be irrelevant to the situation at hand and for the time being. As for chimeras, the require-ments of avoiding the "creation of entities in which human sentience or consciousness might be expected to occur",[722] as well as precluding such chimeric animals from breeding,[723] enable a *seeing as-if* there is no breach to the human versus non-human divide. Even if human pluripotent stem cells have been introduced into non-human animals, these chimeras remain animals and continue to be treated as such, apart from precluding their procreation. The HA Report further creates a sense of regulatory control (as we have discussed) and a notion of free choice, through recognition of the refusal to engage in research involving hybrids and chimeras on the ground of 'conscientious objection'.[724] Hence, while the HA Report may purport

---

[721] Bioethics Advisory Committee, *Human-Animal Combinations in Stem Cell Research.* Singapore: Bioethics Advisory Committee, September 2010, at 3, Recommendation 2.

[722] *Ibid*, Recommendation 3.

[723] *Ibid*, Recommendation 4.

[724] *Ibid*, Recommendation 5.

to address human-animal combinations generally, it is in effect an embodiment of pockets of information in a well-defined (storage) space – resources that could be drawn upon for specific (mainly scientific, ethical and policy) purposes. Not surprisingly, a number of ambiguities remain. Until the enactment of the HBRA in 2015, it was not entirely clear if non-human stem cell may be introduced into a human embryo or foetus, or if 'true' hybrids may be created by mixing human and non-human gametes. In addition, the question of how human sentience could be defined and measured has been left unanswered. There is only a general assurance that *for the time being* a non-human animal with human sentience is unlikely to be produced.

5.13 Bioethical Instauration

When constituted as regulatory objects (and subjects), chimeras and hybrids fall under the power of regulatory control. Earlier on, policy-makers discovered that the construction of the ethico-legal category of the 'pre-embryo'[725] is a means by which human embryo research could be kept off the slippery slope. Arguably, the ability to control 'pre-embryos' as 'things' underscored Baroness Warnock's confidence in a legislative response to human embryo research.[726] As we have also seen, the distinction drawn between research and therapy, the segregation of motives and the requirement of informed consent could all be regarded as ethical and legal 'technologies' by which the object of 'pre-embryo' is carved out of the social bedrock. Although reification may present placeholders like 'pre-embryo', 'hybrid' and 'chimera' to be somewhat free-standing, the exercise has also been instaurative of a script or an account of what it means to be human. These bioethical artefacts restore a conventional and fundamentally anthropocentric script of human nature. For this reason, scholars like

---

725 That is, an 'embryo' from the point of creation up to time the primitive streak appears – which is approximately 14 days for a human embryo.
726 Michael Mulkay. *The Embryo Research Debate: Science and the Politics of Reproduction.* Cambridge: Cambridge University Press, 1997, at 149.

Michael Hauskeller have argued that such a script is nothing more than a myth, because the term 'human' only tells us what should matter, rather than what is 'human' in a human-animal chimera. By Hauskeller's account, the term 'human' is essentially *nomen dignitatis* or dignity-conferring.[727]

But myths are not without value. In the context of criminal justice, Mariana Valverde illustrates their importance by showing the various ways in which film, television and newspapers create unrealistic views of crime and crime control in the minds of the public.[728] Media representations of courtrooms, police departments, prisons and people who populate them must be understood to have an impact on how certain evidence is received and interpreted. More important for present purposes is her observation that signs, meanings and myths are integral components to all social processes, including to those relating to crime and justice.[729] Citing Ferdinand de Saussure, she indicates that meaning is not inherent in words or other signs, but emerges through differentiation from competing signs, as well as association with similar signs. Hence creation of meaning requires system-wide relations of contrast and comparison.[730] She further indicates that Freudian metonymy (or displacement) and metaphors are ways in which associations are made or unmade. Apart from signs, myths also make representations and have meaning. She notes:[731]

---

[727] Michael Hauskeller, Making Sense of What We Are: A Mythological Approach to Human Nature (2009) *Philosophy* 84: 95-109. Hauskeller observes (at 106): "When we embrace a particular conception of human nature we implicitly make a statement about what, in our view, human life is or should be all about, what matters or should matter in life, and what makes a human life good. In that sense, human nature is a myth, by which I don't mean that there is nothing that all humans and only human have in common, but rather that each attempt at defining what we are is the telling of a story that implicitly or explicitly claims to be of prime significant for the way we ought to lead our lives."

[728] Mariana Valverde, *Law and Order: Images, Meanings, Myths.* New Brunswick: Rutgers University Press, 2006.

[729] *Ibid*, at 163.

[730] *Ibid*, at 20-21.

[731] *Ibid*, at 25.

A myth ... is not a lie or a misrepresentation. It is not the opposite of 'truth'. In fact, myths are often conveyed by representations that are not manipulated, tampered with, or posed. There are few myths more powerful than the generic 'happy childhood' that is the common denominator of most baby photos, for instance. And yet the parents are hardly engaging in a conspiracy to disseminate the patriarchal ideology of the nuclear family when they proudly show their relatives pictures of little Jane. The point is that mythical meanings get communicated, sometimes very purposefully but at other times unwittingly or even accidentally, through certain representations whose meanings are not within the control of the person taking the photo or writing the words.

A myth usually resists attempts to reduce it to factual information since it is often representations made by a specific author for a specific audience, and is thus embedded in particular political and cultural relations.[732] Particular ways of representation (such as maps used by the military, graphs by economists and diagrams of the crime scene by lawyers) and visual techniques change the perception of audiences, especially in communicating a certain sense of objectivity in the representation made.[733]

In this chapter, we have considered the ways in which techniques in law has been used in bioethics to construct chimeras and hybrids as 'objects' (and regulatory subjects). These techniques include not only distinguishing between medical therapy and research, but also among different types of research, such as the exclusion of transgenic animals and animal-animal hybrids and chimeras. The avoidance of terms like 'inter-species' is illustrative. Legal and ethical analytics and rules have been applied, on an almost symmetrical basis, to achieve objectification. Timing and the manner of presentation have been integral to the process, along with certain legal and ethical values. Of these, the value of fairness (or impartiality) has been one of

---

732 *Ibid*, at 35.
733 *Ibid*, at 51-52; 55.

the most important. As re-constituted metaphorical placeholders, 'hybrids' and 'chimeras' serve as models of 'Seeing As-If' that enable regulatory control. They are metaphorical for their 'world-conceiving' characteristic.[734] However, it is their temporality and 'open-texture' feature that allows the designation of conceptual frameworks which enable us to communicate with others and engage in the discussion of ideas, impressions and feelings. Although tentative in construct, they are useful as 'pockets' (rather than as some pervasive discourse) of resources that have currency for the time being to achieve more immediate objectives.

Like Bruno Latour, it seems to me that Étienne Souriau's 'instauration' could be another way to explain the bioethical artefacts of chimeras and hybrid (among others) as they are not *res extensa* of the anthropocentric self or society.[735] These artefacts have an independent mode of existence and, arguably, may be judged independently of particular user or use. As this French term *instauration* is based on the Latin verb *instaurare*, Souriau probably did not intend for it to be understood simply as 'instituting' or 'establishing'. Instead, 'instauration' is intended to convey a connotation of restoration or resumption.[736] In effect, the means by which membership to the *homo sapiens* species is conferred has been re-affirmed and restored through the techniques and processes we have considered. The contingency that research involving HACs could give rise to independently living organisms with unclear species membership has to be bracketed and quarantined so that the identity and uniqueness of humankind – an assumption upon which our social and political

---

734 James W Underhill. *Creating Worldviews: Metaphor, Ideology and Language*. Edinburgh: Edinburg University Press, 2011, at 7.

735 Bruno Latour. *An Inquiry into Modes of Existence: An Anthropology of the Moderns*, Catherine Porter (tr.). Cambridge MA: Harvard University Press, 2013.

736 Leonard Lawlor, A Note on the Relation between Étienne Souriau's *L'Instauration philosophique* and Deleuze and Guattari's *What is Philosophy?* (2011) *Deleuze Studies* 5, 3: 400-406. Lawlor observes (at 404): "What Souriau wants to retain from the Latin sense of the word is the idea of doing something over again."

institutions are premised upon – remain secured. But the prospect of this contingency remains, and these endeavours to set ourselves apart as unique living species with full dignity concomitantly give rise to the very risks that now confront us. Instauration further recognises the processes that bring these artefacts into being, essentially through demonstrating the mutual dependency of these artefacts and stem cell researchers.[737] In other words, researchers have power over chimeras and hybrids as their biological tools-of-trade, just as these artefacts have power over the researchers in the intended or desired outcomes.

In this respect, instauration again gives emphasis to the contingency that arises from the biological nature of these artefacts that we do not completely understand or know, and hence relates to outcomes that cannot be predetermined. In other words, instauration makes risks and risk-taking explicit, and it is to these that our focus is turned in the chapter that follows.

---

[737] Catherine Noske, Towards an Existential Pluralism: Reading through the Philosophy of Etienne Souriau, *Cultural Studies Review* (2015) 21, 1: 34-57.

6

Risks in Bioethics

6.1 Risks in the Visibility of Human Eggs

Yan Thomas describes a mechanism deployed by Roman law in constituting *res religiosae* – matters of religious law. Under the *lex Iulia* on public violence, it is an offence to violate a *sepulcher*.[738] However, an empty tomb is not protected under the law unless it qualifies as a *sepulchrum*. By law, a tomb becomes a *sepulchrum* only after a body (or a legally sanctioned representative of it, such as a wax moulding)[739] has been laid within.[740] Once a *sepulchrum*, it is a *res religiosae*, so that the particular area of the soil and the monument built upon it could not be sold, subjected to servitude, claimed as private property, acquired by prescription, used as a basis of a guarantee, seized as security or made the subject matter of a stipulation.[741] By virtue of its inalienability, rules were developed for

---

[738] Yan Thomas, Res Religiosae: on the categories of religion and commerce in Roman law. In Alain Pottage and Martha Mundy (eds.), *Law, Anthropology, and the Constitution of the Social: Making Persons and Things.* Cambridge: Cambridge University Press, 2004, pp 40-72, at 58.

[739] *Ibid*, at 50.

[740] *Ibid*, at 46.

[741] *Ibid*, at 41-42.

the definition of space and body, and to confer on them transformative power.[742]

However, the normative instauration of artefacts like the chimeras and hybrids we considered in the previous chapter is not a *fiat*. It is a dynamic process, as the rules of engagement do not have the immanency of perpetuity, but have varying degrees of durability. For instance, the rules of science, as the scallops of St Brieuc Bay in Michel Callon's study demonstrates,[743] do not necessarily succeed in co-opting these biological constructs into designated roles. Similarly, instauration is responsive to a larger narrative or script for coherence, and it draws support from different levels of social associations and goals for legitimacy and existential currency. I have, for reasons of temporality, historicity and epistemic flux, argued that 'placeholder' is a better description of the artefacts of chimeras and hybrids than 'metaphor'.

As Isabelle Stengers and Bruno Latour read Souriau, to speak of instauration is to prepare the mind to engage. To say that a work of art is 'instaured' when a potter begins to mould a lump of clay is to witness an iteration of work-to-be-made, so that at each interaction, a form that is mutually shaped is re-visited and re-made. From this disposition, to 'instaure' is:[744]

> to prepare oneself to see the potter as one who welcomes, gathers, prepares, explores and invents – just as one "invents" a treasure – the form of the work. If they originate from a sketch, then works ensure, resist and exert themselves – and humans, their authors, must dedicate themselves to them, which is not to say, however, that

---

[742] *Ibid*, at 56 and 66.

[743] Michel Callon, Some Elements of a Sociology of Translation: Domestication of Scallops and the Fishermen of St. Brieuc Bay. In John Law (ed.), *Power, Action and Belief: A New Sociology of Knowledge?* London: Routledge & Kegan Paul, 1986, pp 196-229.

[744] Isabelle Stengers and Bruno Latour, The Sphinx of the Work. In Étienne Souriau (tr. Erik Beranek and Tim Howles), *The Different Modes of Existence*. Minneapolis: Univocal, 2015, at 21.

they serve as a mere conduit for them ... If the sculptor is responsible, it is in the sense of "having to respond to," and it is the confrontation with this lump of clay that he has no idea how to help reach its completion that he must respond to.

Beginning with the human embryo and continuing into oocytes, chimeras and hybrids, the instauration of these artefacts is not creation *ex nihilo*. It has been a matter of governance *ab initio*. As the earlier chapters depict in some detail, bioethics has and continues to respond to human pluripotent stem cell research under conditions of ignorance and uncertainty. The various goals that are at stake give rise to certain risks that require further response. In this engagement, each action produces a counter-action (or ricochet, as Latour describes it) that necessitates a further reaction. When it was assumed that the 14 day limit would lead to closure of the controversy over research involving human embryos, the use of animal oocytes owing to a shortage of human ones resulted in renewed controversy over human-animal combinations. As we have seen in Chapter 2, the appropriate bioethical response to Irving Weissman's proposed human neuron mouse experiment seems to ultimately return us back to the issue of animal welfare. Insoo Hyun explains this nicely:[745]

> It is perhaps an extreme form of arrogance – an unstated moral imperialism connected to human stem cells – to assume that the transfer of human neural matter into nonhuman brains will end up enhancing research animals above their typical species functioning. The more likely result, if our past experience with transgenic animals is a guide, would be a precipitous drop in animal welfare.

But does this mean that it has all been a matter of *plus ça change, plus c'est la même chose*? I think not. Even if the end result in deliberations over the introduction of human pluripotent stem cells into animals

---

[745] Insoo Hyun, *Bioethics and the Future of Stem Cell Research*. Cambridge and New York: Cambridge University Press, 2013, at p 154.

remains a question of animal welfare, processes have been developed and new knowledge has been gained in engaging with the broader challenges of pluralism and non-public reason.[746] More specifically, I argue that the controversy over human-animal combinations has instituted bioethics as a public space for communicative engagement and as an emergent civil epistemology. The latter is reserved for the next chapter. In this chapter, we consider how bioethics has mediated scientific risks and uncertainty in reinforcing elements of *status quo* and in shaping public understanding and attitudes. Bioethics has, at times collaboratively with the news media, played a key role in framing scientific risks and future uncertainties. It has in this capacity created for itself a mediated public sphere, or at a minimum, a space within which public expectations, scientific imperatives and political mandates are negotiated. Where research involving human-animal combinations are concerned, we have already seen how bioethics has been influential in steering a way forward. Here, we consider how the risks and uncertainties of human egg donation have likewise been intermediated through bioethics.

In the winter of 2005, the scandal in South Korea surrounding Professor Hwang Woo-Suk gave emphasis to the shortage of eggs that are needed for research. This scandal contributed to further conservatism on the part of regulators.[747] There has been increasing

---

[746] This description by Hyun illustrates what I understand to be non-public reason: "It appears to me that it is man's 'uneasiness of thought and consciousness' that is under siege in the debate over neurological chimera research, so it should come as little surprise if people's anxieties in this area prove to be the most difficult to mollify through reasoned, philosophical debate." *Ibid*, at 152.

[747] For a discussion on related developments in South Korea, see: Leo Kim, Explaining the Hwang scandal: national scientific culture and its global relevance, *Science as Culture* (2008) 17: 397-415; Sungook Hong, The Hwang Scandal that "shook the world of science", *East Asian Science, Technology and Society: an International Journal* (2008) 2: 1-7; So Yeon Leem and Jin Hee Park, Rethinking women and their bodies in the age of biotechnology: feminist commentaries on the Hwang Affair, *East Asian Science, Technology and Society: an International Journal* (2008) 2: 9-26; Tae-Ho Kim, How could a scientist become a national celebrity: Nationalism and Hwang Woo-Suk scandal, *East Asian Science, Technology and Society: An International Journal* (2008) 2: 27-45.

pressure to find a sustainable source of oocytes for SCNT, and a possibility would be to increase the numbers of oocytes donated by women. One way in which this could be achieved is by offering incentives for women 'at-risk' (i.e. women suffering from infertility) – even healthy women – to contribute to research. The concern going down this route is the possibility of woman being coerced into undergoing a potentially risky procedure of hyper-stimulation and oocyte retrieval with no direct therapeutic benefit. As these risks were considered to be quite distinct from those relating to human-animal combinations, the BAC decided to address the subject of egg donation in a separate report even though they relate to stem cell research. The flow of events that followed is similar to the approaches that the BAC adopted in its deliberation on human tissue and genetics. On 7 November 2007, public consultation commenced with a press conference and public distribution of the ED Consultation Paper.[748] A public meeting was convened on 22 November 2007 just before many Singaporeans would go away during the year-end school holiday. The public consultation ended on 7 January 2008, a day before public consultation on human-animal combinations commenced. On 3 November 2008, a report (the 'ED Report') with recommendations on the subject was published by the BAC.[749] Superficially, egg donation does not appear to be a difficult matter at all. At least, that was how the topic was initially considered, and how the public still largely regards it. But the simplicity masks the many contradictions and paradoxes in the social arrangements as we know them. Developments since the publication of the SC Report in 2002 suggest a learning curve in bioethics governance that is not limited to policy makers, but also for researchers and the broader public. A means by which this 'learning' came about has been in the notion of 'risks' and the mechanisms put in place to assess and address them.

---

[748] Bioethics Advisory Committee. *Donation of Human Eggs for Research: A Consultation Paper*. Singapore: Bioethics Advisory Committee, 2007.

[749] Bioethics Advisory Committee. *Donation of Human Eggs for Research*. Singapore: Bioethics Advisory Committee, 2008.

Iain Wilkinson explains that the concept of risk can be analysed as a cultural prism, as it presents "opportunities to magnify specific contexts of rationalisation so as to detail the social conditions, moral commitments, political movements, institutional arrangements and technical means by which these are made possible and are set upon their course."[750] If one agrees that all knowledge is bound by its social and cultural context, risk is never fully objective but relates to realities that:

> ... involve the reproduction of meaning and knowledges through social interaction and socialization and rely upon shared definitions ... and can be viewed as assemblages of meanings, logics and beliefs cohering around material phenomena, giving these phenomena form and substance.[751]

Following Stephen Hilgartner's study of 'risk objects', a helpful starting point is to examine the construction of 'women' as 'objects', and then as 'risky' when linked to causal attributes of 'safety', 'inducement' and 'payment' as harms or danger in the ED Consultation Paper and the ED Report.[752] Concerns over 'safety' have generated its own category of 'health risks'. In this connection, the policies and ethical guidelines of the NAS (which has the National Research Council (NRC) and the Institute of Medicine (IOM) as its constituent organisations) were important to the BAC, as they have also been in relation to human-animal combinations. Concerns over 'inducement' and 'payment' fall within a broader category of ethical (and 'unquantifiable') risks. Where initially the attempt has been to quantify the risks entailed in egg donation as scientific risks, the inability to do so – not completely anyway – led to a shift in focus to

---

[750] Iain Wilkinson, *Risk, Vulnerability and Everyday Life*. London and New York: Routledge, 2010, at 26.

[751] Deborah Lupton, *Risk*. London and New York: Routledge, 1999, at 29 and 30.

[752] Stephen Hilgartner. The Social Construction of Risk Objects: or, How to Pry Open Networks of Risk. In James F Short and Lee Clarke (eds.), *Organizations, Uncertainties, and Risk*. Boulder, CO: Westview Press, 1992, pp 39-53.

individual choice and the avoidance of exploitation. The inter-mediation of bioethical discourses and institutions is to be noted, as well as the public sphere that has arisen. We first consider the various conceptions of risks, and how they relate to the risk discourse in the BAC's documents on egg donation.

6.2 Risks Object Identification and Issues Framing

From early to mid-2007, work on preparing recommendations on egg donation was in full swing. Since that time, a broad notion of 'risk' has framed much of the discussion, deliberation and communication on the topic. At the outset, the BAC recognised the possibility of heightened public concern arising from the ethical scandal in South Korea involving Professor Hwang Woo-Suk, and was careful to avoid this. The riskiness of the egg retrieval process was a key concern. While everyone understood that some risk to health is entailed in egg donation, a challenge was in quantifying it. An IRB could conceivably have difficulty approving research proposals that entail oocyte donation by women not undergoing fertility treatment, as donors would be put at health risk without any known benefit. It would be even more difficult to expect research participants to be fully informed and voluntarily agree to assume such risks. Between end August to early October 2007, a separate consultation paper on egg donation for research was drafted. The draft ED Consultation Paper comprises six main parts:

(1) An introduction of the issues,

(2) A description of the use of human eggs in research, and especially in somatic cell nuclear transfer technology,

(3) A description of the sources of human eggs,

(4) An analysis of the procedures and risks involved in egg donation,

(5) A description of the legal and regulatory framework, and

(6) A specific treatment of the issue of payment for providing eggs for research.

The draft was crafted in such a way as to set out the costs and benefits of different policy options and to invite public feedback on what would be considered to be an acceptable balance. For instance, an issue presented to the public was whether it would be ethically proper to pay a woman for donating eggs to research with the prospect of potential downside risks. These risks are explained as adverse health consequences to donors and exploitation of women (especially through financial inducement of poor women) in various forms. Should a payment or compensation scheme be allowed, the transnational reach of financial inducement was explicitly indicated as a source of concern, in view of the fact that many foreign women take up low-wage work in Singapore.

The appropriateness in the use of a particular classificatory term such as 'entity' as collective reference to an IVF embryo, a parthenote, and similar artefacts was based on opinions of medical and scientific experts. Medical and scientific opinions have also been heavily relied on in the assessment and articulation of scientific viability and known risks. I provide two illustrations. First, the relative effectiveness of 'fresh' as opposed to 'immature' eggs was based on scientific judgment. In the draft ED Consultation Paper, the replacement of the word 'ineffective' in the fourth line of the following paragraph with 'less effective' was based on medical and scientific opinions obtained:[753]

> In SCNT research, fresh eggs or surplus eggs from women undergoing fertility treatment are preferred to immature eggs or eggs that have failed to fertilise after IVF. Eggs that have failed to fertilise after IVF are ineffective as they have been shown to have limited developmental potential and the resulting embryos contained chromosomal abnormalities.

---

[753] Draft ED Consultation Paper, Fieldnotes, 27 September 2007, at paragraph 16 (emphasis added).

Second, the risk entailed in egg donation was also determined based on existing medical and scientific knowledge. The original paragraph 23 of the draft ED Consultation Paper explicitly highlighted the possible risk connected to hormonal stimulation for the purposes of egg donation:[754]

> There is also a concern that ovarian stimulation may lead to an increased risk of future infertility and cancers of the breast, ovary and uterus. However, there is no scientific evidence to support this. More research is required to determine if there are definite undesirable long-term effects of ovarian stimulation.

A milder language was subsequently adopted to de-emphasise potential risk from egg donation as the claim lacked scientific backing. The last sentence of the paragraph was deleted, and hence revised as:[755]

> While there is also a concern that ovarian stimulation may lead to an increased risk of future infertility and cancers of the breast, ovary and uterus, there is however no scientific evidence to support this.

There was initially uncertainty as to whether this potential risk should be stated in the ED Consultation Paper at all. The ultimate decision was to retain much of paragraph 23, primarily because there has been growing emphasis in ethical norms and legal developments on the importance of risk communication to enable the exercise of autonomous choice. The fact that research was not expected to confer any immediate benefit on research participants was a stronger justification for providing all relevant information, including infor-mation not regarded to be scientifically certain, to the participant. Some degree of agreement over expected level of risk enabled the consolidation of the issues and discussions in the ED Consultation Paper, after various meeting between September and October 2007.

---

[754] *Ibid*, paragraph 23.
[755] Draft ED Consultation Paper, Fieldnotes, 27 September 2007.

By November 2007, the objectives were subsequently systematised as a set of structured questions.

Early discussions on the provision of some form of payment for egg donation revolved around concerns over inducement and the commoditisation of the body. If payment is to be allowed, there was a sense that a regulatory body should be established or designated to ensure that there is no inducement in the procurement of eggs for research. Also recognised were the possible ramifications on organ donation on the one hand, and small-sample tissue donation on the other. The strong stance against the commodification of the body in ethics and in law was a major consideration. In Singapore, discussion on whether the rule against financial compensation for the provision of organs should be relaxed has remained controversial.[756] In a research setting, the BAC has earlier indicated in its report on human tissue research that the giving of tissue (including reproductive materials) for research should be altruistic although reasonable compensation for certain expenses (such as for travel) is permitted.[757]

Three possible policy approaches to financial compensation of women providing eggs for research are developed based on bioethical discourses on the subject, as well as the regulatory approaches of other jurisdictions. They are set out in the ED Consultation Paper as:[758]

---

[756] *Human Organ Transplant Act*, Cap. 131A, 2012 (revised edition), Sections 14 and 15.

[757] Bioethics Advisory Committee, *Human Tissue Research.* Singapore: Bioethics Advisory Committee, 2002, at paragraph 8.6, which states: "Although the donor may make an outright gift of his or her tissue in the sense that she renounces any property rights to or in connection with the tissue, it is entirely open to the donor to stipulate or define the kind of research uses to which the tissue may be applied." In the research context, commercial trading of human tissue is prohibited under Section 32 of the *Human Biomedical Research Act* of 2015.

[758] Paragraph 39 of the ED Consultation Paper, at A-14. These approaches are reiterated in paragraph 4.26 of the ED Report, at 21-22.

(a) No compensation but only reimbursement of expenses incurred;

(b) Reasonable compensation for time, risk and inconvenience, in addition to reimbursement of incurred expenses; and

(c) Substantial compensation that amounts to outright payment of eggs as a commodity.

The ruling out of option (c) was relatively straightforward as there are legal precedents going back several decades that block any donor's proprietary claim over her or his body or derivatives thereof.[759] It also noted a relatively universal agreement that the donor relinquishes all rights to the donated materials at the point of donation. However, the position should be made explicitly clear to donors. A practical rationale for this limitation is that it would be extremely difficult to apportion the value of the cells towards the final product as compared to all the information that researchers would gather and apply to the research. Evaluating this against the four different models of donation which Charis Thompson sets out as consent, 'propertisation', in-kind reciprocity and benefit sharing, a strong reading of the rule against propertisation and commercial-isation leaves only the option of consent model to be pursued.[760]

---

[759] The celebrated decision of the Supreme Court of California in *John Moore v Regents of the University of California et al.*, (1990) 51 Cal. 3d 120, 271 Cal. Rptr, has famously confined the legal discussion on the prospects of ownership over one's body to one on informed consent in common law jurisdictions. While this discussion has more recently been broadened to contractual rights over bodily materials in the English Court of Appeal's decision in *Yearworth v North Bristol NHS Trust* [2010] QB 1, commercial dealing in the body is not legally recognised, if not altogether prohibited. Also see: Shawn H E Harmon and Graeme T Laurie, *Yearworth v. North Bristol NHS Trust*: Property, Principles, Precedents and Paradigms, *Cambridge Law Journal* (2010) 69, 3: 476-493.

[760] Charis Thompson, *Good Science: The Ethical Choreography of Stem Cell Research*. Cambridge MA and London: MIT Press, 2013, at 180-181. An expectation that all contributions to research should be altruistic in a strong sense (i.e. no benefit apart from what is deemed to be 'fair') would preclude benefit-sharing, where donors and commercial firms share profit, or in-kind reciprocity, where donors

On the issue of compensation, it was felt that compensation (if allowed under options (a) and (b)) should be proportionate, although the difficulty in preventing inducement in every situation was acknowledged.[761] Compensation could range from taxi fare, hospital charges to loss of time from work. There would quite possibly be very uneven distribution for compensating loss of time from work, although it might be possible to avoid inducement from a theoretical standpoint, since a donor would not receive more than what she would otherwise gain from working, in contrast to providing a standard compensation, which might be an inducement for very poor women. On the practicality of providing compensation based on earnings, it was noted in a discussion that compensation based on tax returns, for National Servicemen called up for military training, could be an approach for such a scheme. More contentious is the comparator of an often large sum of money paid by pharmaceutical companies or clinical research companies to healthy volunteers for participating in Phase I drug trials. The justification that was presented for the large payment was compensation for the risk of exposing a person to a novel drug. But (as we shall see) egg donation was distinguished as encompassing rather different types of risk. For the purposes of the ED Consultation Paper, it was finally decided that compensation be provided for time, risk and inconvenience, and that the level of compensation should not be such that it amounts to an unreasonable inducement.

A difficulty that I was confronted with in working on the ED Consultation Paper was achieving a sufficiently clear understanding of the extent of the risks posed to donors, and especially the uncertainty of long term risks. Grappling further with the issue, it seems that there is a very deep institutional knowledge of risks. The documents of the NRC and the IOM have been important because

---

could derive non-monetary benefits. As we shall see, the latter in the form of an egg sharing scheme has not been considered to be ethically acceptable in Singapore.

761 Fieldnotes, 13 August 2008.

of the close research and policy relations that local researchers shared with colleagues in the US, as well as the recognition that it is the 'best scientific knowledge of the day' on health risks relating to egg donation. This display of 'trust' was a pragmatic choice, as the standards of good analysis are shared,[762] and it was not considered necessary to 're-invent the wheel' by re-examining the scientific and medical bases and perimeters. However, the NRC did also indicate that even for good qualitative analysis, one should be mindful that procedures tend not to be clear-cut, given the difficulties in validating findings, and that "technical adequacy is a necessary but not sufficient characteristic: analysis must also be relevant to the given risk decision."[763] In the end, these ambiguities did not appear to have a significant impact as the subject matter and target audiences were essentially self-selecting so that the criteria of effectiveness were broadly satisfied. For the public, its reception was mostly uncritical. The documents of the BAC were considered to communicate accurate information and were felt to be balanced.[764] In the section that follows, we consider the genealogy of a technical conception of risk that was adopted in the ED Report.

6.3 Genealogy of Risk

Heather Douglas explains that in the 1970's, a shift in policy stance away from absolute safety in regulatory efforts led to a focus on risk analysis for the determination of risk significance.[765] Fresh uncertainties were introduced into what was considered to be settled

---

[762] The NRC has set out several characteristic features of good quantitative analysis. National Research Council, *Understanding Risk: Informing Decisions in a Democratic Society*. Washington DC: National Academy Press, 1996, at 100-102.

[763] *Ibid*, at 101.

[764] *Ibid*, at 152. In the run-up to the public consultation, the operative criteria have been identified as: (1) getting the science right; (2) getting the right science; (3) getting the right participation; (4) getting the participation right; and (5) developing accurate, balanced and informative synthesis.

[765] Heather E Douglas. *Science, Policy, and the Value-Free Ideal*. Pittsburgh: University of Pittsburgh Press, 2009.

science (Latour's 'ricochet'?). Risk analysis itself is regarded as comprising two distinct parts: risk assessment (where scientific knowledge is relied upon to provide insights on the extent and nature of the risk), and risk management (where determinations are made as to how risk is to be handled in practice). The origins of the risk assessment/risk management distinction was in turn traced to William Lowrance, who according to Douglas wanted to keep the more 'objective' basis of risk assessment from essentially value-based risk management.[766] Douglas considers as advantageous this conceptual insulation of the more science-based part of risk analysis, as risk assessment "*should be* protected from pressures to shift the assessment of risk because the results are politically inconvenient".[767] This is further important in securing scientific integrity, and in summarily setting out current scientific understanding of the risk concerned.[768] From a social constructivist viewpoint however, Iain Wilkinson reminds us that: "... 'objectivity' is a social value and what we accept as 'objective' knowledge about our world is always shaped by the quality of our social commitments and cultural worldviews."[769]

6.3.1 *Risks Objectification*

This risk assessment/risk management distinction has been formally endorsed in a report (called the 'Red Book') of the NRC on risk

---

766 Lowrance attributed four steps to measuring or 'assessing' risks. See William W Lowrance. *Of Acceptable Risk: Science and the Determination of Safety*. Los Altos: W Kaufmann, 1976, at 18; cited by Heather Douglas: *Ibid*, at 140. Douglas indicates that "by separating 'measuring/assessing risk' from 'judging safety', Lowrance intended to separate the scientific component of the process – measuring the risk – from the value-laden social and political component of the process – deciding what to do about the risk": *Ibid*.

767 *Ibid*, at 141 (Emphasis in original).

768 Heather Douglas adds: "one reason for making a distinction between the two phases was to defend the integrity of the first phase, risk assessment, so that science could be protected from political pressure". *Ibid*, at 144.

769 Iain Wilkinson, *Risk, Vulnerability and Everyday Life*. London and New York: Routledge, 2010, at 57.

management by federal agencies. Primarily focused on risk to health presented by toxic substances such as asbestos, risk assessment was taken to be concerned with the characterisation of the potentially adverse health effects of human exposure to environmental hazards.[770] To this effect, four major steps are encompassed in the assessment: hazard identification, dose-response assessment, exposure assessment and risk characterisation.[771] In contrast, risk management is conceptualised as a decision-making process involving the weighing of policy alternatives and selecting the most appropriate regulatory action, in that the results of risk assessment are integrated with (engineering) data, as well as with social, economic and political concerns.[772] Acknowledging that there will inevitably be gaps in scientific knowledge and other limitations (such as limited analytical resources and analytical complexity), a recommendation in the Red Book was for uniform inference guidelines to be developed to ensure that risk assessments are consistently applied by federal agencies and protected from inappropriate policy influences.[773] Although there is a degree of flexibility, and legal authority among different sets of guidelines may differ, the guidelines are desirable as they:

> ... provide a systematic way to meet statutory requirements, to inform the public and regulated industries of agency policies, to stimulate public comment on those policies, to avoid arguing generic questions anew in each specific case, and to foster consistency and continuity of approach.[774]

---

[770] Committee on the Institutional Means for Assessment of Risk to Public Health, Commission on Life Sciences, National Research Council. *Risk Assessment in the Federal Government: Managing the Process*. Washington DC: National Academy Press, 1983, at 18.

[771] *Ibid*, at 19-20.

[772] *Ibid*, at 3.

[773] *Ibid*, at 7-8.

[774] *Ibid*, at 4.

As Douglas observes, the NRC attempts to secure scientific integrity by ensuring that specific economic and social considerations do not have undue influence, even though the risk assessment process is not completely scientific.[775]

This essentially technical approach to risk assessment broadly reflects popular understanding of risk as a calculative reasoning, often applied in the evaluation of acquisitive opportunities. For many, risk has negative connotations.[776] Weber has famously traced the origins of the economic life of modernity in Western Europe by relating a form of calculative reasoning embedded in everyday (religious) routines, to a 'formal rationality' that enables the efficient ordering and resolution of problems through technical rules and procedures in structures of economy, society and state.[777] To satisfy a psychological need to organise the world around an 'imperative of consistency', human beings have relied on this calculative rationality to mediate between their ideal expectations and the brute facts of experience.[778] An institutionalised form of rationality in pre-modernity is religion, which has attempted to provide meaning to all aspects of life and to provide practical solutions to pain and suffering.

6.3.2 *Are Objective Risks Real?*

But how real are 'risks'? Mary Douglas and Aaron Wildavsky think it depends on the institutions by which they are assessed. There are two other important aspects of risk. First, they observe that ideas about

---

775 Heather E. Douglas. *Science, Policy, and the Value-Free Ideal.* Pittsburgh: University of Pittsburgh Press, 2009, at 143.

776 Peter L Bernstein. *Against the Gods: The Remarkable Story of Risk.* New York: John Wiley & Sons, 1998.

777 Max Weber, *The Protestant Ethic and the Spirit of Capitalism.* New York and London: Routledge, 2005.

778 Max Weber, Religious rejections of the world and their directions. In H H Gerth and C W Mills (eds.), *From Max Weber.* London: Routledge, 1948, at 324.

environment pollution are an instrument of control.[779] This idea could be further developed by relating it to a Foucauldian notion of the relationship between power and subjectivity. In studying the impact of 'power relations' on the 'field of possibilities', Foucault shows how the assumption by individuals and groups of particular behaviours as a preferred way of living corresponds with a governmentality that structures the possibilities of action.[780] Here, the language of risk is a primary technique of governance, where risk discourse structures subjectivity and social relations, essentially by directing conduct along a designated course of action and towards particular goals.

The second aspect of risk that Douglas and Wildavsky explicate is positionality. Drawing on the theory of bounded rationality and prospect theory,[781] they observe that in risk perception, humans act less as individuals and more as social beings who have internalised social pressures and delegated their decision-making processes to institutions. They attempt to manage by following social rules on what to ignore when faced with unknown risk, primarily by institutionalising their problem-simplifying devices.[782] The knowledge of danger is necessarily partial and limited, as the kind of guesses about natural experience depends very largely on the kinds of moral education of the people doing the guessing. In contrast to formalistic methods of risk assessments, rational human behaviour does not use

---

[779] Mary Douglas and Aaron Wildavsky, *Risk and Culture: An Essay on the Selection of Technical and Environmental Dangers.* University of California Press: Berkeley and Los Angeles, 1982, at 47. It was noted that when central establishment is strong, it holds the monopoly of explaining the natural order. Its explanations of misfortune make social outcasts carry the stigma of vice and disease.

[780] Michel Foucault, The subject and power. In Hubert Dreyfus and Paul Rabinow (eds.), *Michel Foucault: Beyond Structuralism and Hermeneutics.* Chicago: Chicago University Press, 1982, pp 208-226, at 220-221.

[781] Prospect theory contradicts a generalisation in decision theory that people are generally risk adverse. They show that people are not risk averse for negative prospects, only positive ones. See Mary Douglas and Aaron Wildavsky, *Risk and Culture: An Essay on the Selection of Technical and Environmental Dangers.* University of California Press: Berkeley and Los Angeles, 1982, at 77-78.

[782] Douglas and Wildavksy seem to suggest that there is no intermediate ground between objectivity and subjectivity. *Ibid*, at 80.

elaborate calculations for making crisis decisions nor do they separate out risks one by one. However, the inability to systematise and rationalise all aspects of social life has contributed to more intense encounters with the 'irrationalities' in life, such as suffering and evil.

Building on Weberian analysis, Iain Wilkinson argues that distinct cultures of moral argument, juridical process and political response (with their own tradition of symbolic representation and established patterns of social disclosure and response) shape the courses of rationalisation taken up under the effort to restore order to the world in response to particular instances of catastrophe and human tragedy.[783] Mitchell Dean goes further in arguing that there is no such thing as risk in reality. Perhaps reflecting a degree of Weberian sensibility, risk is regarded as no more than a means of ordering reality and rendering it into a calculable form.[784] Still others have observed a neoliberal agenda in the language of risk as deployed in some manner of governance.[785] These arguments have found some support from developments in the life sciences. An effect of quantifying some aspects of uncertainty under the technical rubric of 'risk assessment' for the purposes of 'risk management' is to bring to light other aspects that are unquantifiable. It seems that those aspects that could be assessed and managed have generally been regarded as

---

[783] Iain Wilkinson, *Risk, Vulnerability and Everyday Life*. London and New York: Routledge, 2010, at 31-32. Iain Wilkinson echoes Weber's concern that even with more refined rationalisation in scientific technical analysis, there will be no guidance in fundamental human concerns relating to the meaning and purpose of life. See Max Weber, Science as a vocation. In H H Gerth and C W Mills (eds.), *From Max Weber*. London: Routledge, 1948.

[784] Mitchell Dean, Risk calculable and incalculable. In Deborah Lupton (ed.), *Risk and Sociocultural Theory: New Directions and Perspectives*. Cambridge: Cambridge University Press, 1999, pp 131-159, at 131-132.

[785] Hazel Kemshall, *Risk, Social Policy and Welfare*. Buckingham: Open University Press, 2002. See also Nikolas Rose, *Powers of Freedom: Reframing Political Thought*. Cambridge: Cambridge University Press, 1999.

scientific or medical risks, whereas those that could not were treated as 'ethical' or 'moral' concerns.

6.3.3 A Matter of Individual Choice

The limitations of technical risk assessment did not elude the attention of policy-makers and their expert advisors. In a subsequent report, the NRC highlighted that risks should be understood relationally, especially between producers and users of scientific information on risks and the ways in which such information is communicated.[786] This communicative aspect of risks was elaborated on by the Presidential/Congressional Commission on Risk Assessment and Risk Management. Taking up a topic identified as a research need in the NRC's 1989 report,[787] the US NRC elucidated on 'risk characterisation' as a means by which it could be improved to better inform decision-making and resolution of controversies over risk, in its 1996 report.[788] It argues that risk characterisation should be a decision-driven activity directed at informing choices and solving problems, and not an activity added at the end of risk analysis.[789] Reflecting on its earlier conceptualisation of risk, the NRC considered that risk characterisation should not only be a representation of

---

[786] Committee on Risk Perception and Communication, National Research Council. *Improving Risk Communication*. Washington, DC: National Academy Press, 1989, at x.

[787] *Ibid*, at 13. The other eight research topics have been identified as risk comparison, role of message intermediaries, pertinence and sufficiency of risk information, psychological stress, the 'mental models' of recipients, risk literacy, retrospective case studies of risk communication and contemporaneous assessment of risk management and risk communication.

[788] National Research Council, *Understanding Risk: Informing Decisions in a Democratic Society*. Washington DC: National Academy Press, 1996, at xi.

[789] *Ibid*, at 2. Risk characterisation as defined in the 1983 report suggests that it is the final step in the process of risk assessment. Commission on the Institutional Means for the Assessment of Risks to Public Health, Commission on Life Sciences, and National Research Council, *Risk Assessment in the Federal Government: Managing the Process*. Washington DC: National Academy Press, 1983, at 20.

existing scientific knowledge.[790] Aside from being decision driven, the process by which risk is characterised should recognise all significant concerns, reflect both analysis and deliberation, drawing on feedback from interested and affected parties, and be appropriate to the decision.[791] Under this expanded framework, the NRC sets out a new definition of:

> ... risk characterization [as] a synthesis and summary of information about a potentially hazardous situation that addresses the needs and interests of decision makers and of interested and affected parties. Risk characterization is a prelude to decision making and depends on an iterative, analytic-deliberative process.[792]

Within this framework, risk decision-making could be undertaken through a set of diagnostic steps.[793]

6.3.4 *Getting the Communication Right*

On the one hand, risk analysis could be a means by which one (especially an expert) could be seen as hiding his or her subjective preferences behind technical jargon and complexity in order to influence individuals, win an argument or push one's agenda. On the other hand, effective risk communication has become a critical means to improve understanding for the purposes of making informed choices. The division between the two has more often than not been difficult to distinguish clearly. A number of difficulties in communicating risks have been highlighted as including:

---

[790] National Research Council, *Understanding Risk: Informing Decisions in a Democratic Society*. Washington DC: National Academy Press, 1996, at 32.

[791] *Ibid*, at 16. Analysis is considered as using "rigorous, replicable methods, evaluated under the agreed protocols of an expert community – such as those of disciplines in the natural, social, or decision sciences, as well as mathematics, logic, and law – to arrive at answers to factual questions" (at 3-4), whereas deliberation is "any formal or informal process for communication and collective consideration of issues" (at 4).

[792] *Ibid*, at 27.

[793] *Ibid*, at 142-149.

(1) Absence of a single overriding problem that can be simply communicated;

(2) People do not all share common interests and values, hence expectations may differ greatly from one person to another;

(3) Values, preferences and information needs may not be determined easily;

(4) Risk management decisions do not affect everyone uniformly as some citizens may be harmed but others benefit; and

(5) Experts may not agree on scientific assessment of risks.[794]

Two other crucial sources of problems in risk communication have been identified as those deriving from institutional and political systems, and those from risk communicators and recipients. Systemic risks – defined by legal considerations, sources of (and fragmented) authority that includes formal (such as the state) and informal (such as peer pressure) ones, and systematic biases – tends to be more difficult to address than the latter. Risk communication is in turn focused on "establishing and recognising credibility, making the messages understandable, preparing messages in an emergency, capturing and focusing attention, and getting information".[795]

The challenges in 'risk communication' reflect the difficulties posed by uncertainties that remain unquantifiable. A direct impact of attempting to address such uncertainties by duly 'informing' the public provides the basis for Ulrich Beck's notion of 'risk society', which could be read as a heightened awareness of risk, and particularly its ubiquity. Beck argues that social classes have given way to individualisation as the implications of society now filter down to every person. Using the Chernobyl incident as a key epistemic event,

---

[794] Committee on Risk Perception and Communication, National Research Council. *Improving Risk Communication.* Washington, DC: National Academy Press, 1989, at 3-4.
[795] *Ibid,* at 6.

he argues that risks generated by industrial society affect everyone. However, the extent of exposure differs so that risk becomes a force that shapes relations rather than capital (or forces of production). Hence, risk is the 'reflexive modernisation' that is re-shaping the relationship between politics and science.[796] Unlike social phenomena like poverty, many types of risk are perceivable only through the intermediation of science. In that way, scientific knowledge constitutes 'persons' by risk profile,[797] but the process itself is abstract and lacks experiential basis. Consequently, the complexity and uncertainty in scientific causal analysis are often not sufficiently appreciated by the public, whereas science is more commonly understood as a means of control and prediction. However, disasters like Chernobyl heighten public awareness of the inability of science to control and predict, and thereby undermines the credibility of scientific expertise. In addition, science, itself a producer of risk, has often been only able to perceive the risk retrospectively.[798] Increased knowledge of risks creates its own sociality but not in the conventional sense of social classes.[799] Instead, Beck considers this sociality to nurture the *cosmopolitanisation* of an individual, this being a multidimensional process that involves:[800]

> ... the formation of multiple loyalties, the spread of transnational lifestyles, the rise of non-state political actors ... and the development of a different (cosmopolitan) globalization involving worldwide recognition of human rights, worker's rights, global protection of the environment, an end to poverty and so on.

---

796 Ulrich Beck. *Risk Society: Towards a New Modernity.* London: Sage Publications, 1992, at 36.
797 *Ibid*, at 59.
798 *Ibid*.
799 *Ibid*, at 47 and 88.
800 Ulrich Beck. Cosmopolitan realism: on the distinction between cosmopolitanism in philosophy and the social science, *Global Networks* (2004) 4, 2: 131-156, at 136.

Like Ulrich Beck, Anthony Giddens regards late modernity as a 'risk culture', characterised by institutional and individual reflexivity that attempt to cope with the expansion of disembedding mechanisms, especially in the forms of expert knowledge and globalisation.[801] Greater knowledge has contributed to greater uncertainty, as well as an awareness that expert knowledges are contingent and subject to revision.[802] More importantly, expert knowledges have become critical resources in construction of the self, which is seen as malleable and a reflective responsibility to be assumed in taking charge of one's life trajectory.[803] Threats are conceptualised as 'risks' rather than as a 'given', and can be subject to 'an essential calculus' to promote certainty and order. Where risk cannot be precisely calculated, the uncertainty could be further managed through the development of various 'scenarios' of risk with different degrees of plausibility.[804] Unlike Beck, Giddens argues that trust continues to be necessary, as 'acceptable' risk is central to sustaining trust and vital to establishing ontological security, or "the confidence that most human beings have in the continuity of their self-identity and in the constancy of the surrounding social and material environments of actions." Without this trust, one would be engulfed by feelings of anxiety and dread, and paralysed by inaction from indeterminacy.[805] Hence, whereas Beck considers a critique of expertise to be reflexivity, Giddens argues that reflexivity arises from trust in expertise.

---

801 Anthony Giddens, Modernity and Self-Identity: Self and Society in the Late Modern Age. Cambridge: Polity Press, 1991, at 3 and 21.
802 *Ibid*, at 20.
803 *Ibid*, at 32-33. Giddens observes (at 7) that the body is seen less as a 'given' but as subject to individual manipulation and will.
804 Ulrich Beck, Anthony Giddens and Scott Lash. *Reflexive modernization: politics, tradition, and aesthetics in the modern social order.* Cambridge: Polity Press, 1994, at 186.
805 Anthony Giddens, *The Consequences of Modernity.* Stanford: Stanford University Press, 1990, at 35 and 92.

6.3.5 *Intermediating Risks in Egg Donation*

An upshot of the elaborate discussion so far is to highlight the incremental development of an institutional risk discourse and communication. As we have noted, Foucauldian tradition makes clear that risk discourses establish social norms and realities, and could themselves be the basis of sociality. More importantly for us, this discursive development as various forms of institutional learning took place over three decades, and it ultimately culminated (somewhat overstated, but worth drawing the connection) in a workshop report by the IOM (which is part of the NRC) on medical risks in egg donation. This was one of the most important documents considered in preparing the ED Consultation Paper and subsequently the ED Report.[806] This report was highlighted by a member of the BAC's International Panel of Expert, Professor Bernard Lo, who was the co-chair of the Scientific and Medical Accountability Standards Working Group of the CIRM, which develops guidelines for stem cell research in California. Aware of the risks that oocyte donation could present, the CIRM contracted with the National Academies to organise a workshop to gather expert opinion on "what is known about these risks, what needs to be known, and what can be done to minimise them".[807] The report provides a summary of the views expressed by participants at the workshop held in San Francisco on 28 September, 2006.

Two different categories of potential risks were identified by the workshop participants: 'acute risks' and 'long-term risks'. The first category of 'acute risks' comprises three sub-categories that are linked to the different stages of the oocyte retrieval process. The risk of ovarian hyperstimulation syndrome (OHSS) is an 'acute risk' that could arise from a regime of hormone shots administered to donors

---

806 Institute of Medicine and National Research Council, Linda Giudice, Eileen Santa and Robert Pool (eds.). *Assessing the Medical Risks of Human Oocyte Donation for Stem Cell Research*. Washington DC: National Academies Press, 2007.

807 *Ibid*, at 1.

to increase the number of eggs that can be retrieved. The symptoms to OHSS include increased ovarian size, nausea and vomiting, accumulation of fluid in the abdomen, breathing difficulties, hemo-concentration and, in the most severe cases, blood clots or kidney failure. It was generally felt that the risk of OHSS for egg donors is lower than for women involved in IVF as a large percentage of the severe complications of OHSS are linked to hormonal changes from accompanying pregnancy. While it is not possible to fully eliminate the risk of OHSS, it could be minimised through a number of precautionary practices including the modification of the hormone treatment regimen to minimise the factors that contribute to hyper-stimulation (such as higher than normal egg follicle count) and the exclusion of certain donors, such as those with irregular menstrual cycles, ovaries with polycystic appearance and possibly those with high levels of androgens.[808]

The other two sub-categories of 'acute risks' are associated with the surgical procedure, including anaesthesia, and psychological disturbances (that could include anxiety, mood swings and post-donation adjustments).[809] Surgery is required to retrieve the eggs from the follicles upon the completion of hormone treatment. A needle is used, penetrating through the vagina and into the ovary, to aspirate individual follicles in the retrieval process. There is a very small risk of vaginal bleeding, intestinal injuries and peritonitis, and only two in every 100,000 cases had complications that required surgery to correct.[810] Complications due to infection and ovarian torsion were also found to be of very low risk. A number of factors could increase the risk of adverse occurrences associated with surgery, but they were considered to be more prevalent among IVF

---

[808] *Ibid*, at 2 and 17-22.
[809] *Ibid*, at 11.
[810] *Ibid*, at 38-39.

patients than healthy oocyte donors.[811] Risks from anaesthesia were also found to be low as egg donors are unlikely to share certain high-risk factors.[812] As for psychological disturbances, a categorical analysis was similarly applied, where psychological risk was associated with the screening process, problems surrounding the donation procedure itself, and post-donation adjustment to the donation.[813] These risks could be ameliorated through a better selection process, and through more effective counselling.

The second category of potential risks is longer-term, and relate to the development of breast, ovarian and endometrial cancers, as well as concerns over its impact on future fertility.[814] An expert (Dr Roberta Ness) indicated that there is some data to suggest that intensive and regular use of fertility drugs could cause an increase in the risk of breast, ovarian and especially endometrial cancers. Studies have been inconclusive as they did not follow their subjects for sufficient durations of time.[815] More research was considered to be necessary to examine the long-term impact that fertility drugs may have on breast and ovarian cancer prevalence rates. For uterine cancer, the possibility of an increased risk from the use of fertility drugs was recognised even though available data did not have statistical significance.[816] As for the impact of fertility drugs on a woman's long-term fertility, this concern was considered to be scientifically unfounded as no evidence was found to support such a claim.[817]

---

811 *Ibid*, at 39; such factors include previous surgeries, a history of pelvic inflammatory disease, endometriosis, and pelvic adhesions.
812 *Ibid*; such factors were indicated as being male, older, obese or having surgery in an emergency setting.
813 *Ibid*, at 48.
814 *Ibid*, at 11.
815 *Ibid*, at 26.
816 *Ibid*, at 29.
817 *Ibid*, at 30.

As a matter of risk communication, it is interesting to note that the experts have cautioned against an unreflective reliance on probabilities. This passage from the report is instructive on the notion of risk as interpreted vis-à-vis a particular type of risk subject:[818]

> Nearly all of the speakers cautioned against relying on probabilities because the most important strategy in collecting oocytes for stem cell research is to be cautious in relying on probabilities, because the most important strategy to minimise the potential risks to oocyte donors is to make decisions based on *common sense on a case-by-case basis*. Of course, physicians try not to subject any of their patients to unnecessary risks, but because research donors represent a special situation – women who are undergoing a procedure not for their own benefit but for the benefit of others – the workshop participants said that *even greater care* should be taken to make sure that these donors do not pay for their altruism with their own health.

This epistemic history of risk assessment, management and communication has been critical to the way that the BAC has categorised the types of donors, and the ethical considerations and requirements that attend to each category. In addition, the BAC has adopted similar proposals to minimise the risk of OHSS and to encourage alternative sources of oocytes to be considered, such as the use of immature eggs (that could be matured *in vitro*), deriving eggs from polycystic-appearing ovaries, and retrieving eggs from cadavers.[819] Neither the ED Consultation Paper nor the ED Report set out the technical information in great depth but relied on referencing and appending such information. Instead, with the benefit of a somewhat pre-fabricated framework for risk assessment and management, the BAC was able to focus on the definition of 'ethical' risks. As we will recall from our discussion above, such risks relate to uncertainties

---

[818] *Ibid*, at 54 (Emphasis Added).
[819] *Ibid*, at 60.

that could not be adequately quantified within existing knowledge systems.

6.3.6 The 'Remainder' Problem

As we have seen, the approach of the NRC and its related bodies (particularly the NAS and the IOM) in studying the link between risk science and policy has been to focus on specific aspects of risk. Subsequent reports have addressed the responsiveness of risk assessment, communicability of risks and how risks could be understood through different means of characterisation. More recent studies have focused on risks generated through specific scientific practices or usage. Other policy bodies have preferred a broader 'framework-like' approach. While acknowledging the usefulness of risk assessment as an analytical process, the Presidential/Congressional Commission explained that this process:

> ... was developed because Congress, regulators, and the public require scientists to go beyond scientific observations of the relationships between exposures to chemicals and pollutants and their effects on people, the environment, or test systems [i.e. risk factors], and to rely on many scientific inferences and assumptions to answer social questions about what is unsafe.[820]

While public expectation might not be simply altered, the Commission considered it more feasible for analysts to provide explicit descriptions of the "assumptions, data sources, sources of uncertainty, and distribution of benefits and costs across society associated with economic analyses, in parallel with the descriptions associated with

---

820 The Presidential/Congressional Commission on Risk Assessment and Risk Management. *Risk Assessment and Risk Management in Regulatory Decision-Making*. Washington DC: The Presidential/Congressional Commission on Risk Assessment and Risk Management, Final Report, Vol. 2, 1997, at iii.

risk assessments."[821] The Commission further perceived a need to re-calibrate regulatory focus from micro-assessment of risk to the overall goal of sustainable development through risk reduction and improved health status.[822] Under its proposed Risk Management Framework, it would be necessary to conceptualise a potential or current problem in the broader context of public or environmental health in order to manage risks more effectively and efficiently.[823]

More recently, the International Risk Governance Council (IRGC) – a private, independent, not-for-profit Foundation based in Geneva – published a White Paper on an integrated, holistic and structured approach (or framework) to risk governance.[824] As with other policy-based conceptualisation of risks, the risk governance framework proposed by the IRGC has, as its 'generic elements', risk assessment, risk management and risk communication. Unlike other relatively mechanistic approaches to risk management however, the IRGC attempts to include societal context to its framework, but taking into account risk perception, interaction among different actors, policy-making and regulatory style, and socio-political impacts. By contextualising the generic elements of risk governance, the IRGC puts forward a risk process as a conceptual tool, or 'risk handling chain'.[825] A key outcome of this risk process is a system of characterisation as simple, complexity-induced, uncertainty-induced or ambiguity-induced. Categorisation can then enable the selection and implementation of an appropriate management strategy, ranging from routine-based risk reduction considerations and practices, to measures that enable systemic risk absorption and conflict

---

[821] *Ibid*, at iv.
[822] *Ibid*, at i-ii.
[823] *Ibid*, at ii to iii.
[824] International Risk Governance Council. *Risk Governance: Towards an Integrative Approach*. Geneva: International Risk Governance Council, September 2005, at 5.
[825] *Ibid*, at 12.

resolution.[826] Risk communication is treated separately as being cyclical in character (like a feedback loop) and recognised as a companion to all four phases of addressing and handling risk.[827] Underlying the framework of risk process and communication are three major value-based premises and assumptions, these being the inclusion of both the 'factual' and the 'socio-cultural' dimension of risk, emphasis on inclusiveness as a critical aspect of the governance process, and implementation of the principles of 'good' governance.[828] Further helpful in its analysis is the recognition that the nature of risk management also depends on regulatory regimes or governmental styles (or, more generally, political culture). The IRGC observes:[829] "Risk management depends, however, not only on scientific input. It rather rests on three components: systematic knowledge, legally prescribed procedures and social values ..."

The already well-established framework in relation to quantifyable risks associated with egg donation was adopted in the ED Consultation Paper. Its gravitational force is to a large degree grounded relationally to various expert communities and to the perception or reputation of doing 'good science'. In this respect, Deborah Lupton seems right to criticise the representations of modernity by Beck and Giddens as being too simplistic for the failure to acknowledge the complexity of responses to expert knowledge. They are also too speculative about structural and organisational processes without sufficient acknowledgement of "the communal, aesthetic and shared symbolic aspects of risk in their focus on

---

826 *Ibid*, at 15-16.
827 Key topics to be addressed in risk communication have been set out by the IRGC, having taken into account major functions of risk communication. *Ibid*, at 54-57.
828 *Ibid*, at 12. The principles of 'good governance' include "transparency, effectiveness and efficiency, accountability, strategic focus, sustainability, equity and fairness, respect for the rule of law and the need for the chosen solution to be politically and legally realisable as well as ethically and publicly acceptable".
829 *Ibid*, at 62.

individualisation."[830] Rather than perceiving risk as 'out there' and directive, Mary Douglas and Aaron Wildavsky have argued that risk is, or otherwise relates to, the 'other' against which blame could be attributed in order to strengthen group unity. Hence even in the face of seemingly ever present risks of human violence, risks from technology or from economic failure, the manner in which they are identified and addressed is never straightforward but settled by a preference among different kinds of favoured social institutions.[831] They suggest that risk could be deployed to maintain unity in the face of eroding group solidarity. Plausibility depends on enough people wanting to believe in the theory, and this depends on enough people being committed to whatever moral principle it protects.[832] Hence, "[p]ollution ideas cluster thickest where cherished values conflict".[833] Even then, unquantifiable risks that fall outside the purview of expert knowledge remain. The potential long term health risks that the egg donation could pose is acknowledged in the ED Consultation Paper, aside from moral concerns over the commodification and commercialisation of the human body and with exploitation. These then became the primary concerns of the ED Consultation Paper and the public consultation.

6.4 Public Consultation on Egg Donation

During the public consultation, the ED consultation paper was sent to 94 research, governmental and healthcare institutions (including 21 fertility clinics) and professional and religious organisations for

---

[830] Deborah Lupton, *Risk*. London and New York: Routledge, 1999, at 82. See also John Tulloch and Deborah Lupton. *Risk and Everyday Life*. London, Thousand Oaks and New Delhi: Sage, 2003.

[831] Mary Douglas and Aaron Wildavsky, *Risk and Culture: An Essay on the Selection of Technical and Environmental Dangers*. University of California Press: Berkeley and Los Angeles, 1982, at 81 and 187.

[832] *Ibid*, at 38.

[833] *Ibid*, at 43.

comment. Members of the public could download a copy of the consultation paper through the BAC's website, and feedback could also be provided through various means including email, an online discussion forum and an e-consultation platform (through a public outreach system called 'REACH'). Feedback from the discussion forum and e-consultation platform was provided by way of responses to questions set out in the context of a factual scenario and in the format below.[834]

Public Consultation on Donation of Human Eggs for Research

The Bioethics Advisory Committee (BAC) has recently released a Consultation Paper on the donation of human eggs for research. [link provided] The Paper raises issues related to the provision of human eggs for research, especially research involving embryonic stem cells. The BAC seeks views from the public on:

- whether healthy women, not undergoing fertility treatment should be allowed to donate eggs for research and if so, under what conditions; and
- whether compensation of egg donors amounts to inducement.

You are also invited to attend a public talk on this topic on 22 November 2007. The details are available on the BAC website: [weblink provided]

You may contribute to the Consultation by:

a.   Providing us your views on the scenario below or any issues in the Consultation Paper by sending an email to contactus@bioethics-singapore.org or by post to:
11 Biopolis Way
#10-12 Helios
Singapore 138667

b.   Setting up a group or using an existing group that meets regularly for a related or unrelated purpose, to discuss these issues. Where there is a significant number of people meeting, and if it is considered helpful, representatives from the BAC Secretariat will make every effort to participate. If you would like the BAC Secretariat to be present at your discussion, you may send an email to contactus@bioethics-singapore.org.

The BAC will be receiving feedback until 7 January 2008.

Figure 6.1.   Public Consultation on Donation of Human Eggs for Research

---

834   The scenario, as well as a summary of responses from REACH Online Discussion Forum and e-Consultation, is set out in the ED Report (at pp D-1 to D-3), although the overall format is reproduced here for completeness.

Scenario

Abi's father suffers from Parkinson's disease. Since his late 40s, her father started to experience muscle rigidity, tremors, memory loss and a slowing of movement. The family is concerned that he may lose physical mobility in a few years. From what she has been told, Parkinson's disease affects the nerve cells in a part of the brain that controls muscle movement. The exact cause is not known and there is also no cure for it.

Abi learnt that her niece, Carol, is part of a research team at Merlion Medical School (MMS) that is conducting embryonic stem cell research that could lead to a cure for the disease in the long run. However, the research is proceeding slowly due to a shortage of human eggs. Abi feels that she should donate her eggs to help advance the research even though the procedures involved are invasive and carries some health risk. While a cure may not be found quickly enough to help her father, future generations may benefit from the research.

Abi discussed her intention with her older cousin, Betty, who will be undergoing in vitro fertilisation (IVF) at Merlion Hospital. IVF is a clinical and laboratory procedure whereby the eggs and sperm from a couple are extracted and fertilised outside their bodies. Such a procedure is a kind of assisted reproduction aimed at increasing the chances of a couple conceiving a baby. After speaking with Abi, Betty is also thinking of contributing some of her eggs not used in her fertility treatment to MMS.

We would like to invite you to provide your views on the following:

(1) Do you think Abi, who is 35 years of age and a mother of three children, should be able to donate eggs to MMS for research? If Abi needs to take time off from her work so that she could donate her eggs, do you think she should be compensated (either fully or in part) for the loss of her income, inconvenience and risk involved? If so, what type of compensation would be acceptable and not amount to an inducement?

(2) Carol, who is 21 years of age, was inspired by her aunt Abi and she wants to donate her eggs to help advance the work of her research team. Do you think she should be allowed to do so? If she is, do you think she should receive any payment for the time, inconvenience and risk involved? Carol is a graduate student at MMS and does not receive an income.

(3) IVF is an expensive procedure, and even then, the couple undergoing the treatment may not be successful in conceiving a child. Eggs that are left over from the treatment may be kept for future use, donated to other infertile couples, donated for research or destroyed. If Betty, decides to donate her "spare" eggs to MMS for research, do you think she should be subsidised by MMS for the cost of her IVF treatment?

Figure 6.1.   (*Continued*)

The aesthetics of the narrative or the way in which it has been presented should be noted in that a strong association is made between the 'public' and an underlying notion of mutual respect and reciprocity. First, the main objectives of the consultation are clearly set out as a public concern. In providing feedback, a respondent is clearly aware that she or he is participating in a public activity. Implicitly, purely personal prejudices or biases are discouraged in favour of considered viewpoints. Second, publicity for the various feedback channels – including the possibility of participation in focus group discussions organised by civic groups – was broadcasted through a press conference and in subsequent media reports, thereby demonstrating an openness or receptiveness to a gathering of views from non-specialist quarters of society. Third, a notion of mutual respect and reciprocity bordering on altruism is implicit in the motives of the women in the narrative who were in a position to contribute eggs for research. A contrast may perhaps be made with the situation in South Korea, where nationalism was perceived to be a driving force behind egg donation for research – at least prior to the unravelling of the scandal around Professor Hwang.[835] It was in this overall setting that respondents were presented with a number of issues that related to the notions of 'compensation',[836] 'spare' eggs, 'inducement' and 'safety'. These issues may be generalised in the following manner:

(a) Whether a middle-aged woman with children should be able to donate eggs for research, and if so, whether she should be compensated for loss of income, inconvenience and risk involved;

---

[835] Leo Kim. Explaining the Hwang scandal: national scientific culture and its global relevance. *Science as Culture* (2008) 17: 397-415, at 408, 410-411.

[836] In the consultation paper, 'compensation' is defined as "recompense for presumptive loss of income and/or risk and inconvenience", whereas reimbursement relates to "repayment for incurred expenses": ED Report at A-20, footnote (3). These definitions have been retained in the ED Report (at 19). See also discussion in Paragraph 4.26 of the ED Report (at 21).

(b) Whether a young healthy woman should be able to donate eggs for research, and if so, whether she should be similarly compensated; and

(c) Whether a woman who contributed her 'spare eggs' from fertility treatment should be subsidised for the cost of her treatment.

At the end of the consultation, 47 entries were made (on an anonymous basis) at the online discussion forum and the e-consultation platform, although at least 12 entries, and possibly up to 20, of which could have been made by a particular individual. This respondent appeared to be supportive of egg donation by women for research, but much concern was expressed over payment that could lead to financial inducement and exploitation. A number of proposals were made, including procedural safeguards against inducement. For instance, a cap was proposed by this respondent on financial compensation if provided, and this amount should be centrally regulated.

On the first issue, the general view was that women should be free to decide whether to donate eggs for research, although there was concern over possible health risks and inducement to donate for monetary gain. As to the subject of compensation (the second issue in the scenario), there was general agreement to some compensation being provided to middle-aged donors as it was felt that these women should not be financially disadvantaged from contributing to the advancement of science, which was seen as a public good. As with the first issue, concerns were expressed over possible health risks and exploitation. In relation to the 21 year-old graduate student, the public was similarly of the view that compensation should be provided although the risk of coercion and inducement was considered to be greater. This may be attributable to the scandal in South Korea, which received wide media coverage. There was no agreement over what donors should be compensated for, but many were in favour of compensation for time. In addition, many respondents were against commercialisation of the human body although a small number voiced support for it. The third issue related to a compensated egg sharing scheme (where researcher could subsidise the IVF treatment of a woman who agreed to contribute some of her eggs or embryos for research), which is allowed in the UK.[837] A majority of the respondents indicated that the cost of fertility treatment of a woman who donated her 'spare' eggs for research should be subsidised, although some strongly rejected this and regarded such a scheme as effectively commercialisation.

The consultation paper did address many of the concerns of respondents, with the exception of:

(1) Privacy of donors and the confidentiality of their personal information,

(2) The provision of proper information to donors and in a manner that is effective in facilitating understanding, and

(3) The availability of medical care for short-term and long-term adverse health consequences arising from the egg donation procedure.

The third point was also raised in written responses from members of the public, including public institutions, to the key issues raised in the consultation paper.[838]

A majority of the respondents was in favour of allowing healthy women to donate eggs for research. Those who opposed were mostly motivated by religious concerns, although some (such as the Singapore Nursing Board) did not consider the benefit to outweigh

---

[837] Human Fertilisation and Embryology Authority. Code of Practice. London: Human Fertilisation and Embryology Authority, 2009 (October 2015, 8th Edition), at 105-111 (Principle 12).

[838] These respondents were Graduates' Christian Fellowship (at C-11 of ED Report), Institute of Mental Health (at C-16 of ED Report), Law Society of Singapore (at C-20 of ED Report), Dr Chuah Khoon Leong (at C-48 of ED Report), Dr Suresh Nair (at C-69 of ED Report) and Professor George Wei (at C-102 of ED Report).

the health risk entailed. Those who considered egg donation to be similar to participation in a clinical trial argued that compensation for risk should be provided. Others were concerned about inducement, and proposed some form of insurance scheme to be implemented as compensation for risk.[839] There was also some support for compensation for inconvenience, and one respondent proposed compensation for emotional and psychological harm.[840] In addition, two respondents proposed incentives to be provided in order to encourage women to donate eggs for research. For instance, one respondent proposed a complimentary oocyte banking scheme to encourage career-minded women to donate unused eggs for research.[841] Compensated egg sharing scheme was supported by four respondents, but was opposed by at least one institution and one individual.[842]

The respondents presented a number of conditions relating to informed consent. One such condition was that consent should be taken by an independent third party. There should be clear discussion on vulnerable groups, which in this case would include not only legal minors and the mentally incapacitated, but also people who are in economically, socially or by employment vulnerable position where there might be some degree of coercion (such as the graduate

---

[839] There was no agreement on whether risk should be compensated as it was supported by two respondents (such as the Institute of Mental Health and Dr Alexis Heng) but opposed by some members of the IRB of the National Dental Centre.

[840] Dr Alexis Heng, Associate Professor Allen Yeoh and some members of the IRB of the National Dental Centre indicated that compensation for inconvenience should be provided. Mr Patrick Goh proposed that compensation should include any emotional or psychological harm (ED Report, at C-50).

[841] Feedback from Dr Suresh Nair: ED Report, at C-4 and C-5.

[842] Prof Christopher Chen (ED Report, at C-8), some members of the IRB of the NDC (ED Report, at C-34), Dr Alexis Heng (ED Report, at C-61 to C-64) and Dr S Nair (ED Report, at C-68 and C-69) expressed support for the 'compensated egg sharing scheme', but this scheme was explicitly opposed by the National Council of Churches of Singapore (ED Report, at C-32) and by Professor Chan Soh Ha (ED Report, at C-47).

students in the South Korean incident). Notwithstanding the research focus, this would be similar to the practice in IVF treatment.[843]

Concerning the sale of eggs, there was unanimity among respondents that commercialisation of any part of the body, including eggs, should be prohibited. Clear regulatory mechanisms were proposed in response to the fourth issue. Members of the legal community indicated that the regulatory scope in 2007 was lacking in its reach, and that it should encompass all biomedical research in Singapore (this concern has been addressed by the HBRA of 2015). It was further proposed that egg donation be limited to Singaporeans and permanent residents in view of the significant socio-economic gap between these classes of women and foreign workers. Other comments included a compensatory mechanism for adverse events, including some form of mandatory no fault based insurance coverage.[844] Feedback from the public consultation suggests that the risk account provided by the BAC has been made 'real', so that public focus shifted to concerns over undue inducement and exploitation.

6.5 The Public Sphere

STS presents a citizen as possessing varied knowledge systems located in particular practices, subjectivities and identities. Such knowledge systems may be specialist ones, non-specialist or lay knowledge systems, or experience-based expertise. While it is recognised that different forms of expertise are not readily combined, scientific knowledge is regarded as effectively cultural in that it "embodies, reflects and projects commitments of a human kind, which also shape human relations and identifies, imagined communities and

---

843 Fieldnotes, 16 January 2008, M7.

844 The Law Society of Singapore (ED Report, at C-21) and Dr Suresh Nair (ED Report, at C-69) suggested that compensation for risk can take the form of mandatory insurance.

ontologies".[845] Practicing citizenship is regarded in turn as a learning process.[846] Limited accessibility here provides an occasion for criticism, but it is questionable if there is any truly neutral deliberative forum that does not within a framework elevate some perspectives or agenda over others.[847] Issues that are raised as a matter of public concern implicate certain actors jointly and antagonistically.[848] There are not many issues that could be framed in such a manner as to be of practical relevance to every member of a society. Neither would it be sensible to consider a society to be 'democratic' only if its members could (and would be willing) to vote on every sort of issue that may have some implication on them.

Furthermore, globalisation has contributed to greater diversity in the framers of issues that relate to stem cell science and technology. Like genetics, stem cells became what Sarah Franklin considers to be a 'global biological', replete with imagery of technological potency, human frailty and future salvation.[849] Given the myriad of interests,

---

[845] Melissa Leach, Ian Scoones and Brian Wynne. Introduction: science, citizenship and globalization. In *Science and citizens: Globalization and the challenge of engagement*, edited by Melissa Leach, Ian Scoones and Brian Wynne. London and New York: Zed Books, 2007, pp 3-14, at 12-13.

[846] *Ibid*, at 30-31.

[847] *Ibid*, at 30.

[848] Noortje Marres, The issues deserve more credit: pragmatist contributions to the study of public involvement in controversy. *Social Studies of Science* (2007) *37*, 759-780, at 772-773. See also Noortje Marres, Front-staging Nonhumans: Publicity as a Constraint on the Political Activity of Things. In Bruce Braun and Sarah J Whatmore (eds.), *Political Matter: Technoscience, Democracy, and Public Life*. Minneapolis and London: University of Minnesota Press, 2010, pp 177-209. Drawing on John Dewey's notion of the 'public', Marres argues that 'green technologies' such as long-life bulbs and energy-efficient domestic appliances act as political mediators of green governmentality on the one hand and of civic practices on the other. Material harm, made 'real' by electric meters and energy standards, contributes to the formation of a 'public' that does not other map neatly with any other social groupings.

[849] Sarah Franklin, Stem cells r us: emergent life forms and the global biological. In Aihwa Ong and Stephen J Collier, *Global Assemblages: Technology, Politics and Ethics as Anthropological Problems*. Singapore: Blackwell Publishing, 2006, pp 59-78, at 61.

meanings, hopes, and concerns – both global and local – that constitute stem cell science and technology, public accessibility has presented significant practical challenges to policy and bioethical bodies like the BAC. Whereas the outreach of the BAC has been broad, the responses elicited appear to comprise a consistent group of core institutions. There could be a few reasons for this. First, many of the social roles that were performed by civic organisations have been progressively subsumed within the various instruments and organs of the state. Second, individual members of society – even highly qualified ones – consider their personal views to be of insignificant weight and would prefer to speak on behalf of, or otherwise as part of, a group or institution. Third, the deliberative 'space' that is created in the consultation papers give emphasis to a notion of citizens as socially embedded and membership within a community. This element is arguably present even in the more generic REACH online consultative platform. Hajer's observation on the performative aspect of decision-making in rebuilding Ground Zero is pertinent: "It is the very stagedness here that creates the power of the deliberative moments: by virtue of being staged they have generated a moment in the public consciousness."[850] Fourth, the state is generally perceived by members of the public as coherent and rational, even if restrictive on issues that are regarded as politically sensitive.[25] But as Stephen Hilgartner notes,[851] champions of transparency sometimes romanticise openness, without adequately considering the merits of institutional procedures or fully recognising the ubiquity and inevitability of information control. He persuasively argues that the fundamental choice is not between the transparent or the opaque, but different systems that shape the role of experts and audience, and different

---

[850] Maarten A Hajer. *Authoritative governance: Policy-making in the Age of Mediatization.* New York: Oxford University Press, 2009, at 185.

[851] Stephen Hilgartner. *Science on stage: expert advice as public drama.* Stanford: Stanford University Press, 2000, at 149-150.

ways in which science is presented on the public stage. Sheila Jasanoff advances a similar point, in her indication that:[852]

> America's particular democratic settlement, in which public claims are continually tested by sceptical citizens and journalists ... the very idea of public demonstrations as a space of experiment is culturally particular, not universal, way of engaging citizens. It assumes that disclosure and transparency are *possible*, and that people have the will, the means, and the competence to evaluate the claims and proofs presented to them.

In East Asia, STS scholars have begun reflecting on the limitations of a deliberative model of public participation that they have enthusiastically promoted.[853] Commenting on three papers that address citizen participation in relatively disparate areas of science and technology, Brian Wynne's observation of the inadequacies of conventional visions and practices of public participation is instructive:[854]

> Not only is it *not* a matter of claiming that publics know as well as experts in their specialist field; we should also not operate in the belief that citizens have well-articulated imaginations about what they believe to be desirable or possible in domains such as health, energy, agriculture and food. Thus to expect such inputs as a currency of participation processes is optimistic, even if searching and salient questions will be posed of experts posing their own such imaginations.

---

852 Sheila Jasanoff. *Designs on nature: science and democracy in Europe and the United States*. Princeton and Oxford: Princeton University Press, 2005, at 263 (emphasis in original).

853 Dung-sheng Chen and Chia-Ling Wu. Introduction: Public Participation in Science and Technology in East Asia. *East Asian Science, Technology and Society: an International Journal* (2007) 1: 15-18, at 18.

854 Brian Wynne. Public Participation in Science and Technology: Performing and Obscuring a Political-Conceptual Category Mistake. *East Asian Science, Technology and Society: an International Journal* (2007) 1: 99-110, at 107.

In the light of these arguments, Massimiano Bucchi and Federico Neresini have attempted to map the different forms of public participation given varying degrees of spontaneity and intensity of participation in the process of knowledge construction. They insightfully observe:[855]

> If the "anaesthetisation" of politics by the massive injection of techno-scientific expertise has not been sufficient to deal with crucial dilemmas, this is not a reason to expect that those same dilemmas will be solved simply by injecting democratic arrangements into science, especially if democracy is defined with its most simplistic meaning of "majority voting".

The 'public' that has emerged from the BAC's work shares certain features with Annelise Riles's PAWORNET (an information sharing network). In her study, Riles observes that networkers did not understand themselves to share a set of values, interests or culture. Instead, they understood themselves to be sharing in their involvement in a certain network that was a form of institutionalised association devoted to information sharing.[856] What defined networkers most of all was the fact that they were personally and institutionally connected or knowledgeable about the world of Pacific institutions and networks. In particular, it was the work of creating documents, organising conferences, or producing funding proposals that generated a set of personal relations that drew people together and also created divisions of its own. The 'public' of the ED Report comprised institutions and a number of individuals – often institutionally connected – that represented a diverse set of values, interests and perhaps culture (construed in terms of their day-to-day practices in

---

855 Massimiano Bucchi and Federico Neresini, Science and Public Participation. In E J Hackett, O Amsterdamska, M Lynch and J Wajcman (eds.), *The Handbook of Science and Technology Studies*. Cambridge MA: MIT Press, 2008, pp 449-472, at 461-464 and 466.

856 Annelise Riles. *The network inside out*. Michigan: University of Michigan Press, 2001, at 58-59, and 68.

the least). This resembles a network in a number of ways (but it is not quite a conventional network, to be sure). They were brought into a particular set of relationship within a deliberative space created in the main by the consultation papers and reinforced through a variety of means that included public meetings, conferences and feedback sessions. Arguably, even individual feedback from REACH encompasses a certain kind of pre-existing (sub-) network that has been formed with a view to soliciting relatively more spontaneous and independent, uninvited forms of civil participatory action. But this 'network' is not a static one and, as far as I am aware, none has been actively sustained. It varies with, but also shapes, the broader phenomenon of science and expectations as to how science ought to be engaged. In this connection, Riles's observation is instructive: "It is not that networks 'reflect' a form of society, therefore, nor that society creates its artefacts ... Rather, it is all within the recursivity of a form that literally speaks about itself".[857] It may be more accurate to consider the BAC's work as subsisting within a 'public sphere', which is a virtual deliberative space where mediated communication on 'bioethical' issues takes place. To be sure, I am not saying that the recursive form of a 'network' is displaced by this 'public sphere'. Rather, the latter is to my mind a more convenient reference to associations of networks that could be highly complex, organic, overlapping and intermeshed. They are sometimes contingent and fleeting, but often difficult to pin down. Yet their impact – those 'nodes' in the networks – may well endure. The idea of a 'public sphere' is intended only to bracket out this communicative space, within which the ideals of reciprocity, inclusiveness, the common good and a public rationality could to varying degrees be attributed.[858] For the BAC, it

---

[857] *Ibid*, at 69.

[858] One possibility is to think of this interactive space as Rawls's 'public political forum', although it is difficult to say if the issues deliberated upon qualify as constitutional essentials or as a basic matter of economic justice. Instead, Habermas's ideal typical notion of a 'public sphere' is loosely applied here, only

is also an avenue where its recommendations could be validated through public scrutiny. I will re-visit this topic in the next chapter.

Perhaps the critical question is not so much that of who constitutes the 'public', but what is being done in the 'public sphere' and why. There are ample studies to show that the 'public' is to a large degree constituted by the intermediary (particularly the mass media) that channels scientific knowledge and 'progress' in biomedical sciences to the larger lay audience. For instance, Eric Jensen has shown that media accounts of therapeutic cloning are almost always affected by many factors beyond the actual research.[859] The difficulty in locating the 'public' may be attributable to the complexities that are entailed in the means and extent to which scientific knowledge is transferred and weaved into everyday life. Implicit in mediated communications is the choice of frames, as well as audience. On this point, the analysis by Joan Haran *et al.* of the HFEA's public consultation in 2006 on the issue of sourcing eggs for SCNT is instructive. They indicated that,[860] despite a seemingly open invitation for feedback, the HFEA's consultation paper has already demarcated the limits of engagement by excluding those who refused to accept the way in which the issues have been framed. It was further noted that egg sourcing through arrangements like egg sharing has already been licensed by the HFEA prior to its public consultation, so that such arrangements may consequently be considered normal in the minds of the public. If the

---

for its emphasis on temporality, intermediation and the ambiguities associated with a rationality that is implicit in open discourses and the relationship between a state (and its appointees) and its public. See: at John Rawls (Samuel Freeman, ed.), *Collected Papers*. Cambridge MA: Harvard University Press, 1999, at 575-576. Jürgen Habermas, *The Structural Transformation of the Public Sphere: An Inquiry into a Category of Bourgeois Society* (translated by Thomas Burger). Cambridge MA: MIT Press, 1991.

859   Eric A Jensen, *The Therapeutic Cloning Debate: Global Science and Journalism in the Public Sphere*. Farnham: Ashgate, 2014.

860   Joan Haran, Jenny Kitzinger, Maureen McNeil and Kate O'Riordan, *Human Cloning in the Media: From science fiction to science practice*. London and New York: Routledge, 2008, pp 95-120.

public consultation was merely performative to an audience already agreeable to the act, did it have any value? Apparently yes, and their explanation is as follows:[861]

> This [public] mobilisation represents a moral authority which becomes, in effect, a supplement to objectivity. In these sciences (rational) public opinion ... operates as the justification for proposed (and, sometimes, already established) practices. ... [C]laims to know the public operate as legitimating practices which provide new arbiters of objectivity and the basis for public decision making about science policy and research.

As we have discussed, there is significant uncertainty over the health implications of egg donation. Within the frame of biomedical science, some aspects of it can be assessed and managed as scientific risks. Quantified risks may be properly communicated, and then accepted or rejected as a matter of rational voluntary choice. In this respect, informed consent has become the all-important requirement. There is however always a remainder because uncertainty implies the existence of 'irrationalities' that cannot be adequately accommodated with the scientific process of standardisation, categorisation and quantification.[862] To add legitimacy to any action that is directed at the remainder, recourse to the public sphere is necessary to transform subjective concerns into objective requirements. If this analysis is

---

861 *Ibid*, at 174.
862 As Violaine Roussel explains: "The discourses of scandal respond to different validity registers depending on the institution – judicial, political, scientific, media – involved. Therefore actors think and act according to social markers that are not standardised or unified. The representations of precaution and risk in medical research refer, for example, to the unavoidable existence of uncontrollable factors, in the context of scientific controversies and uncertainties, whereas other visions of uncertain situations and their effects compel other actors to different behaviours." Violaine Roussel, New Moralities of Risk and Political Responsibility. In Richard V Ericson and Aaron Doyle (eds.), *Risk and Morality*. Toronto, Buffalo and London: University of Toronto Press, 2003, pp 117-144, at 135.

true, it would seem that bioethics as a public concern always engenders a public sphere.

6.6 Allocating Responsibilities

Recommendations that were published by the BAC in the ED Report following the public consultation have since been consolidated into a set of guidelines relating to human gametes and embryos. Considerable emphasis on voluntary informed consent and assurance of non-exploitation is clear from its requirements, which includes the following:[863]

(1) By regulation, written approval from the Director of Medical Services must be obtained for all research involving human oocytes, including those obtained from excised ovarian tissue;

(2) Specific and personal consent from the donors must be obtained before any gametes are to be used for research, and potential donors should be provided with sufficient information to make an informed decision and be given at least a week to decide;

(3) Women wishing to donate eggs specifically for research must be interviewed by an independent panel, which must in turn be satisfied that these donors are of sound mind, clearly understand the nature and consequences of the donation, and have freely given explicit consent, without any inducement, coercion or undue influence;

(4) All egg donors should be informed if their eggs will be used to create embryos, including human-animal combination embryos, which will be destroyed in the process of research, and if any

---

[863] Bioethics Advisory Committee, *Ethics Guidelines for Human Biomedical Research.* Singapore: Bioethics Advisory Committee, 2015, pp 45-46, paragraphs 5.52, 5.26, 5.28, 5.29 and 5.30.

derived cells from the embryos so created will be kept for future research or possible clinical use;

(5) Donors of eggs obtained specifically for research, and not as a result of clinical treatment, may be reimbursed for legitimate expenses incurred, such as cost of transport and childcare services, and actual loss of earnings, as a result of the procedures required to obtain the eggs. Any other payment should not amount to an inducement and should be approved by an IRB; and

(6) If complications occur as a direct and proximate result of the donation, the donor should be provided with prompt and full medical care.[864]

In a few respects, these guidelines are more onerous than similar guidelines issued by the CIRM and ISSCR,[865] which begs the question as to whether this governance approach would itself preclude healthy woman from rationally deciding to donate her oocytes purely for research. In other words, while I agree that these guidelines are ethically robust, they are more likely to preclude a healthy woman from egg donation than to facilitate it. The endeavour to remove the risks of exploitation could arguably be disproportionate given that, as prospective donors for research, these women are compelled to assume the role of moral entrepreneurs of the self.[866] By this logic,

---

[864] The words "direct and proximate" mirrors those of §100095(c) of the CIRM Medical and Ethical Standards Regulations, Title 17, California Code of Regulation 2011.

[865] Sandra A Carson, *et al.*, Proposed oocyte donation guidelines for stem cell research, *Fertility and Sterility* (2010) 94, 7: 2503-2506; International Society for Stem Cell Research, *Guidelines for Stem Cell Science and Clinical Translation*, 2016, at 9-10, Recommendation 2.2.5; and International Society for Stem Cell Research, *Position* Statement on the Provision and Procurement of Human Eggs for Stem Cell Research, *Cell Stem Cell* (2013) 12: 285-291.

[866] Alan Hunt, Risk and Moralization in Everyday Life. In Richard V Ericson and Aaron Doyle (eds.), *Risk and Morality*. Toronto, Buffalo and London: University of Toronto Press, 2003, pp 165-192.

they as stakeholders become critical in the definition of risks and responsibilities.[867] Ironically, people are often neither all-calculative nor fully informed or interested, so that precautionary (public) activities are directed not at reducing risks, but eliminating them, especially where precaution, driven by a permanent state of anxiety and fear, gives emphasis to the possibility of catastrophe.[868]

A key issue considered at some length was whether eggs could be regarded as 'spare' in the way that a tumour that has been surgically extricated could be so considered. If the issue had been decided in the negative, then there could be two implications. First, this would suggest that some form of payment ought to be made to women who contributed eggs for research because these eggs are not 'spare' (and by implication, unwanted) tissue from a medical procedure.[869] Second, it further suggests that these donors ought to be treated no differently from participants in a clinical trial, and in respect of which significant sums of money – to much ethical controversy – have been given to trial subjects. Indeed, this has been the conclusion that was reached by some.[870] For instance, this position was adopted by the European

---

[867] Michael Power, Risk Management and the Responsible Organization. In Richard V Ericson and Aaron Doyle (eds.), *Risk and Morality*. Toronto, Buffalo and London: University of Toronto Press, 2003, pp 145-164.

[868] Kevin D Haggerty, From Risk to Precaution: The Rationalities of Personal Crime Prevention. In Richard V Ericson and Aaron Doyle (eds.), *Risk and Morality*. Toronto, Buffalo and London: University of Toronto Press, 2003, pp 193-214.

[869] Roberts and Throsby argue that 'fresh' eggs are never 'spare' and this could be a justification for the compensated egg sharing scheme, which the UK Human Fertilisation and Embryology Authority has endorsed. The late Anne McLaren shared this position and thereby argued that scarcity of human eggs could be a basis for allowing human-animal combinations such as cytoplasmic hybrids to be created. See Celia Roberts and Karen Throsby. Paid to share: IVF patients, eggs and stem cell research *Social Science & Medicine* (2008) 66:159-169; and Anne McLaren. Free-Range Eggs? *Science* (2007) 316:339.

[870] Ballantyne and Lacey argue that if women are asked to provide eggs for commercial stem cell research, they should be fairly compensated for their contribution. Dickenson (2007:67-82) goes further in proposing some degree of property interest to be conferred as the protection of women's interests in oocyte donation by way of contract alone is considered to lack robustness. See Angela

Society on Human Reproduction and Embryology Task Force on Ethics and Law,[871] and it may have been a justification for some organisations to provide a relatively large sum of money to egg donors for research.[872] The main difficulty with this position is that it brings to the fore the difficulty of distinguishing compensation from inducement, and any decision made in that connection may have serious repercussions on payments that are currently allowed for participation in clinical trials.

The ED Report makes clear that eggs could be 'spare' in that they are surplus to the fertility treatment and, in such a scenario, the giving of eggs for research should not be on a compensated basis. Such a position is consistent with the BAC's view that any contribution of tissue for research should be by way of gifting made altruistically. This further avoids the ethically problems of inducement and commercialisation of the human body. However, the BAC recognises that in a situation where a healthy woman should decide to donate eggs for research, she should be compensated for loss of time and earnings from undergoing the egg retrieval process. As we have noted, the main justification for this stance is one of fairness – the donor should not be financially disadvantaged by the giving.[873] Furthermore,

---

Ballantyne and Sheryl De Lacey. Wanted – Egg donors for research: a research ethics approach to donor recruitment and compensation. *The International Journal of Feminist Approaches to Bioethics* (2008) 1, 145-164; and Donna Dickenson. *Property in the body: feminist perspectives.* Cambridge: Cambridge University Press, 2007.

[871] European Society on Human Reproduction and Embryology Task Force on Ethics and Law. Oocyte donation for non-reproductive purposes. *Human Reproduction* (2007) 22, 1210-1213, at 1213.

[872] Some of the organisations that allow compensation to be paid to donors of eggs for research have been considered by the BAC in its consultation paper: see A-16 and A-17 of ED Report.

[873] The BAC's broader conceptualisation of 'payment' that should be made to healthy donors is arguably not too different from Charis Thompson's recommendation that "we compensate egg donors as a means of minimizing risks to donors, encouraging donations for the right reasons and under the best conditions of informed consent...and preventing trafficking in eggs". See Charis Thompson.

the egg donation procedure is a very invasive one. While the eggs that are given in this context are not 'spare', healthy donors are not regarded as clinical trial subjects because the risks associated with the procedure are quantified (whereas there is greater uncertainty from participation in clinical trials)[874] and researchers are required to insure these donors against any complications that occur as a direct and proximate result of the donation. While there may be a residual long term risk that is as yet not quantified or is indeed unquantifiable, altruism requires that such a risk be borne by the donor, who has not acted under any compulsion. It may be argued that rather than focusing on particular health risks, the BAC has instead directed its attention to addressing more generally the safety of donors as a welfare concern. As we have seen at the start of this section, the risks-based construction of 'safety', 'spare' eggs and 'inducement' has in turned led to a particular set of procedures on consent taking.[875]

This development lends support to the argument of Michael Power and others that 'risks' relate to individualisation (through abstract-tion, instauration, and so on), particularly when potential harm to personal, legal and reputational interests are envisaged.[876] Rather than attributing this superficially to conditions in a highly legalised

---

Why we should, in fact, pay for egg donation. *Regenerative Medicine* (2007) 2, 203-209.

[874] The US NRC and IOM suggest that medical risks of human egg donation are quantifiable and manageable. This view is not shared by others who argue that there is residual risk that could be unquantifiable and significant (see for example Dickenson and Idiakez). It should also be noted that some members of the public indicated in their feedback that compensation for risks would not be adequate. See National Research Council and Institute of Medicine. *Assessing the Medical Risks of Human Oocyte Donation for Stem Cell Research: Workshop Report.* Washington DC, 2007; and Donna Dickenson and Itziar A. Idiakez. Ova Donation for stem cell research: an international perspective. *The International Journal of Feminist Approaches to Bioethics* (2007) 1, 125-144.

[875] A relatively comprehensive discussion was taken up in the ED Report that culminated in Recommendations 2 to 4; see pp 12-15 of the ED Report.

[876] Michael Power, *The Risk Management of Everything: Rethinking the politics of uncertainty.* London: Demas, 2004, at 13-14.

society, Power considers the problem to relate more fundamentally to responsibility aversity – a critical manifestation of cultural conditions that encourage "a high appetite for risk, because of the attraction of positive outcomes, and a low appetite for responsibility and blame in the face of negative outcomes".[877] Power observes that defensive proceduralism arises when the 'risk game' becomes a 'blame game'. He further points out that defensive preoccupation with reputational and legal risks has little to do with any direct possibility of legal action. Instead "legal and other norms get embedded into organizational routines not because the real risks of litigation are well understood, but because the mere possibility creates a defensive orientation towards the need to justify decisions in retrospect".[878] Such a phenomenon becomes even more problematic as those (such as accountants, lawyers and even policy makers) whose responsibility relates directly to risk management are themselves preoccupied with reducing risks to themselves.[879] Michael Power is particularly

---

[877] *Ibid*, at 45.

[878] *Ibid*, at 46-7.

[879] *Ibid*, at 48. Barbara Vis's study of the politics of welfare state reform in the Netherlands suggests that policy-makers (as well as voters) will avoid risk if they consider themselves to be in a domain of gains and when they see their status quo as still acceptable or tolerable. In contrast, they are more likely to opt for gamble when they view their current situation as a loss. She sets this out summarily as: "Governments in a gains domain pursue absolute gains and are unwilling to engage in risky reform efforts, while governments in a losses domain pursue relative gains and are more willing to accept the risks of reform." See: Barbara Vis, *Politics of Risk-taking: Welfare State Reform in Advanced Democracies*. Amsterdam: Amsterdam University Press, 2011, at 125. Representing four possible outcomes as a four-cell grid in applying this reasoning, Vis indicates (at 126-127) that (1) governments will only undertake welfare state reform with risky electoral repercussions if they consider the status quo a loss; (2) if governments pursue reform, the implementation of the reform will be relatively easy if voters are reform-friendly (i.e. if they are also in a losses domain) or relatively difficult if voters are reform-hostile (i.e. if they are in a gains domain); (3) if governments consider the status quo to be a fain, they will not undertake electorally risky reform; and (4) if governments do not favour reform, there will be no conflict if voters consider the status quo as a gain, but conflict may arise if voters consider status quo to be a loss.

concerned that this overwhelming focus on risk management is a threat to democracy and public life, as democratic processes and government become subsumed within administrative paradigms. He refers to Mary Douglas for a counter-intuitive observation. Where risks suggest inevitability or absence of choice, Douglas has indicated that "we choose what to fear in order to support our way of life".[880] To counter what he perceives to be a negative development, Power's proposals include, first, a re-characterisation of risk management as a form of learning and experimentation rather than rule-based processes, thus placing stronger reliance on human capabilities to imagine alternative futures instead of quantitative ambitions to predict the future; and second, counter the individualisation process by developing public understandings and 'civic epistemologies' of how risk issues are processed and potentially amplified by the institutions of media and law. A broader political culture must communicate an understanding that not every risk is controllable and that expert opinions are not infallible. It should also provide the necessary institutional conditions or 'safe haven' for the exercise of professional and expert judgments in honest and reasonable decision-making.[881]

It is a debatable issue as to whether the BAC's approach in engaging with the bioethical challenges of human egg donation is consistent with Power's proposals. Evaluating the public consultation component in particular, including its subsequent impact on the BAC's recommendations and guidelines, as well as on the regulations on assisted reproduction services and the HBRA (discussed in Chapter 2), it is reasonable to say that public engagement has been more than a mere 'white-washing' process.[882] This was a concern raised by

---

880 *Ibid*, at 55-56 and 60.
881 *Ibid*, at 61-65.
882 Corporate law in the UK and in Singapore provides for a 'white-washing' procedure whereby financial assistance by a company for the purpose of acquiring its own shares or the shares of its holding company becomes

Kerry Holden and David Demeritt, as they considered Singapore's 'developmental state' political culture to stand in contradiction to a climate of liberal democracy within which the scientific enterprise is said to have thrived. While observing that 'good science' now also depends on being seen to observe certain ethical terms and conditions, they suggest that Singapore's standard of governance is primarily directed at economic gain.[883] While their claim in respect of Singapore may be easily contested, they are correct in their observation that 'good science' necessitates scientific rigour and ethical vitality. Devising such a research culture has been described by Charis Thompson as a 'choreography' of ethics and science, where science cannot proceed without ethical accounting.[884] While she leave open the question as to whom or what such a choreographer might be, Thompson insightfully observes that 'good science' cannot be achieved or legislated once and for all, but must be an ongoing and iterative enterprise, involving many different kinds of contributors.[885]

My argument here is that bioethics, and more specifically, bioethical bodies have and should continue to assume the role of a choreographer, as well as to serve as a 'dance venue' in terms of a public sphere, broadly conceived. Returning to the BAC, it was not established primarily to engage the public; public involvement was subsequently seen to be vital for reasons that include the filling of epistemic 'gaps' in institutional knowledge, and to secure broader legitimacy on an initiative that will not yield immediate benefit to the public. Arguably, a civic epistemology has taken shape since 2001,

---

permissible after complying with a number of procedural requirements, including the publication of a notice setting out certain requisite information in a major newspaper. Section 76, *Companies Act*, Chapter 50 of Singapore Statutes (2006 Revised Edition). See also *Public Prosecutor v Lew Syn Pau and Another* [2006] SCHC 16.

[883] Kerry Holden and David Demeritt. Democratising science? The politics of promoting biomedicine in Singapore's developmental state. *Environment and Planning D: Society and Space* (2008) *26*, 68-86, at 80.

[884] Charis Thompson, *Good Science: The Ethical Choreography of Stem Cell Research*. Cambridge MA and London: MIT Press, 2013, at 64.

[885] *Ibid*, at 225.

particularly in a public sphere initially developed as a moderate gradualist platform that was grounded in certain values regarded by the BAC as critical to facilitate participation. This initiative contributed to the formation of a 'public' in that a set of social relations emerged in the way that the BAC interacted with a diverse constituency of respondents. Artefacts (like 'embryo' and 'egg') and language (centred around a notion of 'respect for persons') became essential components of a recursive form of an emergent civic epistemology, or a generally accepted or recognised basis by which the 'public' would think about and engage stem cell science and technology. Events leading up the BAC's recommendations for egg donation contributed to the development, as well as refinement, of ethical language. A 'learning curve' (not confined to policy-makers and regulators, as considered in Chapters 3 and 4) was also evident in that a number of respondents, especially those from religious groups, felt that they were better able to engage in ethical deliberation outside of their particular belief systems. As noted earlier, a number of respondents to the consultation on egg donation voiced the need to explicitly provide for privacy safeguards. The BAC might have considered an explicit mention to be unnecessary as the concern would have been addressed in an earlier report,[886] although its mention and subsequent incorporation into the ED Report reflects communicative engagement. It is accordingly insufficient to consider the BAC's public consultation exercise as only a 'white-washing' process, but necessarily the component of a broader and emergent civic epistemology. This is a dynamic and iterative process, as is our knowledge of 'risk' and 'public'.

---

[886] Bioethics Advisory Committee, *Personal Information in Biomedical Research.* Singapore: Bioethics Advisory Committee, 2007.

7

An Emergent Civic Epistemology

7.1 Introduction

The HA Report and its recommendations were officially made public at a press conference held on 22 September 2010. This seventh report of the BAC was published after an embargo of almost a year from the time it was accepted by the government. A reason for this delay is the lack of clarity as to which government agency should assume regulatory responsibility over research involving human-animal combinations. Another concern was over possibly adverse public reaction towards the government's endorsement of the research, especially by a number of vocal religious groups. An informant mentioned that this concern was especially pertinent as Singapore's 16th Parliamentary general election was expected to take place soon (the election took place some time later, on 7 May 2011).[887] To allay this worry, a copy of the report was sent ahead of the press conference to leaders of the main religious groups, with an invitation to meet with the BAC on 15 September 2010. The purpose of this meeting was to explain the BAC's position, which differed from that of some religious viewpoints largely due to fundamental disagreements over the ethics of human embryo research. While the BAC did not anticipate any new grounds

---

[887] Interview, 3 March 2010, MT.

of concerns to be raised, it did not rule out the option of a further delay to the public release of its recommendations should this meeting turn out badly.

The meeting did not ultimately draw many religious group leaders, although representatives from the most active respondents during the public consultation (i.e. National Council of Churches in Singapore (NCCS), the Catholic Medical Guild and the Islamic Religious Council of Singapore (MUIS)) were present. Feedback from this meeting did not differ from a previous meeting, also with religious group leaders, on 13 September 2008. However, the ambience was more reconciliatory at this meeting, even though certain religious objections to the research were reiterated. The presence of representatives from MUIS was important as it was not fundamentally opposed to the research, provided that certain (mainly regulatory) safeguards were met. This difference in religious viewpoint appeared to have an effect in shifting the attention to more pragmatic (as opposed to dogmatic) concerns. The meeting itself appears to validate the experiences of CIRM on the importance of public engagement. In my interviews with Professor Bernard Lo and Dr Geoffrey Lomax,[888] both of them emphasised the importance of engaging with the public even though the CIRM need not accept all the comments from the public. Responding to comments from the public, and where applicable, explaining why the CIRM has adopted a different viewpoint or stance, or the reasons for its disagreement with public opinion were modes of inclusiveness. These practices helped to set the tone for reasonable engagement among parties with very different views and experiences.[889]

Given the relatively calm reception by the religious group leaders of the recommendations, the BAC went ahead with the scheduled release of the HA Report. The press conference was attended by

---

[888] Interview with Professor Bernard Lo (on 16 August 2008) and Dr Geoffrey Lomax (on 12 May 2009).

[889] Feedback to this effect was received in my interviews with religious group leaders who were present.

reporters from local newspapers and a regional news agency. No foreign press was present even though invitations have been sent to them. This was unlike the release of the BAC's recommendations for hESC research in 2002, when media hype on the subject was at a peak, or the release of its recommendations on genetic testing in 2005, around the time when news of the scandal in South Korea broke out. In its press release, the BAC highlighted that its deliberation on research involving human-animal combinations was motivated by a desire to:

> update its recommendations for human stem cell research, especially in the light of recent developments ..., [and it further reiterated that it] expects stem cell research to have considerable potential in the treatment of currently incurable diseases ..., [also noting that c]linical trials of stem cell treatments are beginning in a number of countries.[890]

These points were captured in the press reports that followed; all of which highlighted public concern over possible breach of perceived differences between humans and animals, the benefits that could be derived from stem cell science and technology, as well as the ability to circumvent ethical challenges and to harness the benefits through reliance on sound and effective regulation by a national body on stem cell research.[891] Similar sentiments were articulated by the

---

[890] Bioethics Advisory Committee, *Press Release: Human-Animal Combinations in Stem Cell Research*, 22 September 2010, at paragraph 4.

[891] Claire Huang Jingyi, Bioethics advisory panel proposes national body to monitor stem-cell research: one of 5 recommendations following 2-year consultation exercise, *TODAY*, 23 September 2010; BAC recommends setting up a body to monitor stem cell research, *Channel News Asia*, 22 September 2010; Grace Chua, Call for national body on stem cell research: It should review research involving human-animal combination of cells, *The Straits Times*, 23 September 2010; Xu Xiang Yu, Mouse with Consciousness, Pig with Feelings: Human-Animal Combinations; There will be Chaos in the World, *Joint Evening Newspaper*, 22 September 2010; Chua Huiling, Bioethics Advisory Committee: Establish National Body to Control Human-Animal Stem Cell Research, *Joint Morning Newspaper*, 23

then-Minister for Health Mr Khaw Boon Wan (now Coordinating Minister for Infrastructure and the Minister for Transportation), who wrote on his blog that rational assessment is needed in considering how to move forward with the technology:[892]

> I remember the movie, "The Fly", in which a research project went awry and the scientist involved acquired fly-like capabilities and yucky eating habits. He tried desperately to reverse the experiment but never succeeded. It was a popular movie theme and "The Fly" was remade by different Directors. I have at least watched two different versions of it. Scientists will want to push the boundary, to discover, to invent, to benefit mankind. Rogue scientists are rare and we need rules to rein them in, without stifling genuine research with good potential. The easiest thing, as a regulator, is to say "No" to all such pursuits. But we will be missing out on opportunities that can benefit us all. In any case, sweeping things under the carpet does not prevent rogue scientists from pushing the boundary in perverse ways ... MOH is studying their recommendations and will respond to them. Personally, I find the proposed BAC approach practical: allow some research, but limit it to a narrow area where the potential for benefits is significant and real, and regulate such research tightly. As for the potentially yucky stuff, continue to prohibit it.

Several days later, the MOH announced its formal acceptance of the BAC's recommendations, adding that a new legislation to regulate bio-medical research was being prepared. In addition, the MOH indicated that it would work with the Ministry of National Development and the AVA to establish a "robust framework to ensure compliance with

---

September 2010; Oleh Samshul Jangarodin, Penubuhan badan semak dan pantau kerja penyelidikan sel induk disaran [Proposed establishment of monitoring body for stem cell research], *Berita Harian* [Daily News], 23 September 2010.

[892] Blog post by Ministry of Health on 23 September 2010, and subsequently reported in The Straits Times: *Allow for genuine research, leave out the yucky stuff*, 24 September 2010.

BAC's recommendations".[893] Shortly after, the research community was surprised by a circular issued by the AVA on 1 October 2010 to strongly advise the IACUC against approving research involving the creation of cytoplasmic hybrid embryos and the introduction of human stem cells into animals until such time when the BAC's recommendations are implemented.[894] This development was unanticipated as it is explicitly provided in the BAC's HA Report that existing arrangements relating to the IACUC to ensure the welfare of laboratory animal should continue to apply, particularly where there is no serious risk of the research animal developing human sentience or consciousness. As a consequence of the circular, clarification was sought from the BAC, and *status quo* was reinstated through the issuance of a follow-on clarification circular.

A separate and distinct network animates the 'state' or 'government' in the context of biomedical research. There are divergent interests and responsibilities, most directly represented by the different ministries that constitute this network. There are also advisory bodies and coordinating agencies that may be difficult to situate. For highly technical areas like policies on human pluripotent stem cell research, the 'government' did not present itself in the form of a paternalistic, all-knowing and repressive developmental state. This does not imply an absence of political agenda or coercive power, but the relationship between the different modalities of power has a rather more peculiar character. We find agency to reposit in different localities within, as well as along the boundaries of, inter-relational power and knowledge structures. Within this network, the BAC served as an assemblage point and outlet in terms of public engagement and policy action. It has also been the primary intermediator among the various stakeholders of biomedical research, as well as with the broader public. At this stage (and akin to an

---

[893] Ministry of Health, Press Release: MOH accepts Bioethics Advisory Committee's recommendations on Human-Animal Combinations in Stem Cell Research, 27 September 2010.

[894] Fieldnotes (including communication with Dr Lim Bing), 30 October 2010.

adjudicative structure), the reliability of state power to avert or otherwise manage the risks of harm, variously construed, has become so convincing that neither the religious group representatives (even those opposed to the research) nor members of the public appeared to be particularly perturbed. From a practical viewpoint, the governance framework put forward by the BAC appeared to have gained legitimacy and a level of social acceptance.

7.2 The BAC as a Pseudo-Juridical Entity

Although the BAC is constituted as an independent advisory body to the Singaporean government, it functions in many ways like a pseudo-juridical entity. In 'pseudo', I mean that it is not juridical in a literal or formal sense (i.e. political recognition to that effect). To most people both within and outside of Singapore, the BAC is seen as governmental in the sense that it is appointed by the government and serves as a national body on bioethics. Of importance is that its emergence initiated a relatively novel approach to governance and signalled a changing role of the state within this governance framework. Here, I argue that the BAC bears pseudo-juridical features in at least five respects:

    (a) Real links to state and juridical institutions;

    (b) Pervasive use of legal norms, rationalities, techniques and language;

    (c) Institutional forms which are characteristics of juridical institutions;

    (d) Sociality that is legally informed; and

    (e) Integration through intermediation.

7.2.1 *Links to State and Juridical Institutions*

The BAC is proximate to state power in having a direct communicative link to the SCLS (whose then-chairperson has since been elected the

President of the Republic of Singapore), but it is not itself a state entity. While the recommendations and guidelines of the BAC may not have the formal force of law, they have influence over regulatory arrangements and practices: first, they prescribe standards of conduct and generate expectations that shape practices and conduct; second, they present measures that are introduced for the containment of 'unethical' behaviour – whether in relation to research ethics or research integrity – and constitute the 'good' and the 'acceptable'; third, there may be punitive consequences (not necessarily legal) for non-compliance; and fourth, they were mostly meta-law and now form the substantive basis of the HBRA. It is presently unclear what impact this legislation will have on the BAC, but its role in pronouncing or declaring normative standards and meta-law requirements is unlikely to change.

7.2.2 Legal Norms, Rationalities, Techniques and Language

In the previous chapters, I have attempted to explicate the legal rationales, techniques and practices that have been deployed in the policy construction of artefacts like 'hybrids' and 'chimeras' as metaphorical placeholders; in constituting documents to establish relationalities and for scripting; and to visualise risks and the 'common good' (variously construed) to enable engagement and action. From my study, a relatively prevalent view is that legislation should be generic and not readily revisable. Legislation appears to have the character of making explicit certain 'truths', and is hence enduring. In contrast to legislation, regulations and policies are not seen as subject to this constraint. This is somewhat of a surprise to me, as I had understood legislation in a more functional and hence time-bound manner. At first blush, juridification in the deployment of legal norms, rationalities, techniques and language may be difficult to detect. But on deeper analysis, what seems to emerge is the slow halting advancement that Latour considers to be the critical means by which these constructs initially intended to operate 'in the meantime' become social facts.[895] In this sense, the BAC bears some semblance to juridical bodies like Latour's account of the *Conseil d'État*, also in that it is effectively a mixed political-regulatory body.

7.2.3 Juridical Forms

Taking a broader view, the policy setup centred around the BAC (not to mention its operations) resembles a judicial structure. As we have seen, normative prescriptions from the BAC are practically binding on all IRBs in Singapore. IRBs in turn adjudicate on the ethical acceptability of research proposals. There is at present no appeal mechanism to the BAC, but this has been debated in the BAC and elsewhere.[896] From my interviews on this issue, it seems that the main obstacle to implementing such a mechanism is more a matter of resource limitations. In terms of inputs into the work of the BAC, it is difficult to deny the very fundamental influence of officers of the law. The key sub-committees and working groups that have been responsible for all its reports to date were chaired by either a senior judge or a law professor.[897] Judge Richard Magnus, who was responsible for the BAC's SC Report, has since succeeded Professor Lim Pin as the second Chairman of the BAC from 2011. All legally trained members of the BAC have indicated that legal skills in mediation, adjudication and securing a reasonable outcome to ethical contentions have been important to meeting their responsibilities on the Committee.

---

[895] Bruno Latour, *La fabrique du droit: Une ethnographie du conseil d'État* [The factory of law: an ethnography of the Conseil d'État]. Paris: La Découverte, 2002, at 80.

[896] The *Human Biomedical Research Act* of 2015 allows for appeal against the decision of an IRB, although the precise mechanism is yet to be worked out at the time of writing. It is unlikely that the BAC will have an adjudicative function within this legislative framework.

[897] Both Senior District Judge Richard Magnus (interview on 18 April 2009), who chaired the Human Stem Cell Research Sub-Committee, and Professor Terry Kaan (interview on 16 June 2009), who chaired the Human Genetics Sub-Committee, said that the legal training has enabled them to mediate differences in an impartial manner.

I have also attempted to present the ways in which the BAC made representation, provided opportunities to be heard, gave demonstrations of evidence, recorded narratives and reported on outcomes. Most evidently, its construction and framing of duties in terms of rights and responsibilities have a strong corollary in law. All of these are commonplace features of a courtroom and consistent with the requirements of legal norms. In his study of a report of the NAS relating to diet, nutrition and cancer, Stephen Hilgartner argues that various means of information control are entailed in the creation and management of a stage. Such controls are akin to frame selection in effect. Institutions and their work procedures regulate access to information much like a backstage that manages the flow of persons, speech and documents. More importantly, they serve to structure relations between experts and publics, and are devices "of *constituting* performers and audiences with particular capabilities (and enforced inabilities) of speech and perception."[898] In a sense, the consultation papers may perhaps be likened to a stage (or courtroom?) upon which one narrative of pluripotent stem cell science and technology is presented to a diversely composed audience. In the context of our discussion, the BAC (and its institutional procedures relating to the consultative process and its documents) has been instrumental in co-producing a public vis-à-vis pluripotent stem cell science and technology. It may be further argued that, just as the enactment of a stage and performance would precede an audience, the BAC, through the instrumentality of its consultation papers, played a critical part in producing a 'public sphere' through engagement. The entire process from the initial construction of a bioethics narrative, to the justifications for its recommendations, and ultimately in public engagement and pronouncement, has generally been mandated by constitutional norms, and informed by legal due progress. The BAC is, in this regard, pseudo-juridical in form.

---

[898] Stephen Hilgartner, *Science on stage: expert advice as public drama*. Stanford: Stanford University Press, 2000, at 147 (emphasis in original).

7.2.4 Sociality

Unlike a courthouse, the BAC is not primarily concerned with dispute resolution. Institutionally, the BAC may be more comfortable with indeterminacies and paradoxes.[899] For instance, in soliciting feedback from the public, the accounts provided by the BAC in its HA Consultation Paper are quite different from the sort of narratives that have been used to argue for strong investment in science and technology. In other words, it is a narrative somewhat different from the futuristic deterministic account such as the 'greyist' narrative deployed to push for institutional reform.[900] Instead, they are more open-ended, positive and deployed as means by which members of the public could contribute creatively to technological assessment, more similar to the 'science fictions' that Clark Miller and Ira Bennett envisage.[901] The BAC's approach follows a broader trend of public engagement of similar bodies in the US and Europe, and such 'science fiction'-like narratives are tools that help the public engage more positively and intimately with scientific and technological futures;[902] in addition, the UK government's 'GM Nation' exercise has been described as occasions "where writers might be asked to develop

---

[899] If one agrees with the account of law as autopoietic, Teubner explains that the components of a legal system (being actions, norms, processes, identity, legal reality) are seen as cyclically linked with each other in multifarious ways. Self-reference, paradoxes and indeterminacies are overcome by declaring the circularity to be a problem of legal practice, rather than legal thought, thereby ensuring the independence of its cognition. Gunther Teubner, And God Laughed ... Indeterminacy, Self-Reference and Paradox in Law, *German Law Journal* (2011) 12: 376-406, at 385-386.

[900] Martijn van der Steen, Ageing or silvering? Political debate about ageing in the Netherlands, *Science and Public Policy* (October 2008) 35, 8: 575-583.

[901] Clark A Miller and Ira Bennett, Thinking longer term about technology: is there value in science fiction-inspired approaches to constructing futures? *Science and Public Policy* (October 2008) 35, 8: 567-606.

[902] Miller and Bennett observe: "... the US government has built public comment periods and public hearings into regulatory decision-making processes, while European governments and universities have pioneered novel forms of public engagement such as consensus conferences and *cafés scientifiques*": *Ibid*, at 599.

multiple stories and dialogues that could be shared with the public alongside more technical reports" to be used when citizens "meet and dialogue about their preferences with regard to genetically modified organisms".[903]

Rather than attempt to isolate the 'law' from bioethics as a composite, I have moved away from the study of law an object. While some degree of essentialism is unavoidable, I have attempted to study how juridification has operated on the periphery, rather than as a field of habitual knowledge[904] or as an autopoietic institution.[905] In many ways, bioethics is similar to governance of financial derivatives in Annelise Riles's study.[906] As a lawyer working in the area of bioethics, legal rationalities, techniques and norms are everywhere, and nowhere. This is perhaps most evident as bioethicists remain divided as to whether the law *is* bioethics or otherwise totally separable.[907] In the analytic of juridification, I have attempted to illustrate how the law has been capable of being other to itself, and in hybridisation with other modalities of power. As Ben Golder and Peter Fitzpatrick have observed elsewhere:

> Law is central to an experience of modernity ... [and] represents a key modality of our sociality, of our continuate being with each other. Through its ability to combine iteratively a determinate securing of limits and a responsive regard to the disruption of those limits and their re-formulation, law provides an opening to futurity.[908]

---

903 *Ibid*, at 605.

904 Pierre Bourdieu, The Force of Law: Toward a Sociology of the Juridical Field (translated by Richard Terdiman), *Hastings Law Journal* (1987) 38:805-853.

905 Niklas Luhmann (tr. E King and M Albrow), *A sociological theory of law*. London: Routledge and Kegan Paul, 1985.

906 Annelise Riles, *Collateral Knowledge: Legal Reasoning in the Global Financial Markets*. Chicago and London: University of Chicago Press, 2011.

907 Tom L Beauchamp, Informed Consent: Its History, Meaning, and Present Challenges, *Cambridge Quarterly of Healthcare Ethics* (2011) 20: 515-523, at 518.

908 Ben Golder and Peter Fitzpatrick, *Foucault's Law*. London and New York: Routledge, 2009, at 125.

The focus of this study has not been to critique law or to advocate for its further inclusion or exclusion in bioethics. Instead, I have attempted to demonstrate how the law as a social technology has contributed to the production of bioethical knowledge and practices within a public policy setting, through means that include rendering the future knowable and calculable. [909] The symbols, concepts and techniques in law have also been instrumental in constituting bioethics as a system of governance. In Singapore, it began with the juridification of nascent life – the 'embryo' and 'pre-embryo'. Bioethical knowledge has since advanced, from when 'personhood' begins, to what makes a 'person'. The process has encapsulated collaborative linkages across different social systems and powers, including law.

7.2.5 *Integration through Intermediation*

It is generally recognised that robust science and sound ethics are essentially components to a responsible research culture. It is probably too much of a stretch to say that the BAC has been a 'choreographer' (discussed in the previous chapter), but it has at least served as an intermediator between the state and, first and foremost, the biomedical research community, as well as other key stakeholders including professional and governance bodies of various sorts (e.g. NAS, CIRM, AMS, DCE and ISSCR), regulators, research institutions and funders, the bioethics community and the wider public. This proactive initiative of policymakers and regulators in dealing with the

---

[909] As José Julián López and Janet Lunau explain: "Whereas the other disciplines might be able to speak to the ethical, legal or social implications in isolation, law can speak to the medical-ethical-legal-social thing in tis compound thingness. Juridification, after all, refers to 'a form of reasoning that subjects the plural disciplines and identities of social life to the homogenous and hierarchical norms of a self-defining and increasingly asocial discourse of law.'" José Julián López and Janet Lunau, ELSIfication in Canada: Legal Modes of Reasoning, *Science as Culture* (March 2012) 21, 1: 77-99, at 82.

complexities that could potentially arise from the social, ethical and cultural dimensions of hESC research has been observed to promote a higher level of public trust.[910] It may be a reason why the role of bioethical discourses as the mediator between science and society has also been observed to have expanded dramatically.[911] Whether more could or should be done to promote effective and fair governance remains a difficult question, particularly in an international environment. The role of international law in the governance of issues on global health and biomedical research has been limited.[912] This has for the main part been attributed to the narrow focus of international law on state sovereignty and interactions among states. Consequently, it has limited effect on individuals and non-state entities. Principles of sound governance like transparency, engagement and accountability are seemingly ineffectual without a 'choreographer' that could convene together a diverse range of actors and to galvanise action in meeting key governance challenges.[913] For the time being, the prevailing policy viewpoint favours integration through intermediation, so that any direct state intervention (apart from public funding) in the practice of science should be limited, if not avoided. Even where the legislative framework established by the HBRA is concerned, the regulatory intent is essentially described as a 'light-touch' approach. How much this continues to hold true as the legislation comes into effect remains to be seen. At the present time however, the Mertonian principles of universalism and disinterestedness hold sway.[914] Any role that the state is to have should be limited to the background, so

---

[910] Herbert Gottweis, Brian Salter and Catherine Waldby, *The Global Politics of Human Embryonic Stem Cell Science: Regenerative Medicine in Transition*. Basingstoke: Palgrave Macmillan, 2009.

[911] *Ibid.*

[912] Lawrence O Gostin, *Global Health Law*. Cambridge MA: Harvard University Press, 2014, at 61-64.

[913] Gostin explains that the initial failings of international institutions like the WHO and the World Bank have given rise to a complex and multiplicity of global health institutions. *Ibid*, at 132-172.

[914] Robert K Merton (Norman W Storer, ed.), *The Sociology of Science: theoretical and empirical investigations*. Chicago: University of Chicago Press, 1973, at 270-278.

that science could be maintained as an independent and politically disinterested enterprise as much as practicable.

7.3 The State – Decentred but not Disinterested

In the previous chapter, we have considered the constitutive power of risk discourses. Perceptions of risk have been a ground of sociality, and a legitimising force for policy decisions that shape social arrangements. To the extent that the recommendations of the BAC address risk concerns and the allocation of responsibilities, its work is an intricate part of a broader political culture of precaution and preparedness. As we have considered, 'risks' have operated in various forms and at different levels to motivate and justify policy development. In this section, we broaden our consideration to the non-consequentialist character of 'risks'. In particular, we consider their affective qualities that appeal to solidarity (or 'communities of fate', as will be discussed below). These are arguably the qualities that secure durability in socio-political arrangements, beyond purely utilitarian calculations. By linking life sciences initiatives to the long term survival prospect of Singapore, bioethics has become a *raison d'être* for (as well as, of) government. As a tiny nation-state, policy-makers have been especially conscious of Singapore's vulnerability. The trauma of expulsion from the federation of Malaysia in the short space of about two years of achieving independence from colonial rule may have further etched this vulnerability into the national psyche. Not surprisingly, a journalist asked the late Mr Lee Kuan Yew (the architect of modern Singapore) in an interview if the nation-state should be "always living in fear of a catastrophe".[915]

Through what has been described as a developmental state model, the state-led industrialisation of Singapore between the late 1960's to 1990's capitalised on the nation state's locational and infrastructural

---

915 Han Fook Kwang, Zuraidah Ibrahim, Chua Mui Hoong, Lydia Lim, Ignatius Low, Rachel Lin and Robin Chan, *Lee Kuan Yew: Hard Truths to Keep Singapore Going*. Singapore: Straits Times Press, 2011, at 25.

strengths to attract transnational corporations. This strategy has been relatively successful in enabling Singapore's capabilities in back-end manufacturing, consumer electronics and a variety of financial and distributional services, which have in turn generated economic returns and a crucial source of legitimacy for the state. The rule of law has often been regarded as intrinsic to this developmental strategy. The assurance that the state will 'stick to the law' has been considered to be critical in securing stable relations with transnational corporations and ensuring continued foreign direct investment. By this formulation, the rule of law amounts in effect to the security of persons, property rights and contract enforcement. Such a conception of law could be traced to Friedrich Hayek, whose preference for a minimal state has attributed to the Common Law a spontaneous (rather than engineered) origin and a prioritisation of the rule of law ahead of development. Reflecting on the development experiences of East Asian nations, Francis Fukuyama takes a different view in arguing that the rule of law is but a distinct dimension of development, and not a precondition.[916] Referring to the industrialisation of South Korea between 1954 and 1990, he observes that state building has led to economic growth, and economic prosperity has led to rule of law, greater legitimacy of the state and social mobilisation in terms of people forming interest groups in civil society thereby gaining access to politics.[917] However, state building does not necessarily lead to the development of the rule of law. Fukuyama notes that while China was among the first to have adopted state building, it failed to develop rule of law and political accountability. However, this legacy of state building was a basis for highly-qualified authoritarian governments,

---

[916] Francis Fukuyama, *The Origins of Political Order: From Prehuman Times to the French Revolution.* New York: Farrar, Straus and Giroux, 2011, at 470.

[917] *Ibid*, at 474-475. Fukuyama observes (at 473) that the governments of Singapore and Malaysia have been able to maintain popular support despite of lack of liberal democracy due to rapid economic growth, which has served to legitimise government policies. In contrast, the Indonesian state lost legitimacy when its economic growth faltered during the financial crisis of 1997 to 1998.

as exemplified in successful authoritarian modernisers including South Korea, Taiwan, Singapore and modern China itself. The success of these countries is attributable not so much to political institutions, but to cultural commitment towards science, learning and innovation. Consequently, economic success has been achieved even though the rule of law and political accountability are relatively underdeveloped in many East Asian countries.[918]

To be sure, Fukuyama's point is *not* that the rule of law is unimportant. Effective legal institutions are difficult to construct as they require physical facilities and huge investments in the training of lawyers, judges and other officers of the court, including law enforcement officers.[919] When developed, the rule of law is an important component of political order that enables political accountability, and this in turn provides a peaceful path toward institutional adaptation.[920] Of importance to our discussion here is his observation that the state must intentionally and systematically adopt the rule of law. This is perhaps most evident in his argument that the Common Law was intimately associated with the rise of the early English state and dependent on state power for its eventual dominance.[921] To understand biotechnology in Asia, Aihwa Ong emphasises the need to take the role of the state seriously. Through the analytic of global assemblages, she argues that the notions of the state, its people and their collective interests are re-created in biotechnologies:[922]

---

[918] *Ibid*, at 317.

[919] *Ibid*, at 247.

[920] *Ibid*, at 482-3.

[921] *Ibid*, at 253, 256-257. Fukuyama observes that the early monarchs like William I and Henry I had an interest in acting as a court of appeals in cases where subjects were not satisfied with the justice dispensed by the local seigeurial or manor courts. The monarchy earned a fee for services relating to dispensation of justice, and this further increased the prestige of the king, and in turn undermined the authority of local lord when his opinion was overturned.

[922] Aihwa Ong, An Analytics of Biotechnology and Ethics at Multiple Scales. In Aihwa Ong and Nancy N Chen (eds.), *Asian Biotech: Ethics and Communities of Fate*. Durham and London: Duke University Press, 2010, pp 1-51, at 15-16.

Contrary to popular perceptions, the regulation of biotech flows is managed not only by pharmaceutical companies and global health agencies, but also by nationalist states that increasingly shape and patrol flows of human tissues and biotech products. In contrast to market-state systems, emergent players in the field of biotechnology and biomedicine are situated in political environments with robust sovereignty and paternalist rule. Having laid the foundation for capitalist development, Asian states are turning to biotechnologies as a mechanism of regeneration, not only of the economy and of the people, but also of national prestige.

Different forms of biotechnology have been used to generate and influence corporeal and affective interests, or 'communities of fate', which refers "not to elements of a global civil society but to the network of collectivities that become connected as a result of diverse ethical decisions and feelings associated with technological innovations."[923] Taken together, Ong sets out 'Asian biotech' as referring to "an assemblage of science, politics, and collective concerns that configures a realm of transcendent imaginary in which sciences in tandem with ethics shape political identities."[924] Of especial pertinence to us is the anthropology of 'situated ethics' that Ong puts forward. As she explains:

[This notion] rejects the common assumption that moral reasoning can be simply determined by class location, or reduced to the scale of the isolated individual ... [Instead,] it is more fruitful to locate moral reasoning at the intersection of overlapping scales of risk and ethics.[925]

---

[923] *Ibid*, at 20.
[924] *Ibid*, at 21. Ong (at 43) generalises "Asia" as "a region of political and ethical contradictions, of population surplus and bio-insecurity, of economic backwardness and full-throttle capitalism, of memories of colonial humiliations and the cumulative force of resurgent nationalism".
[925] *Ibid*, at 34.

As in South Korea and Japan, policymakers in Singapore have deployed regenerative medicine as apparatus of biosecurity in the production of:

> ... a new idiom of ethics that is bringing to life communities of shared corporeal needs and vulnerabilities. Biotech and biomedical procedures thus trigger emotional maps of belonging and collective fate, enhancing an awareness of the scientific and raising the security stakes of being modern Asian subjects.[926]

Through this observation, Ong argues that 'communities of fate' combines the rationalities of market and science with the 'irrationalities' of feeling and identity in a manner that displaces a strict binary of nature versus culture.

Many scholars have pointed to a distinctive openness to Singapore's approach. Together with Hong Kong, William Keller and Richard Samuels label this 'techno-globalist' given the nation-state's subscription to a political philosophy of free trade within an open international economy with unfettered capital mobility and a relatively laissez-faire regulatory system.[927] In contrast, the approaches of Japan and South Korea are regarded as 'techno-nationalism' under this schema, as there have been stronger tendencies to exert domestic control over production processes and less reliance on foreign direct investment.[928] Taiwan falls in between the two groups, in an approach that represents 'techno-hybridity'.[929] Charis Thompson similarly

---

[926] *Ibid*, at 34-35.

[927] William W Keller and Richard J Samuels, Innovation and the Asian economies. In William W Keller and Richard J Samuels (eds.), *Crisis and Innovation in Asian Technology*. Cambridge: Cambridge University Press, 2003, pp 1-22, at 11. Keller and Samuels recognise that their ideal-typical schema does not provide a complete (and possibly inaccurate) portrayal of the technological regimes in East Asian countries, but their explicit goal is to put forward states as the primary units of analysis.

[928] *Ibid*, at 10.

[929] *Ibid*, at 12. This categorisation has found some degree of support in a recent ethnographic study: Jennifer Liu, Asian Regeneration? Technohybridity in

observes Singapore's strategy to be 'internationalist', with policies that include the "serial kidnapping" of leading biomedical researchers from around the world to further its nationalistic goals.[930] Her ethnographic study that compares Singapore with South Korea clearly distinguishes the two regimes:[931]

> Singapore built and began to fill a facility devoted to a lifestyle of integrated research that embodied both the bench-to-bedside trajectory and the convergence of business, information, and biosciences, while taking care of all the living needs of its civic entrepreneurs. [Referring to South Korea's Dr Hwang Woo Suk before his fall from grace] The prize of one was, or could have been glory ... [Referring to Singapore] The prize of the other is its potential to be Asia's, if not the "world's easiest place to do business," thanks to its stable legal, political, and economic environment. While Singapore has led the way in regional intellectual property law and finance reform, South Korea has been urged by the European Union and others to strengthen its intellectual property regimes. While Singapore continues to pay foreign faculty more than its nationals and to recruit superstars from prestigious universities overseas, South Korea saw one of its own nationals become a household name around the world, and boasts the most successful education system in the world. Both represent different ways of being Asian Tigers.

Joseph Wong attributes Singapore's 'internationalism' to its historical linkages with multinational firms, including big pharmaceutical companies, as well as its locational advantages.[932] However, he is

---

Taiwan's biotech? *East Asian Science Technology and Society International Journal* (2012) 6, 3: 401-414.

930 Charis Thompson, Asian Regeneration? Nationalism and Internationalism in Stem Cell Research in South Korea and Singapore. In Aihwa Ong and Nancy N Chen (eds.), *Asian Biotech: Ethics and Communities of Fate*. Durham and London: Duke University Press, 2010, pp 95-117, at 112.

931 *Ibid*, at 113-114.

932 Joseph Wong, Betting on Biotech: Innovation and the Limits of Asia's Developmental State. Ithaca and London: Cornell University Press, 2011, at 2.

correct in observing that investment in biotechnology involves 'different kinds of bets', in view of uncertainties as to technological viability, economic (and, particularly commercial) value, and temporal range (as the "distance between laboratory and market continues to be very long, unpredictable, and fraught with unforeseeable snags along the way, including regulatory constraints, clinical obstacles, and market uncertainties").[933] More importantly, Singapore (like Taiwan and South Korea) recognises its own vulnerabilities, particularly its small economy and lack of experience with the development and commercialisation of technological innovation.[934] But what I hope to show through my ethnographic study is that the state has not retreated into obscurity, but has adapted its policy strategies to address and manage the uncertainties in the life sciences in a novel way. This is a development that is inconsistent with neoliberalism, which puts forward the view that it is in the public interest to reduce government intervention and allow the operation of the market to benefit as many 'consumers' as possible.[935] A neoliberal agenda directed at creating a 'market society' could lead to a failure of public

---

[933] *Ibid*, at 7.

[934] Wong observes: "Like most other advanced economies, Korea, Taiwan, and Singapore are rich but relatively small, so their prospects in commercializing biotech will depend on global markets, investment, and R&D collaboration. Like many others, they are late entrants into the life sciences field, and relatively inexperienced. They are also without the scale advantages we see in the United States, and emerging giants such as China and India. As a result, decision makers in these three economies, like those in other places, must make strategic choices about how to allocate resources, coordinate disparate actors, and manage the uncertainties of long-term biotech innovation." *Ibid*, at 15.

[935] Warwick Funnell, Robert Jupe and Jane Andrew, *In Government We Trust: Market Failure and the Delusions of Privatisation*. London: Pluto Press, 2009, at 17. Neoliberal thinking was traced to the 1970s when liberal democracies abruptly turned away from what was perceived to be the unchecked growth of the welfare state to public sector reform that forced the retreat of government from the provision of social services. This phenomenon may be further attributed to the inability of Keynesian economics to deal with the 'stagflation' of the 1970s (at 12-16).

life,[936] and is not necessarily consistent with the ideals of democratic society.[937] Neoliberal thinking has been impactful on policymaking, and it has contributed to the privatisation of many state-owned enterprises from the 1990's. In spite of this, the state has retained its ability to channel private initiatives into areas of state priority, and to structure and use state power for development.[938]

An important observation advanced by Wong, and consistent with my ethnographic study, is the emergence of a "multiple stakeholder state", responsible for promoting research and development on the one hand, but also for the protection of human subjects that are involved in research on the other.[939] As these competing goals immediately make clear, regulatory policies are contested among different actors, including within government by different ministerial interests, and consequently uncertain. The state itself has multiple roles, as a mediator and broker, having to reconcile these competing interests, values and perspectives. The inherent uncertainties of regulatory policies relating to the life sciences, and the challenges of asymmetric information, limit the ability of the state to impose a single viewpoint or regulatory stance. Apart from brokerage and mediation, the state further functions as both a market and premarket

---

[936] Anthony Giddens, *The Third Way and its Critics*. Cambridge: Polity Press, 2000, at 51.

[937] Funnell, Jupe and Andrew, I think, correctly observe that concern over the ability of public servants to influence resource allocation decisions in ways that are detrimental to public interests is not necessarily addressed by re-assigning such decisions to the market, for instance. Warwick Funnell, Robert Jupe and Jane Andrew, *In Government We Trust: Market Failure and the Delusions of Privatisation*. London: Pluto Press, 2009, at 273-274.

[938] Atul Kohli's comparative analysis of the state as an economic actor in developing countries is helpful in highlighting the "key issue ... [as] how elites structure use state power for development ... power to define goals clearly and narrowly and power to pursue those goals effectively." Atul Kohli, *State-Directed Development: Political Power and Industrialization in the Global Periphery*. New York: Cambridge University Press, 2004, at 385-386 (Emphasis added). See also at 10-12.

[939] Joseph Wong, *Betting on Biotech: Innovation and the Limits of Asia's Developmental State*. Ithaca and London: Cornell University Press, 2011, at 148-150.

regulatory gatekeeper, especially because the biotech and healthcare sectors "are not constituted solely by consumer demand and industry supply ... [but] by the regulatory functions of the state that shape market access for biotechnological innovations."[940] In addition, the state, as the monopsonistic purchaser of care also affects in some way the price of all health care products and services.[941] Putting this more generally, the state not only defines the regulatory space, but deploy science and technology as regulatory tools to further social and political goals.[942] Link and Link goes further to argue that the government has been and should act as entrepreneur in the provision of technology infrastructure when its involvement is both innovative and characterised by entrepreneurial risk. In the context of the US, they highlight six policy action frameworks, and using a nonlinear model of innovation, show how positive impact has been created when the government acted as entrepreneur on the economy and on society.[943] Specific examples of the US government having acted as entrepreneur, primarily through public-private partnerships, include establishing research joint ventures, the National Institute of Standards and Technology, and university research parks.[944] Hence, contrary to neoliberal thinking of a limited state, the generation of corporeal and affective interests, or 'communities of fate', and the

---

[940] *Ibid*, at 156, and 151.

[941] *Ibid*, at 158.

[942] Roger Brownsword and Karen Yeung, Regulating Technologies: Tools, Targets and Thematics. In Roger Brownsword and Karen Yeung (eds.), *Regulating Technologies: Legal Futures, Regulatory Frames and Technological Fixes*. Oxford and Portland: Hart Publishing, 2008, pp 3-22, at 8-9.

[943] The six frameworks are set out as *National Cooperative Research Act* of 1984, the *Omnibus Trade and Competitiveness Act* of 1988, the *Organic Act* of 1901, the *Biomass Research and Development Act* of 2000 as amended by the *Food, Conservation, and Energy Act* of 2008, the *Building a Stronger America Act* (pending) and the Small Business Innovation Development Act of 1982. Each of these resulted in a public/private partnership that had the economic objective of leveraging either public-sector R&D or private sector R&D, or both. Albert N Link and Jamie R Link, *Government as Entrepreneur*. New York: Oxford University Press, 2009, at 157.

[944] *Ibid*, at 158-160.

management of uncertainties are some of the rationales for state involvement, even if in a less direct and overt manner where bio-ethical governance of biomedical research is concerned.

7.4 Risk and Precaution

Do risks provide a sufficient justification for direct state intervention? How 'real' are these risks? These are some of the often and repeatedly asked question throughout the course of the ED and the HAC projects. Deborah Lupton describes how the different approaches to analysing the role of risk in subjectivity and social relations could relate to one another along an epistemological continuum that spans from the realist position at one end to 'strong' constructionist (or relativist) position at the other end.[945] For a realist, risk is an objective hazard, threat or danger that can be measured independently of social and cultural processes, but may be distorted or biased through social and cultural frameworks of interpretation. Key questions that a realist would ask include: What risks exist? How should we manage them? How do people respond cognitively to risks? In contrast, a 'strong' constructionist takes the position that nothing is a risk in itself, since risk is a product of historically, socially and politically contin-gent 'ways of seeing'. The 'governmentality' and post-structuralist perspectives are examples of this disposition, and their primary interest is in determining how the discourses and practices around risk operate in the construction of subjectivity and social life. An intermediate position is occupied by a 'weak' constructionist, taking risk as an objective hazard, threat or danger that is inevitably mediated through social and cultural processes and can never be known in isolation from these processes. The ('risk society') ap-proaches of Beck and Giddens (discussed in the previous chapter), as well as the 'cultural', structuralist and phenomenological perspectives, are categorised in this position. However, whereas the 'risk society'

---

[945] Deborah Lupton, *Risk*. London and New York: Routledge, 1999, at 35.

approaches would focus on the relationship of risk to the structures and processes of late modernity and its meaning in different sociocultural contexts, the other 'weak' constructionist perspectives consider the choice of certain dangers as risks over others, the ways in which risk operates as a symbolic boundary, and the context in which risk is situated.

Broadly speaking, the reports of the BAC presents risk in a 'weak' constructionist sense. Certain risks, such as the onset of OHSS, are generally felt to be 'real'. Other risks that are associated with long-term adverse health effects, commercialisation and humanising nonhuman animals are regarded as relatively more value-based or cultural, but no less important or 'real'. The latter should not be surprising as they are 'uncertain risks' that are either not quantified or unquantifiable. Uncertain risks reveal the limits of science owing to a number of reasons including complex causalities, length of time, scale and durability of impact, among others. Any decision that pertains to them must be premised on social and political values. Consequently, uncertain risks also have a more pronounced political character, quite aside from their perceived potential to undermine public trust or social stability. One standard approach to an uncertain risk is to react only when its imminent occurrence renders it more certain. However, the precautionary principle or approach, first articulated in the 1992 *Rio Declaration on Environment and Development*,[946] brought about a new way of engaging with uncertain risks. Precaution is meta-legal in that it allows "legal provisions to incorporate

---

[946] United Nations, *Rio Declaration on Environment and Development*, UN Doc. A/CONF.151/26, vol I, annex I, 1992. Paragraph 15 states: "In order to protect the environment, the precautionary approach shall be widely applied by States according to their capabilities. Where there are threats of serious or irreversible damage, lack of full scientific certainty shall not be used as a reason for postponing cost-effective measures to prevent environmental degradation."

considerations beyond those resulting from strictly positive law."[947] In other words, the precautionary principle recognises the impossibility of establishing absolute safety, but instead enables action through the determination of four criteria:[948]

(1) Risk typification and assessment, encompassing the categories of risks (i.e. risks that are 'unacceptable', 'residual' or 'uncertain'), and the components of a precautionary risk assessment;

(2) Damage, or impact which could be severe and irreversible;

(3) Scientific uncertainty, which generally relates to a minimum level of knowledge; and

(4) Different capacities, in recognition of the fact that the states concerned have different capabilities in dealing with a challenge.

Apart from these criteria, the values of democracy and transparency are embedded in many international instruments, including the *Rio Declaration* (in Principle 10), so that public participation is fundamental to the precautionary process.[949] It is important to emphasise here that the four criteria that substantively define precaution denote processes that would often already be encapsulated in democratic organisations and institutions. In addition, these processes that embody the precautionary principle re-balances knowledge systems, such as the interaction between legal politics and science, so that "science would be sought for the suspicions and doubts that it raises rather than for the knowledge it offers."[950] To put this differently, science is not seen as presenting indisputable truths (in

---

[947] Laurence Boisson de Chazournes, New Technologies, the Precautionary Principle, and Public Participation. In Thérèse Murphy (ed.), *New Technologies and Human Rights*. Oxford: Oxford University Press, 2009, pp 161-194, at 163.

[948] *Ibid*, at 168-178.

[949] *Ibid*, at 178-179.

[950] *Ibid*, at 192.

the light of the uncertain risks) but nevertheless has an important role in framing and constraining the debate.

Precaution has not found uniform application however. Through an extensive comparative study of policy orientations toward the precautionary principle in the US and in the European Union, Jonathan Wiener found that:[951]

> From the 1970s through the 1980s, both the United States and Europe adopted precaution in particular laws, and then in international agreements. In the 1990s, Europe – at both the level of the EU and in key Member States – then adopted the PP [Precautionary Principle] as the formal overarching basis for risk regulation, while the United States did not.

Despite this difference, Wiener did not find the US and Europe as growing progressively more precautionary over time. Instead, Europe appeared to be more precautionary in relation to certain risks (such as genetically modified food, toxic chemicals, teenage use of marijuana and other drugs, and guns) whereas the US was more precautionary towards other risks (such as new drug approval and adverse side effects, embryonic stem cell research, cigarette smoking and teenage use of alcohol).[952] These differences were attributable

---

951 Jonathan Wiener, The Rhetoric of Precaution. In Jonathan B Wiener, Michael D Rogers, James K Hammitt and Peter H Sand (eds.), *The Reality of Precaution: Comparing Risk Regulation in the United States and Europe*. Washington DC and London: RFF Press, 2011, pp 3-35, at 12. The comparative approach combines two comparative methodologies: a set of case studies of specific risks and policies, and a quantitative analysis of a sample of 100 risks drawn from a database of nearly 3,000 risks: see Jonathan Wiener, The Real Pattern of Precaution. In Jonathan B Wiener, Michael D Rogers, James K Hammitt and Peter H Sand (eds.), *The Reality of Precaution: Comparing Risk Regulation in the United States and Europe*. Washington DC and London: RFF Press, 2011, pp 519-565, at 524.

952 Jonathan Wiener, The Real Pattern of Precaution. In Jonathan B. Wiener, Michael D. Rogers, James K Hammitt and Peter H Sand (eds.), *The Reality of Precaution: Comparing Risk Regulation in the United States and Europe*. Washington DC and London: RFF Press, 2011, pp 519-565, at 524-526. Wiener observes (at 526): "Simplistic contrasts – that "Americans are risk-takers while Europeans are

to the occurrence of crisis events, availability heuristics and processes of social amplification, and political responses.[953] As for the general character of risk regulation in the US and Europe, Wiener indicated that neither the case studies nor the quantitative study provided support for the hypotheses of US-Europe convergence, divergence or reversal (flip-flop) in relative precaution over the past four decades.[954] However, the research did show significant interconnectedness and transnational exchange in the diffusion, borrowing and 'hybridisation' of regulatory systems.[955]

In addition, precaution is not always referred to in the implementation of risk containment measures. Frances Miller observes that most patient safety initiatives in the US and Europe have not been addressed in precautionary principle terminology. She explains that differences arise mainly owing to events that are largely circumstantial or economic:[956]

> ... under pressure from medical activists for faster access to experimental drugs and from the pharmaceutical industry for accelerated approval policies as the drug industry globalizes, the FDA has relaxed its comparatively rigorous regulatory barriers. At the same time, the EU has increasingly centralized its drug approval processes, tightening the standards in use by some of the less safety-focused Member States, but it has not appreciably raised the level of rigor already in effect in others.

---

risk-averse" – are not supported by actual regulatory experience. Nor are claims that "Americans are individualistic and antiregulation, while Europeans are collectivist and proregulation," in the face of greater U.S. precaution in regulatory policies that restrict the freedom to smoke and that limit freedom and privacy in order to combat terrorism."

953 *Ibid*, at 540-541.

954 *Ibid*, at 533.

955 *Ibid*, at 541-544.

956 Frances H Miller, Medical Errors, New Drug Approval, and Patient Safety. In Jonathan B Wiener, Michael D Rogers, James K Hammitt and Peter H Sand (eds.), *The Reality of Precaution: Comparing Risk Regulation in the United States and Europe*. Washington DC and London: RFF Press, 2011, pp 257-284, at 277.

Instead, the main risks often associated with biomedical research are risks of physical or psychological harm to participants, risks to the objectivity and scientific integrity of research (mainly from conflicts of interests) and risks to other social values, such as public trust.[957] These risks have in turn been scrutinised for potential 'gaps' in 'real world' risk assessment, calibration errors (due to lack of information or multiple variables for instance), different values in risk assessment and evaluation, and different attitudes towards risks.[958] The problem with a strong version of the precautionary principle – as Jonathan Wiener observes – is that it negates other important considerations such as cost, innovation, false positives and risk-risk trade-offs. Instead, the 'Better Regulation' initiative (further discussed below), with focus on impact assessment, selection among risks and executive oversight, is preferred as a more moderate approach for less extreme risks.[959] The precautionary principle has a less direct but no less important function in public policy however. It is what Michelle Everson and Ellen Vos argue to be:[960]

> ... a 'high-level policy', which political actors must use to elaborate particular rules to apply to particular fact-finding procedures. The legal contextualisation of the principle underlines its relational status. Precaution and the evidential basis for precaution alter in the

---

[957] Duff R Waring and Trudo Lemmens, Integrating Values in Risk Analysis of Biomedical Research: The Case for Regulatory and Law Reform. In Law Commission of Canada, *Law and Risk*. Vancouver and Toronto: University of British Columbia Press, 2005, pp 156-200, at 157.

[958] *Ibid*, at 160-166.

[959] Jonathan Wiener, The Real Pattern of Precaution. In Jonathan B Wiener, Michael D Rogers, James K Hammitt and Peter H Sand (eds.), *The Reality of Precaution: Comparing Risk Regulation in the United States and Europe*. Washington DC and London: RFF Press, 2011, pp 519-565, at 551. Wiener indicates that strong form precautionary principle remains applicable towards extreme catastrophic risks.

[960] Michelle Everson and Ellen Vos, The scientification of politics and the politicisation of science. In Michelle Everson and Ellen Vos (eds.), *Uncertain Risks Regulated*. Abingdon and New York: Routledge, 2009, pp 1-17, at 7.

light of the particular circumstances of production, the socio-economic features of particular production processes, as well as with regard to the legal culture within which evidence for precaution must be established.

Arguably, it is this precautionary disposition that not only creates relevance for, but perhaps even necessitates, bioethics as a public policy tool in addressing the challenges of uncertain risks thrown up by novel biotechnologies.[961] In this respect, the intermediary role of bioethics is crucial due to the perceived impropriety for the state to meddle directly in scientific affairs. At this point, a few remarks may be made about why a purely legal response to uncertain risks is felt to be inappropriate. The law is assumed to be more concerned with prevention than precaution, and tends to preclude risks on an all-or-nothing basis (i.e. in the binary of 'allowed' or 'prohibited'). Along a similar trajectory, the law is considered to be most pertinent when harm arises, in which case it has a restitutive or reparative function. In contrast, a less directive and more flexible bioethical framework has broadly been considered to be more appropriate than a legal one in the governance of 'emergent' or 'new' biotechnologies. A further reason for this has been consistently based on the view that novel biotechnologies progress much faster than law, so that the latter must always (but can never quite) catch up with the former.[962] Such a view

---

[961] In the bioethics and STS literature, there appears to be an inclination to re-frame precaution as vulnerability. It is beyond the scope of this study to consider the increasingly rich discourse on vulnerability, and this development is noted here for completeness. As illustration of works in this genre, see the collection of papers in: Catherine Mackenzie, Wendy Rogers and Susan Dodds (eds.), *Vulnerability: New Essays in Ethics and Feminist Philosophy*. Oxford: Oxford University Press, 2013; Anique Hommels, Jessica Mesman and Wiebe E Bijker (eds.), *Vulnerability in Technological Cultures: New Directions in Research and Governance*. Cambridge MA: MIT Press, 2014.

[962] For instance, Clarence Davis writes: "A regulatory system that takes two years to issue a rule cannot deal with an economy where project lines typically change every six months. A regulatory law focused on types of chemicals cannot deal with something like nanomaterials, where often the same chemical substance can have

considers the law to be always reactive to the risks that have become 'real'. Interestingly, a concomitant concern over the efficacy of bioethical governance has contributed to hybridised legal and quasi-legal arrangements that continue to be justified by precaution. To be sure, there are clearly merits in the broader bioethical response to risks, and this book argues in favour of this development. However, these pronounced assumptions of the law should be questioned.

Let us first consider the claim that the law always lags behind scientific development, and would hence be unable to respond appropriately to risks. This may be correct in respect of legal formalities, but it fails to appreciate that the law is often relied upon to make risks 'real'. For instance, regulatory bodies established through legislation make explicit the types of risk that they attempt to control or ameliorate. In the US, government agencies like the DHHS make apparent a wide range of risks that affect human health and safety, and the environment. More importantly, it is arguably difficult, if not impossible, to understand risks as distinct from legal and other regulatory processes. For 'emerging' areas like nanotechnology, regulatory procedures have enabled policymakers to manage uncertainty through institutional and regulatory design. Hence the question of what to regulate may not be so different from how to regulate, since the risk envisaged may be indistinguishable from the appropriate regulatory instrument that relates to it.[963] The study presented in this book shows how legal rationalities, techniques and practices have

---

radically different effects depending on small changes in its shape or the method by which it is manufactured." J Clarence Davis, Foreword: Nanotechnology, Risk, and Governance. In Christopher J Bosso (ed.), *Governing Uncertainty: Environmental Regulation in the Age of Nanotechnology*. Washington DC and London: RFF Press, 2010, pp xii to xviii, at xvii.

963 Marc Allen Eisner, Institutional Evolution or Intelligent Design? Constructing a Regulatory Regime for Nanotechnology. In Christopher J Bosso (ed.), *Governing Uncertainty: Environmental Regulation in the Age of Nanotechnology*. Washington DC and London: RFF Press, 2010, pp 28-45.

been applied in various ways to make risk explicit by giving it form and substance.

In addition, it is erroneous to think of law as a closed knowledge system. Legal and regulatory rules relate the regulator to the regulated, although this relationship could well be collaborative due to asymmetric information, where the regulated is likely to be far more knowledgeable than the regulator on the 'risks' envisaged.[964] Graeme Laurie *et al.* have, through the metaphor of 'legal foresighting', argued that law can be a means of creating pathways into the unknown technological future, and this could mean "a fundamental re-visioning of the legal setting itself, its instruments, institutions, and regulatory or governance mechanisms."[965] For such foresighting exercises to be effective, the law must work towards the discovery of share values, the development of shared lexicons, forging of a common vision of the future, and take steps to realise that vision with the understanding that this is being done from a position of partial knowledge about the present.[966] In a nutshell, the law must reach beyond itself to be effective in achieving the outcomes that are considered desirable by itself as a purposeful social institution. Mariana Valverde *et al.* illustrate how legal processes are inherent to understanding the risk of a repeat sexual offence under 'Megan's Law',[967] which encompasses the US community notification statute relating to sexual offenders. Comprising three tiers, this risk assessment process determines the scope of community notification. In examining the constitutional basis of Megan's Law, they observe

---

964 Cary Coglianese, Engaging Business in the Regulation of Nanotechnology. In Christopher J Bosso (ed.), *Governing Uncertainty: Environmental Regulation in the Age of Nanotechnology.* Washington DC and London: RFF Press, 2010, pp 46-79.

965 Graeme Laurie, Shawn H E Harmon and Fabiana Arzuaga, Foresighting Futures: Law, New Technologies, and the Challenges of Regulating for Uncertainty, *Law, Innovation and Technology* (2012) 4, 1: 1-33, at 3.

966 *Ibid*, 11-27. A reflexive approach involving five foundational considerations and a three-dimensional master matrix are proposed.

967 *Jacob Wetterling Crimes Against Children and Sexually Violent Offender Registration Act* of 1994, Pub. L. No. 104-145.

that "the courts have emphasized the scientific expertise that is said to be behind the registrant risk assessment scale (RRAS) in order to argue that Megan's Law is not a tool of punishment but rather an objective measure to regulate a social problem." However, reliance on Megan's Law as grounded in 'objective' scientific knowledge has given rise to an "intermediary knowledge in which legal actors – prosecutors and judges '– are said not only to be more fair but even more reliable and accurate in determining a registrant's risk of re-offence."[968] Such intermediary knowledge illustrates a cross-pollination between scientific knowledge and legal ones. Taking a position that differs from that of Niklas Luhmann and Gunther Teubner, Valverde *et al.* present the 'law' as cognitively and normatively open, whilst highlighting that an institutional or structural arrangement like the court may enable the creation of a "more or less common fund of knowledges" by which conceptions of 'risks' materialise:[969]

> [I]t is important to note that the swapping of knowledge is not simply a result of one-time social interactions between actors with different training. The swapping is built into the very structure of the court. In an interview, the judge explained that he is not himself an expert on addiction. Rather, the team structure of the court ... allows everyone in the court to use the same knowledges ... The use of the term "team" is quite purposeful since it erases the institutional distinctions that would in other situations not only divide people but set them at cross-purposes.

Initiatives like 'Better Regulation' mentioned earlier add impetus to introducing greater reflexivity and openness to law-making and

---

968 Mariana Valverde, Ron Levi and Dawn Moore, Legal Knowledges of Risk. In Law Commission of Canada, *Law and Risk*. Vancouver and Toronto: University of British Columbia Press, 2005, pp 86-120, at 103 and 106.

969 *Ibid*, at 115. Luhmann and Teubner are said to conceptualize the law as "cognitively open but is normatively closed" (at 94).

implementation.[970] Although presently limited to OECD countries, 'Better Regulation' illustrates measures taken to encourage and enable states to improve legal quality. Notably, this initiative is not driven by a crisis, and is markedly different from deregulation. Significant emphasis is placed on the integration of stakeholder engagement into each step of the rule-making cycle, and ultimately, as part of the day-to-day work of policy makers and citizens. Taking stakeholder inputs seriously and continuously evaluating engagement practices are expected to improve the effectiveness of regulations. Essentially, the current trend is a shift away from privileging one knowledge system over another, but to recognise that they could all contribute in important ways to knowledge-generation in public policy and governance.[971] This is sensible because each knowledge system has its own biases and 'blind spots'. Although I agree with the view that law is not epistemically exclusive, it nevertheless prioritises and emphasises certain requirements over others. For instance, Roger Brownsword and Morag Goodwin set out what the law must achieve in response to novel and transnational technological activities:[972]

(1) Maintain continuity, stability and the rule of law;

---

[970] OECD, *OECD Regulatory Policy Outlook 2015*. Paris: OECD Publishing, 2015. See also '*Better Regulation in Europe – The EU 15 project*' at: http://www.oecd.org/gov/regref/eu15

[971] Sheila Jasanoff has argued for the recognition of law and science as knowledge-generating institutions, although fact-finding serves different functions in these two settings. For the courts, its concern is less about the science than rendering justice under conditions of uncertain risks. Sheila Jasanoff, Law's Knowledge: Science for Justice in Legal Settings, *American Journal of Public Health* (2005) 95, S1: S49-S58.

[972] Roger Brownsword and Morag Goodwin, *Law and the Technologies of the Twenty-First Century*. Cambridge: Cambridge University Press, at 23. See also the five foundational considerations of law in mapping out technological futures: Graeme Laurie, Shawn H E Harmon and Fabiana Arzuaga, Foresighting Futures: Law, New Technologies, and the Challenges of Regulating for Uncertainty, *Law, Innovation and Technology* (2012) 4, 1: 1-33, at 11.

(2) Minimise anticipated risks and maximise expected benefits; and

(3) Safeguard fundamental values of communities, such as respect for human rights and human dignity.

In view of the fact that the law or some other knowledge system will amplify some concerns and omit others, inclusivity is the best and possibly only means of devising a holistic approach. Here again, Michelle Everson and Ellen Vos put across the rationale for public engagement nicely:[973]

> ... participation does not simply serve abstract normative goals of government such as enhancing trust or meeting democratic requirements, but also acts as part of knowledge creation itself, as a material contribution to the evidential bases for the assessment and management of risk. In this way, participation thus aims to enhance the quality both of scientific opinion and of the management decision. ... allowing citizens and/or stakeholders to participate in management decision making may also enhance the quality of final decisions, as they are then able to express themselves on the management options/preferences at issue, thus augmenting the knowledge-base for decision making.

There is a further justification for greater stakeholder and/or public engagement. Apart from the unquantified risks that arise from the technology itself, uncertainty is compounded by the anticipatory nature of bioethical deliberation and governance. From an STS standpoint at least, key questions include: Who gets to shape the future direction of the technology? Which are the parties most likely to benefit, and at the expense of whom? What are the justifications? When and how should precautionary measures be implemented?

---

[973] Michelle Everson and Ellen Vos, The scientification of politics and the politicisation of science. In Michelle Everson and Ellen Vos (eds.), *Uncertain Risks Regulated*. Abingdon and New York: Routledge, 2009, pp. 1-17, at 8.

7.5 Anticipatory Knowledge and Governance

All accounts of risks are to varying degrees anticipatory.[974] In contemporary societies, Andrew Lakoff and Stephen Collier illustrate how the vulnerability of critical infrastructure (such as water, electricity, communication and transportation) has become an object of knowledge for security experts in the US. Threats that include natural disasters, terrorist attacks, technical malfunction and novel pathogens not only endanger infrastructure, but also, collective life which it enables and sustains. Consistent with our considerations so far, it is the responses to these threats (or risks) that relate more directly to knowledge production than the 'object' itself. Arguably this is all the more so, where the 'object' of knowledge is not something tangible, but a consortium of societal ideals. Many of these risks have yet to materialise, and are made 'real' mainly through the imaginative enactment of certain types of events, or through what Lakoff and Collier refer to as a 'political technology of preparedness'. These responses or interventions have epistemic basis when applied to a problem of collective life and could even constitute a knowledge system to varying degrees.[975]

To pick up on Michael Power's point on addressing 'risk' as a form of learning and experimentation rather than rule-based processes (in the previous chapter), the construction of artefacts like embryos, chimeras and hybrids as 'risky objects' and the articulation of possible

---

[974] We conclude by working through an analytical framework put forward by Nelson, Geltzer and Hilgartner: Nicole Nelson, Anna Geltzer and Stephen Hilgartner, Introduction: the anticipatory state: making policy-relevant knowledge about the future, *Science and Public Policy* (October 2008) 35, 8: 546-550, at 547.

[975] Andrew Lakoff and Stephen J Collier, Infrastructure and Event: The Political Technology of Preparedness. In Bruce Braun and Sarah J Whatmore (eds.), *Political Matter: Technoscience, Democracy, and Public Life*. Minneapolis and London: University of Minnesota Press, 2010, pp 243-266, at 244. Lakoff and Collier illustrate how institutionalised knowledge was developed in the United States Civil Defense in the 1950's as a form of vulnerability mapping in the event of a surprise nuclear attack by the Soviet Union (at 249-255).

harms and dangers as 'risks' involve the generation of 'anticipatory' knowledge', or "social mechanisms and institutional capacities involved in producing, disseminating, and using such forms [as] ... forecasts, models, scenarios, foresight exercises, threat assessments, and narratives about possible technological and societal futures." In other words, they are connected with knowledge-making about the future.[976] Drawing inspiration from Ian Hacking's 'looping effect', where knowledge of psychiatric diagnosis may alter the patient's psychological experience, Nicole Nelson *et al.* observe that anticipatory knowledge does not merely represent the future, but inevitably intervenes in it.[977] As we have seen, the consistency of public concerns with those identified by the BAC may well reflect the 'Thomas theorem', where real consequences follow when something (albeit imaginary) is treated as real.[978]

Hugh Gusterson conceptualises anticipatory knowledge as a means to gap-filling (we considered earlier that public consultation has this function). In his study of the Reliable Replacement Warhead (RRW) program, US weapons laboratories could design new and highly reliable nuclear weapons that are considered to be safe to manufacture and maintain. Initiated by the US Congress in 2004, Gusterson shows that struggle over the RRW occurred across four intersecting "plateaus of nuclear calculations" – geopolitical, strategic, enviropolitical and technoscientific – each with its own contending narratives of the future. He observes that "advocates must stabilize and align anticipatory knowledge from each plateau of calculation into a coherent-enough narrative of the future in the face of opponents seeking to generate and secure alternative anticipatory

---

[976] Nicole Nelson, Anna Geltzer and Stephen Hilgartner, Introduction: the anticipatory state: making policy-relevant knowledge about the future, *Science and Public Policy* (October 2008) 35, 8: 546-550, at 546.

[977] *Ibid*, at 547 and 550.

[978] William I Thomas and Dorothy S Thomas. *The child in America: Behaviour problems and programs.* New York: Knopf, 1928, at 571-572.

knowledges."[979] Hence the *interconnectedness* of the four plateaus of calculation, including the tradeoffs entailed, was evident in the production of anticipatory knowledge vis-à-vis the RRW program.[980] Gusterson further observes that being craft items, no two nuclear weapons are exactly alike. However, the proscription of testing through detonation meant that both performativity and ambiguity (referred to as 'social construction of ambiguity') over reliability become matters of speculation, determined through extrapolation from the past to fill knowledge 'gaps' in the present and future. This attempt at anticipatory knowledge creation also prescribed a form that the future was to take.[981] Although anticipatory knowledge as foreknowledge can be a useful tool for international organisations and national policymakers to cope with lack of information, conflict could arise over the generalisability of foreknowledge. Manjari Mahajan shows this in the contention between international health organisations and Indian bureaucrats over the actual epidemiological risks posed by AIDS in India. Foreknowledge as what is already conceptualised and "equipped with prior models, categories and information" leaves little room for the unexpected.[982] It could thereby privilege a globalised anticipatory knowledge over national policy-making, even if the former might not be true or appropriate in a particular location.

---

[979] Hugh Gusterson, Nuclear futures: anticipatory knowledge, expert judgment, and the lack that cannot be filled. *Science and Public Policy* (October 2008) 35, 8: 551-560, at 553.

[980] *Ibid*, at 558-559.

[981] *Ibid*, at 558-559 (footnote). Gusterson observes: "Anticipation, then, takes on a Heisenbergian dimension as a form of knowledge that not only guesses about events in the world but directs them in unintended but unavoidable ways. In such a situation, the knowing guess is never innocent. The natural inclination to 'play it safe'…may end up, through the feedback loops that connect the anticipated with the actual, enacting the less safe world against which playing it safe was a hedge. The search for insurance against disaster may become insurance of disaster."

[982] Manjari Mahajan, Designing epidemics: models, policy-making, and global foreknowledge in India's AIDS epidemic, *Science and Public Policy* (October 2008) 35, 8: 585-596, at 594.

Ongoing discussions on anticipatory knowledge and governance are helpful in facilitating a more critical evaluation of the BAC's reports and public engagements, particularly where they are anticipatory of a number of challenges envisaged. In its ED Report, the BAC was concerned that in adopting a more liberal attitude towards payment for eggs, it would be moving in the direction of commercialising the human body. More immediately, the BAC was concerned with the exploitation of under-privileged women. This account is an 'anticipatory knowledge' strategically deployed to counter competing (primarily neoliberal) knowledge claims of proponents for the greater monetisation of research.[983] But being a placeholder-type of foreknowledge that falls outside of its constituent 'expertise', there is a greater need for transparency and clarity, mainly to secure its legitimacy. More generally, the frequent lack of transparency and clarity over anticipatory assumptions and objectives is a well-recognised problem in the construction of anticipatory knowledge. Kathleen Vogel illustrates how the quasi-journalistic reporting of gathered intelligence led to an erroneous assessment of Iraq's bioweapons capability.[984] Being critically reflective of the cumulative (temporal and material) effect of anticipatory frames and the practices undergirding them is necessary in order to understand

---

[983] This version of 'anticipatory knowledge' as knowledge marshalled by political teams in anticipation of the knowledge claims of rival teams is proposed by Tara Schwegler. Tara A Schwegler, Take it from the top (down)? Rethinking neoliberalism and political hierarchy in Mexico, *American Ethnologist* (November 2008) 35, 4: 682-700.

[984] Kathleen M Vogel, 'Iraqi Winnebagos™ of death': imagined and realized futures of US bioweapons threat assessments, *Science and Public Policy* (October 2008) 35, 8: 561-573, at 568. While drawing of mobile labs may be the 'immutable mobiles' in Vogel's paper, they take on more varied forms in my research, including images of 'chimeras' and 'hybrids', and more importantly ethical principles that critically define the almost unquestionable disciplined space within which bioethical facticity arises.

and mitigate intelligence failures.[985] Iain Wilkinson similarly observes that risk discourse in the technical domain:[986]

> ... largely concerns the identification of criteria for upholding an 'objective' account of the probable occurrence of specific events of adversity...[and one] should be careful to pay heed to the extent to which the agendas for risk research are determined by sectorial interest groups that have no desire to pursue questions relating to who has the legitimate power to decide which risks should be prioritised and how issues of 'social benefit' and 'technological progress' should be defined.

While transparency and inclusivity are clearly necessary to prevent anticipatory knowledge (and any governance practice that is informed by it) from foreclosing legitimate technological futures, positional reflexivity and critical distance are equally necessary.[987] Public engagement may not ultimately be a productive exercise unless its members have the societal capacity to articulate and apply public values in the context of emergent technologies. Similarly, researchers may not appreciate the social conditions of the technology of interest, and hence fail to recognise the need for dialogue and reflexive decision making. In other words, engagement is not purely performative, but must necessarily be supported by social and institutional arrangements and practices that promote public reasoning for accountability and legitimacy.

---

[985] *Ibid*, at 571. Vogel notes further (at 572): "... one needs to be reflective of the social processes comprising knowledge production, to see how different organizational frames and practices can lead to particular kinds of knowledge being produced to inform the prediction of future threats".

[986] Iain Wilkinson, *Risk, Vulnerability and Everyday Life*. London and New York: Routledge, 2010, at 92-93, and 95.

[987] David H Guston, Understanding 'anticipatory governance', *Social Studies of Science* (2014) 44, 2: 218-242, at 231-234.

7.6 Bioethics as Public Reason and an Emergent Civic Epistemology

A question that has been central to the study presented in this book is concerned with whether research involving the human embryo and pluripotent stem cells should be allowed in the light of the risks of harm that it presents to the moral status of a person and to human dignity. If it is to be allowed, how should it be legitimately governed in view of the uncertain risks that the research entails? As we have seen, the debate that these and related issues have generated is characterised by a diversity of opposing and irreconcilable religious, philosophical and moral doctrines. Scientific knowledge and reasoning have been helpful in framing the discussion by outlining the technical feasibilities, but no satisfactory response could be provided in purely scientific terms. The challenges that these issues present are essentially a more particular manifestation of a critical question that John Rawls presents in *Political Liberalism*:[988] "[I]s it possible for there to exist over time a just and stable society of free and equal citizens who remain profoundly divided by reasonable religious, philosophical, and moral doctrines?" Rawls tells us that such a political order is most likely to be realised through liberal neutrality, premised on the 'liberal principle of legitimacy', which requires the exercise of political power to be publicly justifiable to the citizens (as subjects of this power) through public reason.[989] Rawls explains that public reason is premised on the moral ideals of mutual respect and reciprocity, as it is only through reasoning from this premise that fair terms of cooperation may be derived. Public reason imposes a moral 'duty of civility', where citizens are bound to listen to others and to be fair-minded in deciding when views other than their own should reasonably be accommodated. In exercising public reason, citizens should not base their decision merely on their respective comprehensive conceptions of the good and the right, or otherwise only to

---

[988] John Rawls, *Political Liberalism*. New York: Columbia University Press, 1993, at 4.
[989] *Ibid*, at 217.

advance their own personal interests, but should instead decide on reasons that they can expect their fellow citizens to share, with a view to minimising their differences. According to Rawls, such an expectation is reasonable only in relation to decisions on constitutional essentials and on matters of basic justice.[990] A point worth noting about public reason is that it is not deterministic or univocal, but encompasses many types of disagreement that arise from its constituent 'freestanding' concepts, principles and arguments of the political conception.[991]

In view of the political nature of bioethical governance within a public policy framework, it may be asked if public reason should apply in bioethical decision-making. Herlinde Pauer-Studer explains that public reason should apply to constitutional and parliamentary debates about bioethical issues as they are clearly within the context of a bounded, liberal and democratic political society that Rawls has confined its application to.[992] When policymakers or judges have to deal with a bioethical issue as a constitutional concern, they should set aside their personal comprehensive doctrines and instead apply political values that are stated in the constitution. Public reason should similarly apply to debates on bioethical issues in parliament that relate to constitutional rights and questions of basic justice. However, she goes further to argue that public reason should also apply to the work of ethics committees where proposals for legal regulations are deliberated. In this role, ethics committees have a public function and so its members should not decide based on comprehensive moral and religious doctrines. But reference to freestanding arguments that go beyond the meaning of the basic

---

[990] *Ibid*, at 214 and 227. Rawls explicit states that the limits imposed by public reason do not apply to all political questions.

[991] John Rawls, *The Law of Peoples*. Cambridge MA: Harvard University Press, 1999, at 140-143.

[992] Herlinde Pauer-Studer, Public Reason and Bioethics, Medscape General Medicine (2006) 8, 4: 13-21, at 16.

political values should be acceptable as their validity does not depend on comprehensive doctrines.[993]

On the nature of public reason, Pauer-Studer argues that the Rawlsian conception has the strength of being more inclusive over other conceptions, notably Habermas's. As she explains, Habermas's discourse-based conception ultimately requires a particular normative claim to be selected through argumentation conducted in accordance with the principles of impartiality and fairness.[994] Others have argued in favour of Habermas's less restrictive conception of public reason. Adela Cortina, for instance, argues that bioethics should be a discursive space where moral judgments can be shaped and discovered.[995] By her assessment, a discourse-based public reason should apply to any institution whose activities have public consequences. She further argues that bodies like bioethics commissions could serve as 'authentic laboratories of bioethics', provided that members of the commission debate issues based on 'civil ethics' and in good faith, and for the purpose of reaching a dialogical decision, which is revisable, open and reasonable.[996] Not specific to bioethics, Onora O'Neill similarly recognises merit to a broader conception of public reason than Rawls's: first, it allows for the justness of particular institutional arrangements to be evaluated, and second, it does not exclude the non-citizens.[997] In proposing a relatively more discourse-based approach, O'Neill observes that all communications are ultimately constrained by institutional structures and ideological content in order to be intelligible, assessable and relational. When a communication that is intelligible and assessable is also universal (or law-like) in form, it acquires normative character. Combined with

---

[993] *Ibid*, at 17-18.

[994] *Ibid*, at 15.

[995] Adela Cortina, Bioethics and Public Reason: A Report on Ethics and Public Discourse in Spain, *Cambridge Quarterly of Healthcare Ethics* (2009) 18: 241-250.

[996] *Ibid*, at 249.

[997] Onora O'Neill, Changing Constructions. In Thom Brooks and Martha C Nussbaum, *Rawls's Political Liberalism*. New York: Columbia University Press, 2015, pp 57-72, at 66.

universal scope (i.e. capable of being justified to an unrestricted audience), it presents itself as a broader conception of public reasoning. In other words, public reasoning could be re-constructed more broadly as reasoning designed to reach an unrestricted audience with an intent "to ensure that all can understand them, and assess them, and see their point and perhaps, more, even if they find and foresee little current prospect of living by them."[998]

If we are prepared to accept a degree of flexibility to conceptualising public reason in terms of its form and scope,[999] it is difficult to deny its application in the decisions and recommendations of bioethical bodies we have considered in this study (principally the BAC, NAS, AMS, DCE and GEC). None of these bodies have appealed to particular or sectorial interests, and all have attempted to provide justifications based on some notion of common interests and common good. The narratives presented for the purposes of public consultation mostly reflected mixed judgments, which are typical of bioethical decisions because they are based on a series of partial answers to descriptive and prognostic questions, and justified in different disciplines and discourses.[1000] For this reason, none of them are generated with a view to being truly universal in scope, and some of which are explicit expressed as pragmatic in nature. While it is not always clear if the issues are of constitutional significance or relate to basic justice, the spirit of law is implicit in the constitutionality of the approach adopted. All recommendations that have been proposed,

---

998   *Ibid*, at 69. Onora O'Neill also observes that it is necessary to ask which principles (such as principles of violence or deception) cannot be universally adopted, as their adoption, even by some, would be expressed and reflected in action that would disable or prevent at least some others from similar action.

999   For instance, Kim argues that Confucian perfectionist goods can be incorporated as the core elements of public reason with which citizens can justify their arguments to one another and the state can justifiably exercise its public authority to reasonable citizens. Sungmoon Kim, Public Reason Confucianism: A Construction, *American Political Science Review* (2015) 109, 1: 187-200.

1000 Marcus Düwell, *Bioethics: Methods, Theories, Domains*. London and New York: Routledge, 2013, at 9.

especially where they relate to governance practices, respect the rule of law in being non-arbitrary, prospective and impersonal.[1001] Even if, as we have considered above, there should be state interest in promoting biomedical research for reasons of nationalism or economic gain, the initiative of (in the case of the BAC) setting apart bioethical evaluation as an independent mechanism has been mostly effective in keeping direct state interests at arms-length. Most critically, public engagement has not been purely performative or otherwise directed solely at promoting a national agenda. I base my assessment on this test that Albert Weale has put forward:[1002] "for any putative piece of public reasoning, how likely is it that any member of the public with sufficient skill and time could follow the train of reasoning that led to a practical policy conclusion without finding logical fault, as distinct from differing in assumptions?" The key thought – as he explains – is that in a democracy, anyone, in principle, ought to be able to replicate the same conclusion for a given set of premises and body of evidence. For present purposes, we are able to sidestep the question of whether we should leave behind the boundedness of public reason under the Rawlsian formulation. None of the bodies considered in this study have attempted to do so. However, there are good reasons, as Onora O'Neill observes, to examine the justness of institutional arrangements by which these bodies have constructed the narratives on human pluripotent stem cell research as anticipatory knowledge. It seems to me that such an initiative is encapsulated in the notion of civic epistemology in STS.

Civic epistemology refers to the "social and institutional practices by which political communities construct, review, validate, and deliberate politically relevant knowledge ... [and includes] the styles of reasoning, modes of argumentation, standards of evidence, and

---

1001 Lon L Fuller, *The Morality of Law*. New Haven: Yale University Press, 1964.

1002 Albert Weale, New Modes of Governance, Political Accountability and Public Reason, *Government and Opposition* (2011) 46, 1: 58-80, at 76.

norms of expertise that characterize public deliberation and political institutions."[1003] In other words, civic epistemology relates to the ways by which policy issues are reasoned and understood (i.e. knowledge making) through an organised political order (what Miller terms 'knowledge-order').[1004] Here, knowledge is product of complex judgments involving a variety of means by which multiple forms of evidence are assessed for their credibility and meaning, weighed and integrated. These complex judgments are in turn products of particular knowledge claims that are valued and selected through a dynamic social processes. Within a knowledge-order, knowledge and social processes mutually shape each other.

My sense is that civic epistemology is a helpful way to think about bioethics, particularly within a public policy context and applied as governance practice. Drawing on different knowledge systems, including law, bioethics has developed its own epistemology on research involving the human embryo and human pluripotent stem cell research. We can perhaps debate if its epistemic quality is anticipatory knowledge or amenable to be applied as anticipatory governance, but from a precautionary policy perspective, bioethics appears to be recognised as such. As the study reported in this book shows, public perception is similarly so. The knowledge-order of bioethics and its dynamism are more difficult to depict. To take the analogy of weaving a straw mat, this study on juridification seeks to trace the intricate ways in which law in terms of its rationalities,

---

[1003] Clark Miller, Civic Epistemologies: Constituting Knowledge and Order in Political Communities, *Sociology Compass* (2008) 2, 6: 1896-1919, at 1896. Miller distinguishes (at 1908) civic epistemology from other constructivist approaches in the former's focus on sociological transformations, on how competing epistemic and ontological forms of reasoning and argumentation are grounded in strong social and institutional arrangements for making and validating knowledge; and the central role of knowledge institutions and networks in securing and opposing particular framing of issues. See also Sheila Jasanoff, *Designs on Nature: Science and Democracy in Europe and the United States.* Princeton: Princeton University Press, 2005, at 15.

[1004] Clark Miller, Civic Epistemologies: Constituting Knowledge and Order in Political Communities, *Sociology Compass* (2008) 2, 6: 1896-1919, at 1898.

concepts, language, techniques and practices has been paired with different knowledge strands. Where Singapore is concerned, the legal strands are most clearly represented in the HCOPA and the HBRA, but neither may be said to constitute all of bioethics governance. The limitation of this analogy is that it does not sufficiently account for the contributions of the political order.

In this chapter, I have attempted to show that where juridification is concerned, the political order is implicit in (for the BAC) the pseudo-juridical form of bioethics bodies within a 'bioethics-as-public-policy' framework, in their exercise of public reason and in their engagements in the public sphere. This dimension is clearly important for at least three reasons. It confers legitimacy and is an avenue by which legitimacy is recognised. This is particularly important where political compromises are entailed in issues that draw a diversity of opposing and irreconcilable religious, philosophical and moral views. As we have seen in Chapter 4, this may be a reason why bioethics as a national knowledge-order proved to be viable in the US, UK, Denmark, Germany and Japan, among others, but not at the level of the United Nations. As Clark Miller explains, the diversity of national civic epistemologies in international governance can be a difficult hurdle to surmount.[1005] Within a national knowledge-order, political and legal standards, institutions and processes govern the production of knowledge and expertise, and secure for them legitimacy. There are no comparable arrangements in international governance. Another reason that underscores the importance of the political order is that it precludes juridification from 'crowding out' other social and

---

[1005] *Ibid*, at 1911. Miller explains: "These differences stem from variances in processes for warranting the credibility of policy-relevant knowledge, notions of what counts as expertise and what kinds of expertise are most appropriate for policy purposes, normative expectations regarding the delivery of expert advice (e.g., standards of transparency, accountability, legitimacy, etc.), as well as the constitutional frameworks and political institutions to whom knowledge and advice are being offered. While these expectations typically remain implicit in national affairs, they have given rise to explicit conflict in international politics."

political norms – the key concern that was discussed in Chapter 1. Still, this prospect of juridification as legal pollution seems convincing for some. At a recent public session on the HBRA in Singapore, a researcher vehemently lamented this legislative approach. [1006] He seemed convinced that this would be the death knell of biomedical research endeavours here. Curious enough, it is already an explicit requirement for all human biomedical research in Singapore to undergo some form of ethics review. The HBRA has mostly inscribed existing ethical requirements into law. While some researchers still complain that the process of ethics review is a burden to research, most have accepted it as a 'necessary evil'.

For other researchers, this and other studies suggest that ethical and regulatory guidance is very much intrinsic to how they think about their scientific work and its value. In Japan, Margaret Sleeboom-Faulkner[1007] indicates that strict and 'rather un-transparent' regulation might have been a cause of the slow rate of the advance of Japanese hESC research and SCNT, compared to other areas of research like mouse genomics. As we have considered in Chapter 2, researchers in Japan did not rush into hESC research even though there was no religious objection to hESC research. Instead, they succeeded in improvising iPSC technology that produced human pluripotent cells without causing the destruction of an embryo. Admittedly, navigating through bioethics governance has become a complex exercise. This is no less the case with working within a 'bioethics-as-public-policy' framework or with bioethics as governance practice.[1008] As John Gillott observes, the approach of contemporary

---

[1006] Fieldnotes, 22 April 2016.

[1007] Margaret Sleeboom-Faulkner, Debates on human embryonic stem cell research in Japan: minority voices and their political amplifiers, *Science as Culture* (2008) 17: 85-97.

[1008] A challenge of juridification in bioethics is to, as Graeme Laurie *et al.* suggest, improve value clarity, objective clarity, duty-clarity and oversight in order to enhance effectiveness and responsiveness. Graeme Laurie, Shawn H E Harmon and Fabiana Arzuaga, Foresighting Futures: Law, New Technologies, and the

governments to the governance of biomedical research is a hybrid in many respects.[1009] We have considered this in Chapters 3 to 5. The complexity has conferred on bioethics decisions the reputation of being mixed judgments, for instance. In the light of this and for reasons set out in this chapter, I think it is appropriate to regard bioethics as an 'emergent' civic epistemology. It seems unlikely that bioethics or any governance practice that stems from it will achieve complete internal coherence. This is the third reason why its embeddedness in a political order is important. To my mind, the 'emergent' quality of bioethics as civic epistemology is a merit, and not one that it should outlive.

Challenges of Regulating for Uncertainty, *Law, Innovation and Technology* (2012) 4, 1: 1-33, at 33.

[1009] In his review of the governance of biosciences in the UK and elsewhere, John Gillott observes: "Contemporary governments' approach to the governance of bioscience research can be considered a hybrid ... It is defined by engagement, rhetorically, performatively and substantively, with the Democratic Model, a model informed by themes linked to SSK [Sociology of Scientific Knowledge] and other strands of social science. There are of course other processes in play. In practice, there is overlap in government's and others' treatment of distinct trend reflecting mixed understandings, pragmatism and disparate aims at governmental level." See: John Gillott, *Bioscience, Governance and Politics*. Basingstoke: Palgrave Macmillan, 2014, at 180.

Methodology: Ethnography and Actor-Network-Theory

Fieldwork and Ethnography

The critical episode of my ethnographic research has been between August 2007 to December 2012,[1010] although the events (not exclusive to Singapore) that are studied stretch from the time that the BAC was formed (in 2000) to the enactment of the Human Biomedical Research Act (in 2015). On fieldwork, Carol Greenhouse defines it as a relational practice linking knowledge production to the historical and local specificity of experience. In this connection, she considers field studies of law to make a broad subject because of their quantity and variety, as well as the mutual embeddedness of legal and social concepts.[1011] Ethnography is a means by which the mutual embeddedness of scientific and social concepts has been studied by social scientists. For instance, Jeanette Edwards, Penny Harvey and Peter Wade indicate that anthropologists "work ethnographically, looking

---

[1010] Initial and subsequent annual approvals for this study entitled "Ethnographic Study of Policy Development on Biomedical Research Involving Human-Animal Combination" were obtained from the Institutional Review Board for Human Participants of Cornell University, Ithaca, New York, as Protocol ID#: 0907000514.

[1011] Carol J Greenhouse, Fieldwork on Law. *Annual Review of Law and Social Sciences* (2006) 2: 187-210, at 187.

at how connections are made and unmade between persons, on what terms and with what effects."[1012] Ethnography is my methodology. As a means of open-ended inquiry, it has the capacity to represent complexity in a manner that is least reductionist, and thereby maximises interpretive flexibility.[1013] Rose, O'Malley and Valverde indicate that ethnography is aptly suited for analysing governmentality by virtue of these characteristics.[1014] Cris Shore adds that the ethnographic method is effective for the study of 'elites' because they form parts of wider encompassing culture but are not readily accessible.[1015] In addition, he indicates that:

> when studying elites we should be cautious about generalizing from the micro to the macro. What happens at the local level is not a microcosm of, or synecdoche for, processes and formations occurring at the national or global levels. Even within a shared social system or political culture, elites and masses occupy a very different habitus.[1016]

Law as a key constituent of 'bioethics' qualifies as a distinct elite culture. During the period of my research, I have worked as a legal researcher with the Secretariat of the BAC. In this role, my primary responsibilities could be segregated into three main categories: conduct research into laws and regulatory policies of Singapore and select jurisdictions, produce analytical reports and facilitate the formulation of recommendations, and discharge general administrative duties, which include arranging and organising meetings. I had

---

1012 Jeanette Edwards, Penny Harvey and Peter Wade. *Anthropology and Science: Epistemologies in Practice.* Oxford: Berg, 2007, at 6.

1013 Marilyn Strathern, Accountability...and ethnography. In Marilyn Strathern (ed.), *Audit Cultures: Anthropological studies in accountability, ethics and the academy.* London: Routledge, 2000, pp 279-304, at 285.

1014 Nikolas Rose, Pat O'Malley and Mariana Valverde, Governmentality. *Annual Review of Law and Social Sciences* (2006) 2: 83-104, at 92.

1015 Cris Shore, Introduction. In Stephen Nugent and Cris Shore, *Elite Cultures: Anthropological Perspectives.* London and New York: Routledge, 2002, at 9.

1016 *Ibid*, at 6.

four colleagues: a medically trained head of the Secretariat, a psychology professor, a junior scientist (with a strong interest in STS), and an administrator. Whether working within the Secretariat or with the BAC, we constantly endeavoured to translate among, as well as associate, different knowledge systems. While these systems and the more specific scientific agenda are driven by public interests, the issues grappled with were often far beyond day-to-day concerns of ordinary people. This study is in this sense about the work of 'high priests'. More specifically, it attempts to provide some insights on:

(a) The historical context by which elites can be meaningfully understood,

(b) The external conditions and interests that promote and sustain local or national elites matched with the norms, values and shared interests that characterise or unite such elites,

(c) Strategies they use to reproduce themselves over time, and

(d) The language and practices through which elites represent themselves and the techniques they use to legitimise their position.[1017]

I have focused on the 'high priests' largely because 'bioethics-as-public-policy' is seen by some to assume this role in relation to biomedical sciences in Singapore and elsewhere. As Annelise Riles explains, ethnography is especially suited for such a study, where actors are guarded.[1018]

[1017] *Ibid*, at 12-13.

[1018] Annelise Riles. *Collateral Knowledge: Legal Reasoning in the Global Financial Markets.* Chicago and London: University of Chicago Press, 2011, at 13. Riles explains: "An anthropologist specializes in understanding what is so important, so fundamental, so much a part of the taken-for-granted agreed bases of social life that from the point of view of one's subjects it goes largely unnoticed. If the actor could simply tell you about the symbolic structures underlying their kinship, for example, you wouldn't need ethnography; you could simply conduct a telephone survey."

This study attempts to provide an account of the relatively more anecdotal or social aspect of knowledge systems operating within bioethics. This "rather oblique form of knowledge practice" has been described by Douglas Holmes and George Marcus as having "a keen discursive character whereby information is endowed with social perspective and meaning".[1019] The BAC members have intuitions and insights based on their observations, relationships and experience. However, such 'knowledge' does not count in 'serious' or 'academic' ethical analysis, even though it has been profoundly influential in steering the direction of bioethical policies. In attempting to represent this somewhat anecdotal bioethical knowledge, I provide an account of the 'para-ethnographic'; or substantive, methodological and theoretical considerations in the marginal ways of knowing within bioethics.[1020]

During my interviews with the BAC members, they consistently indicated that in operating 'outside' of government, their appointment on the BAC was not an extension of their official positions. Instead, their role has been to determine and guide the actions of government in ways that meet the requirements of 'good science', primarily through the provision of advice. The advisory nature of the BAC's work should not be under-estimated as it reinforced the

---

[1019] Douglas R Holmes and George E Marcus, Fast Capitalism: Para-Ethnography and the Rise of the Symbolic Analyst. In Melissa S Fisher and Greg Downey (eds.), *Frontiers of Capital: Ethnographic Reflections on the New Economy.* Durham and London: Duke University Press, 2006, pp 33-57, at 38.

[1020] Douglas R Holmes and George E Marcus, Cultures of Expertise and the Management of Globalization: Toward the Re-Functioning of Ethnography. In Aihwa Ong and Stephen J Collier (eds.), *Global Assemblages: Technology, Politics and Ethics as Anthropological Problems.* Singapore: Blackwell Publishing, 2005, pp 235-252, at 240-241. As a methodology, they argue that para-ethnography is a means to re-functioning ethnography as "a way of dealing with contradiction, exception, facts that are fugitive, and that suggest a social realm not in alignment with the representations generated ... Making ethnography from para-ethnography redefines the status of the subject or informant, asks what different accounts one wants from such key figures in the fieldwork process, and indeed questions what the ethnography of experts means within a broad, multi-sited design of research". *Ibid*, at 236-237.

intended independence. Since any advice of the BAC would not be technically binding on the government, the members did not consider themselves to be doing or influencing 'politics'. At the same time, they also did not consider themselves to be technicians (or technocrats) in that no member (save one) considered himself or herself to be a professional ethicist. This is not to say that the BAC members were unfamiliar with ethical discourses, rationales and practices, or that their contributions have been insignificant. Even then, many BAC members considered their contributions to be 'trivial'. There may be a number of reasons for such a sentiment. First, the Secretariat has been mainly responsible in crafting the proposed recommendations with the working group and the BAC Chairperson. Second, the work of the BAC did not draw directly on the individual expertise of the members, or only tangentially at best. Third, no grand theories were discussed nor was there any deep and intense philosophising in any of the BAC's meetings. It was not uncommon that the information exchanged within the BAC, and between the BAC and its Secretariat, both in and outside of formal meetings, had an anecdotal character.

Far from trivial, the Secretariat depended heavily on such anecdotal information in steering both the orientation and substance of the work. Each BAC member was deeply embedded in their respective communities, both locally and overseas. For instance, leading physicians on the BAC have been well attuned to research sentiments on the ground from their day-to-day interactions with patients and their colleagues in the biomedical research community. Similarly, researchers on the BAC have provided insightful 'real time' information on challenges that confronted the research community, such as the bureaucratisation of research or the greater emphasis on industrial collaboration.[1021] While the BAC members were very aware of the ethical requirements and what the ethical environment ought

---

[1021] Annelise Riles, Real Time: Unwinding Technocratic and Anthropological Knowledge. In Melissa S Fisher and Greg Downey (eds.), *Frontiers of Capital: Ethnographic Reflections on the New Economy*. Durham and London: Duke University Press, 2006, pp 86-107.

to look like, they also understood the reality of practical challenges and constraints. I find this description of Alan Greenspan by Douglas Holmes and George Marcus could apply to many of the BAC members (in a biomedical rather than economic context): "someone shaped in sensibility and habitus by the routines of economic discipline, partial to its formalities, yet distinctively in rebellion to its conventional wisdom and guidance".[1022] A similar set of sensibilities, intuitions (or habitus) and relationalities underscore the tremendous experiential value of anecdotal information provided by the BAC members, as Holmes and Marcus have observed in regulating financial markets:[1023]

> ... from their [i.e. bureaucratically power officials like Greenspan] privileged networks of relationships these subjects can construct representations of the economy, drawn from experiential material that is fundamentally different from those representations that arise through the application of the statistical modes of analysis. Again, what makes these anecdotal accounts something more than merely another form of 'information' or 'data' is their social character – mediated through networks of interlocutors – conferring on these accounts distinctive authority can inform policy formulation and action.

This research corroborates the finding of ethnographers like Douglas Holmes, George Marcus and Annelise Riles in their works on financial markets that anecdotal information is critically important to understand tacit knowledge in governance,[1024] and further illustrates the value of ethnography as a methodology.

1022 Douglas R Holmes and George E Marcus, Cultures of Expertise and the Management of Globalization: Toward the Re-Functioning of Ethnography. In Aihwa Ong and Stephen J Collier (eds.), *Global Assemblages: Technology, Politics and Ethics as Anthropological Problems*. Singapore: Blackwell Publishing, 2005, pp 235-252, at 240.

1023 *Ibid*, at 246.

1024 Douglas R Holmes and George E Marcus, Fast Capitalism: Para-Ethnography and the Rise of the Symbolic Analyst. In Melissa S Fisher and Greg Downey (eds.),

Reflexivity in ethnographic writing is important as conscious self-examination of the "interpretive nature of fieldwork, the construction of ethnographic authority, the interdependence of ethnographer and informant, and the involvement of the ethnographer's self in fieldwork."[1025] It is employed to realise the overarching interests of ethnography in "meaning, interpretation, subjectivity, intersubjectivity, thick description, dialogics, and polyphony".[1026] Arguably, reflexivity is a means by which to overcome the possible lack of distance between myself – the observer – and the observed. In view of my involvement in the work of the BAC, Pierre Bourdieu indicates that 'objectivity' may be compromised in that I would not be able to "objectify the objectifying distance and the social conditions that make it possible" to study the observed logic of practices.[1027] George Marcus considers Bourdieu's view of 'objective' distance to be too restrictive. He argues that:

> Bourdieu's account is tone-deaf to the inevitable moments of subjective criticism that have always occurred in even the most scientific ethnography. By denying or ignoring this integral dimension of the most objectifying methods, Bourdieu misses the

---

Frontiers of Capital: Ethnographic Reflections on the New Economy. Durham and London: Duke University Press, 2006, pp 33-57; and Annelise Riles, Real Time: Unwinding Technocratic and Anthropological Knowledge. In Melissa S Fisher and Greg Downey (eds.), *Frontiers of Capital: Ethnographic Reflections on the New Economy.* Durham and London: Duke University Press, 2006, pp 86-107.

[1025] Antonius C G M Robben, Reflexive Ethnography. In Antonius C G M Robben and Jeffrey A Sluka (eds.), *Ethnographic Fieldwork: An Anthropological Reader.* Singapore: Blackwell, 2007, pp 443-446, at 443.

[1026] *Ibid,* at 446.

[1027] Pierre Bourdieu. *The Logic of Practice,* trans. Richard Nice. Stanford CA: Stanford University Press, 1990, at 14. Bourdieu explains (at 26) that "[o]bjectivism, which sets out to establish objective regularities (structures, laws, systems of relationships, etc.) independent of individual consciousness and wills, introduces a radical discontinuity between theoretical knowledge and practical knowledge ..."

sorts of tensions that propel the ethnographer toward reflexivity in the first place ...[1028]

Associating Bourdieu's constrained reflexivity as sociological reflexivity, Marcus adds that there are other styles of less limiting reflexivity in anthropology and feminist scholarship. Anthropological reflexivity is "one that emphasizes the intertextual or diverse fields of representation that any contemporary project of ethnography enters and crosses in order to establish its own subject and to define its own voice."[1029] Objectification through representation of the social phenomenon being studied as social facts depends not only on the discourse of the ethnographer, but also her literal position in relation to the subjects. The importance of positioning is given further emphasis in feminist reflexivity.[1030] Donna Haraway's notion of 'situated knowledge' is helpful here.[1031]

In working collaboratively in the field, my sense is that ethnography that encompasses interactive engagement is ethically more defensible since the ethnographer does *not* assume a more privileged position than her subjects. I am constantly aware that my account of law, bioethics, or juridification in bioethics is partial and hence not the last word on the subject. It also reflects ethnographic method as based on a "long-term commitment to research based on intensive and on-going relationships with informants, a mix of participant observation and open-ended interviews."[1032] In addition, reflexivity is practiced both at the level of the BAC and also the Secretariat. Perhaps attributable to a number of conditions that include the reality and proximity of power relations, the indirect or tangential relevance

---

1028 George E Marcus. *Ethnography Through Thick and Thin*. Princeton NJ: Princeton University Press, 1998, at 195.

1029 *Ibid*, at 196.

1030 *Ibid*, at 198.

1031 Donna Haraway. *The Haraway Reader*. New York and London: Routledge, 2004, at 316-317.

1032 Annelise Riles. *Collateral Knowledge: Legal Reasoning in the Global Financial Markets*. Chicago and London: University of Chicago Press, 2011, at 14.

of personal expertise of the BAC members and the Secretariat, and the evaluative nature of ethical work, reflexivity is encouraged in going:

> ... beyond calculative problem solving toward exploring tensions and recognising the ephemeral nature of our identities and social experience ... to question and explore how we contribute to the construction of social and organizational realities, how we relate with others, and how we construct our ways of being in the world.[1033]

In other words, neither BAC members nor the Secretariat could be conceptualised as purely rational creatures of expertise, but they have been "desiring, relating, doubting, anxious, contentious and affective".[1034] This may also explain why learning in policy work, whether bioethics or not, could be metaphorically described as *bricolage*, and the policy-maker, a *bricoleur*.[1035]

Reflexivity is also practised through speaking to people outside of the Secretariat and through writing. In relation to the former, the people whom I have interviewed include members of the BAC and its working groups, policymakers, regulators and researchers. I have also conducted interviews – both formal and informal – with policymakers, researches and bioethicists outside of Singapore. This aspect of my research serves to identify any sites of knowledge production that I might have missed. In 'unwinding' of my own position, I sought to determine new modes of relationship and expression.[1036] To

---

[1033] Ann L Cunliffe and Jong S Jun, The Need for Reflexivity in Public Administration, *Administration & Society* (May 2005) 37, 2: 225-242, at 228.

[1034] Dominic Boyer, Thinking through the Anthropology of Experts, *Anthropology in Action* (2008) 15, 2: 38-46, at 38.

[1035] Richard Freeman, Epistemological Bricolage: How Practitioners Make Sense of Learning, *Administration & Society* (July 2007) 39, 4: 476-496.

[1036] Annelise Riles, Real time: Unwinding technocratic and anthropological knowledge. *American Ethnologist* (2004) 31, 3: 392-405.

these, I add that ethnographic writing itself requires self-critical reflexivity,[1037] and non-dualism.[1038] On this point, Marilyn Strathern provides instructive observation:[1039] "Writing is much more ... than the recording of facts and observations. Consequently, the ethnographer can no longer pretend to be a neutral vector for the conveying of information; her or his own participation in the constructed narrative must be made explicit." I find the experience of Brian Moeran to be helpful, and it reflects that 'front-stage' versus 'back-stage' differential in Stephen Hilgartner's work.[1040] Drawing from his long-term fieldwork in a Japanese advertising agency, Moeran expresses reservation over the effectiveness of 'objective' fieldwork through participant observation and interviews, as "everyone knew who I was and could therefore approach or avoid me".[1041] However, he was able to move from 'front-stage impression management' to 'back-stage' when he helped the agency win a multi-million dollar account from a prestigious Japanese electronics firm called Frontier. At that point, he was no longer regarded exclusively as a visiting foreign researcher.[1042] Moeran had gained access to back-stage reality

---

1037 Liisa H Malkki, Tradition and Improvisation in Ethnographic Field Research. In Allaine Cerwonka and Liisa H Malkki (eds.), *Improvising Theory: Process and Temporality in Ethnographic Fieldwork*. Chicago: University of Chicago Press, 2007, pp 162-187, at 177.

1038 Evens argues for 'nondualism' in that although there is still an object-subject distinction, it is a relative rather than an absolute one. The ethnographic enterprise is observed to be "ontological to its very core". See Terry M S Evens. *Anthropology as Ethics: Nondualism and the Conduct of Sacrifice*. New York and Oxford: Berghahn Books, 2009, at 3.

1039 Marilyn Strathern. *Partial Connections*. Savage ML: Rowman & Littlefield Publishers, 1991, at 7.

1040 Stephen Hilgartner. *Science on Stage: Expert Advice as Public Drama*. Stanford: Stanford University Press, 2000. See especially Chapter 2.

1041 Brian Moeran, From participant observation to observant participation. In Sierk Ybema, Dvora Yanow, Harry Wels and Frans Kamsteeg (eds.), *Organizational Ethnography: Studying the Complexities of Everyday Life*. Chennai India: Sage Publications, 2009, pp 137-155, at 153.

1042 *Ibid* at 146-147. As Antony Puddephatt and others observe, it is often a major benefit for an ethnographer to work in an environment where she or he is

and discovered that what the organisation actually does is very different from what its employees tell you. Given this, it is important for researchers to try to move from 'front-stage' to 'back-stage'. Loïc Wacquant similarly considers his own insider status as an apprentice boxer as a benefit. By experiencing the boxing gym first hand, he was better able to link the social organisation and the shared experiences with the embodied dimensions of individual experience. But in 'going native', Moeran points out that one's 'objectivity' could be compromised for failing to achieve the required detachment for analytical purposes. For him, he states that returning to one's 'home base' at an academic institution is a means of re-gaining the analytical distance.[1043] Similarly, Wacquant emphasises the importance of re-flexivity in situating one's own deeply personal experiences within more systematic theoretical understandings.[1044] For my research, I started from the 'back-stage' of the organisation. However, there is a constant awareness of the 'front-stage' when dealing with the press, at public meetings and most certainly in preparing the reports of the BAC.

---

embedded, as the ethnographer would already be familiar with the dynamics of social organisation and its hidden meanings. See: Antony Puddephatt, William Shaffir and Steven Kleinknecht, Exercises in reflexivity: situating theory in practice. In Antony J Puddephatt, William Shaffir and Steven W Kleinknecht (eds.), *Ethnographies revisited: constructing theory in the field*. London and New York: Routledge, 2009, pp 1-34, at 16-17.

[1043] *Ibid*, at 154.

[1044] Loïc Wacquant, Habitus as Topic and Tool: Reflections on becoming a prizefighter. In Antony J Puddephatt, William Shaffir and Steven W Kleinknecht (eds.), *Ethnographies revisited: constructing theory in the field*. London and New York: Routledge, 2009, pp 137-151. As Wacquant explains (at 149): "Whether the investigator is aware of it or not, theory is always driving inquiry...And it must of necessity engage observation in order to convert itself into propositions about an empirically existing entity. This applies to habitus, which, like every concept, is not an answer to a research question, but an organised manner of asking questions about the social world – in the case recounted here, a methodological plan to vivisect the social fabrication of pugilists in their workaday environment."

Lack of clear distance from my ethnographic subject(s) did result in a number of constraints, particularly in determining what to analyse and to what extent. In getting to know and understand the ideals, rationalities and idioms that my informants and research subjects live by, as well as in appreciating the many practical difficulties and uncertainties in 'hands-on' policy work, these constraints often present themselves as double binds in deciding what and how to represent ethnographically, and what is ethically responsible to critique.[1045] Experiences of other ethnographers show that double binds are ubiquitous. Kim Furton describes a double bind situation in terms of its multiplicity and complexity of messages, their interrelations and reciprocal qualifications, which must be interpreted all at once. Hence, it creates persistent mismatch that forces us to 'dream up' new ways of understanding and engaging the world.[1046] Her study of the Bhopal gas leak disaster in 1984 provides ample illustrations of situational double bind. The choice of a forum for litigation and a decision as to whether grassroots organisations should engage in legal battles represent two instances of double bind. On the former, there were as many reasons for the litigation to take place in the US as there were in India. Litigation in the US would serve to send a clear signal to multinational corporations (Union Carbide Corporation being the parent company of the fertiliser manufacturer

---

1045 As Anthony Wilden and Tim Wilson explained some time back, the phenomenon of 'double bind' is not simply a dilemma arising from a choice between two evils (of 'damned if you do, and damned if you don't'). Rather, it requires a choice between two states which are equally valued. See: Anthony Wilden and Tim Wilson, The Double Bind: Logic, Magic and Economics. In Carlos Sluzki and Donald Ransom (eds.), *Double Bind: The Foundation of the Communicational Approach to the Family*. New York: Grune and Stratton, 1976, pp 263-286. As they define it (at 276): "A true double bind – or a situation set up or perceived as one – requires a choice between two states which are equally valued and so equally insufficient that a self-perpetuating oscillation is engendered by any act of choice between them ... It is the fact that one must choose, and moreover choose between incompatible alternatives."

1046 Kim Fortun, *Advocacy after Bhopal: Environmentalism, Disaster, New Global Orders*. Chicago and London: University of Chicago Press, 2001, at 13.

in India) that they have responsibilities vis-à-vis their foreign subsidiaries. The capability of the courts in India to adjudicate disputes that concerned its citizens was a message no less important, and one that litigation in India would effectively convey. On the latter, grassroots organisations has to decide whether to prioritise initiatives to build institutional structures for local decision-making or to engage in legal battles, given that "[t]he law can create a space for grassroots organizations to work, while undermining the very modes of sociality such space was to protect."[1047] Andrea Timmer observes a similar double bind in the discursive strategies of European non-governmental organisations (NGOs) that construct the Roma as problems that require attention. NGOs have to frame their activities in a manner that will encourage continued support from external government and funding agencies. However, the general standards prescribed as funding conditions could become an obstacle to the particular situational challenges that NGOs have to address.[1048] In the context of law, Jacque Derrida has observed a double bind in the attempt to relate generality (such as a norm, rule or value) to particularity, especially in view of the possibility that the latter may be an outcome that is inconsistent with the former.[1049] Derrida's

---

[1047] *Ibid.* Fortun identifies environmentalism as another double bind, as it relates to a political strategy that brings people together, but at the same time encompassed a "politics of fissure, rather than harmony" (at 16).

[1048] Andria D Timmer, Constructing the "Needy Subject": NGO Discourses of Roma Need, *Political and Legal Anthropology Review* (November 2010) 33, 2: 264-281, at 267. For instance, funding was denied to an NGO because its work was not directed specifically at addressing the 'Roma problem', but related to both Roma and non-Roma, as the main goal was to help integrate the former with the latter (at 268).

[1049] Jacques Derrida, Force of Law: The mystical foundation of authority. *Cardozo Law Review* (1990) 11: 920-1045, at 949 and 951. He observes: "To address oneself to the other in the language of the other is, it seems, the condition of all possible justice, but apparently, in all rigor, it is not only impossible ... but even excluded by justice as law (*droit*), inasmuch as justice as right seems to imply an element of universality, the appeal to a third party who suspends the unilaterality or singularity of the idioms ... It is unjust to judge someone who does not understand the language in which the law is inscribed or the judgment pronounced ..."

critique is pertinent to much of the work of the BAC in having to relate particular biomedical expectations and practices to broader principles, so much so that it has not always been clear to me if the latter became more important than the research subjects and broader public whose interests are to be safeguarded. In addition, there was almost always an inherent conflict in having to choose between promoting biomedical research and human subjects protection, where other considerations (especially those that relate to scientific knowledge as securing for the nation a competitive – often commercial – advantage) greatly confound earnest attempts at ethical valuation.

In discussing the life work of Gregory Bateson, his daughter Mary Catherine Bateson argues that as double bind is endemic in human life, it should not be perceived only as crippling (in creating psychopathologies for instance), but also occasions that provoke resolution or creativity.[1050] Rather than think of double bind as a discrete thing or event, it is relational in its nature as "an abstract pattern of relationships that might show up in particular exchanges", and expression within a broader context.[1051] Paradoxes and dilemmas that relationality creates are also opportunities to learn and grow. Bateson graphically illustrates this relationality as one that "we cannot leave and cannot do without, a relationship which must finally be one of love."[1052] In review of Furton's work, Amy Levine observes that ethnography itself functions as a double bind.[1053] Furton recognises this throughout the course of her study.[1054] In having to choose

---

[1050] Mary Catherine Bateson, The Double Bind: Pathology and Creativity, *Cybernetics and Human Knowledge* (2005) 12, 1-2: 11-21, at 18-19.

[1051] *Ibid*, at 12.

[1052] *Ibid*, at 20.

[1053] Amy Levine, Book Review - Advocacy After Bhopal: Environmentalism, Disaster, New Global Order, *Political and Legal Anthropology Review* (2003) 26, 2: 171-175, at 174.

[1054] As Furton observes: "Competing demands would structure the work: Demands to acknowledge the unfigurability of disaster alongside demands for category-

between different sources of data and orderings, the necessity of selective representation in ethnography precludes any claim to full mastery over one's data. Given the inevitability of exclusion (and informational loss), a key challenge has been to state as clearly as practicable the selection basis and its consequences. [1055] For this reason, an ethnographic work is always unsettled and open to ethical evaluation.[1056] But if Bateson is right, the function of ethnography is more than a double bind. It could also serve as a nurturing response to the distressing challenges that one finds in the relationalities that one is embedded in. As Furton also recognises, ethnography of double binds also creates a space for advocacy.[1057] Like Derrida, Margaret Radin acknowledges that double bind is omnipresent in the pursuit of justice. However, she proposes active engagement, either in considering ways of changing the circumstances or to choose a regime for the meantime in addressing particular problems separately.[1058] Ethnographic research inevitably has political implications.[1059] I take June Nash's point that there is a risk of confusing representation of

---

ization ... Demands to acknowledge both the contingent particularity of example and the universally valid ... Demands for words that upheld entrenched regimes of power, alongside demands for words that disassemble ... Demands to respect both past and future, embodied in the need to remember Bhopal so that we may forget, staging a future less determined by the force of repetition." See: Kim Fortun, *Advocacy after Bhopal: Environmentalism, Disaster, New Global Orders.* Chicago and London: University of Chicago Press, 2001, at 53.

1055 *Ibid*, at 6.

1056 *Ibid*, at 350: "An ethnography of Bhopal should not work toward final synthesis ... The result can never be comprehensive. Expertise itself becomes a paradox, as does ethics. One is always confronted with more to understand and more to address than is possible. One must chose a focus, knowing that responding well to one problem ignores another ... Asking questions about what is most valued won't work ... But one must move, without fully understanding the complex systems in which one works. Ethics happen within such movement. Ethics play out in ways that cannot be controlled."

1057 *Ibid*, at 175.

1058 Margaret Jane Radin, *Contested Commodities.* Cambridge MA and London: Harvard University Press, 1996, at 122.

1059 June C Nash. *Practicing Ethnography in a Globalizing World.* New York: Alta Mira Press, 2007, at 29.

one's finding with advocacy, but this is arguably an inherent risk in all ethnographic works.[1060]

As a legal scholar, my main distress in the field has been to confront the many 'myths' about the law that pervade the policy environment – that the law is slow to respond, legal requirements are unduly limiting, the law impedes scientific progress, etc. In working with the Secretariat, it has also been a dilemma in deciding the extent that the law needs to be presented on a formal basis. The ethnographic representations that I make are to a large degree a response to this distress, and to show what I regard as legitimate and indispensable contribution of law in policy work. More importantly, the critical standpoint that I adopt has been and remains relationally embedded, since criticism from a secure position of traditional ethnographic distance could understandably be regarded as arrogant and irrelevant. This relational viewpoint is further consistent with a rationale in pragmatism. Pragmatists argue that knowledge is contextual, social and inseparable from purposeful action. Ideas arise from experiences that are often encapsulated in social institutions.[1061] In linking ethnography to pragmatism, Murray Leaf explains that there is no distinction in pragmatism between collecting data and analysis.[1062] It follows from the situatedness of knowledge that it is unrealistic to believe that ethnographers can be a 'fly on the wall' in often antiseptic policy environments. Just as important is the nature of my

---

1060 Marilyn Strathern indicates that reality should be grasped through a medium that already has a form of its own. In order to be true to human interlocution, the ethnographer must invite the reader to participate in what she or he participates, which is discourse. Rather than represent another society or culture, she or he should provide the reader with a connection to it. See: Marilyn Strathern, *Partial Connections*. Savage ML: Rowman & Littlefield Publishers, 1991, at 7 and 15.

1061 Alfonso Morales, Forward – Pragmatism as a Discipline: (Re)Introducing Pragmatist Philosophy to Law and Social Science. In Alfonso Morales (ed.), *Renascent Pragmatism: Studies in Law and Social Science*. Cornwall: Ashgate Publishing, 2003, pp xi-xxiv.

1062 Murray J Leaf, Ethnography and Pragmatism. In Alfonso Morales (ed.), *Renascent Pragmatism: Studies in Law and Social Science*. Cornwall: Ashgate Publishing, 2003, pp 92-117, at 102. See also 99.

ethnographic endeavour. It is not intended to be critical as its sole or even primary goal. But as Bateson indicates, ethnography is my attempt to depict opportunities to learn and grow.

Organisations, Documents and Meetings

'Bioethics' as a policy discourse is embodied in, transmitted and shaped by the BAC. As such, an ethnographic study of 'bioethics' in Singapore is very much an ethnographic account of the BAC as an organisation (or institution in an epistemological sense). In organisational ethnography, Sierk Ybema *et al.* provide a number of key features which I adopt here as a framework for discussing my ethnographic study.[1063]

Combined fieldwork methods are used in the form of participant observation, formal interviews and close reading of documentary sources. The close reading of documentary sources has been a critical aspect of my research. It is a means of recognising the recurring linguistic and conceptual conventions and expectations. Mitchel Lasser's explanation in relation to the close reading of legal texts is instructive:[1064]

> The basic idea is to approach the documents or arguments produced by a legal system as if they were serious literary works, and thus treat them with a similar degree of careful, detailed, and almost exhaustive attention. The underlying assumption, of course, is that

---

[1063] Sierk Ybema, Dvora Yanow, Harry Wels and Frans Kamsteeg, Studying everyday organizational life. In Sierk Ybema, Dvora Yanow, Harry Wels and Frans Kamsteeg (eds.), *Organizational Ethnography: Studying the Complexities of Everyday Life*. Chennai India: Sage Publications, 2009, pp 1-20, at 6-9. The seven key characteristics of interpretive organizational ethnography are listed as: (1) combined fieldwork methods, (2) at the scene, (3) hidden and harsh dimensions: power and emotions, (4) context-sensitive and actor-centred analysis, (5) meaning-making; (6) multivocality, and (7) reflexivity and positionality.

[1064] Mitchel de S-O-l'E Lasser. *Judicial Deliberations: A Comparative Analysis of Judicial Transparency and Legitimacy*. Oxford and New York: Oxford University Press, 2004, at 11-12.

these legal texts are meaningful in some way that transcends their already important substantive attributes ... the methodology affirms that legal texts express an implicit conceptual universe that can fruitfully, if imperfectly, be made explicit by meticulous literary analysis.

My ethnographic study is intended to register the postmodern processes at work in everyday life – these postmodernist *'processes of pastiche'*. Pastiche allows for the thorough mixing of modes, meanings, styles. What remains rooted, or of momentary stability, are the processes and relations which connect locales; the sorts of factors, in other words, which shape pastiche, in any locale. It seeks to explore new ways of thinking about contemporary conditions.[1065] In explaining the new legal realism, Sally Engle Merry associates this philosophy with methodologies that includes "transnational and multi-sited ethnographic research that tracks the flow of people, ideas, laws, and institutions across national boundaries and examines particular nodes and sites within this field of transnational circulation".[1066] It is also accompanied by an expansion of the dimensions of legality to include "legal consciousness and emerging legal technologies that constructs and sediment forms of legal knowledge and practice".[1067] Also noteworthy is her description of an approach to doing deterritorialised ethnography, by locating sites where global, national, and local processes are revealed in the social life of small groups.[1068] Christine Hine provides a further illustration of the multi-sited-ness of her study relating to the use of information and communication technologies (ICTs) in biological systematics, and exploring how these

---

[1065] George E Marcus. *Ethnography Through Thick and Thin.* Princeton NJ: Princeton University Press, 1998, at 53-54.

[1066] Sally Engle Merry, New Legal Realism and the Ethnography of Transnational Law, *Law & Social Inquiry* (2006) 31, 4: 975-995, at 976

[1067] *Ibid*, at 980-982.

[1068] *Ibid*, at 981.

developments make sense to those involved in diverse situations.[1069] These 'sites' include online discussion forums, museums, botanic gardens and herbaria, policy documents and web sites, journals, conferences, interviews, emails and informal conversations. The research is multi-sited in that she studied many different places to explore different aspects of a phenomenon.[1070]

Like many other policy organisations, meetings and documents are essential materials for the BAC's work. Part of the work of the Secretariat entails the preparation of meetings and documents for a variety of purposes and audiences. The essential output of the BAC is recommendations published in the form of reports to the government on particular issues in the life sciences. In my research, I examine how certain documents are important representations of institutional thinking and sense-making, and how they enable knowledge transfer or 'cross-pollination'.[1071] Anthropologists have used documents to study the distinction between the 'text' and 'context'. For instance, in his ethnography of the International Monetary Fund, Harper shows the multiple relationships and meanings that texts conceal by looking at the different 'careers' that the same document take.[1072] Don Brenneis employs the term 'career' of forms to illustrate how mundane forms in activities such as writing recommendations and evaluating research proposals constitute academic life in often subtle but concrete ways. As such, 'career' may be seen as the very tangible effect that 'artefacts' may have on

---

[1069] Christine Hine, Multi-sited Ethnography as Middle-Range Methodology for Contemporary STS. *Science, Technology, and Human Values* (2007) 32, 6: 652-671, at 666-667.

[1070] *Ibid* at 668.

[1071] Kyle McGee, *Bruno Latour: The Normativity of Networks*. London and New York: Routledge, 2014, at 90-97.

[1072] Richard Harper, Inside the IMF: An Ethnography of Documents, Technology and Organisational Action. London: Academic Press, 1998.

macrocosmic phenomenon.[1073] My recourse to documents is different
from the studies of Harper and Brenneis. The production of reports
on particular issues, such as egg donation and human-animal combinations, is the central preoccupation of the BAC. In that sense,
it is analogous to a phenomenon that Annelise Riles refers to as:
"Progress was internal to the document", so that the wider progressive scale of the BAC's endeavours does not rest in the larger pro-
gression of conferences and documents however, but in an emergent
discourse on 'bioethics' both within and outside of Singapore.[1074] The
ways that documents mediate among different knowledge systems is
a key focus of my research. Documents are thereby central to the
movement of ideas. As Dorothy Smith argues, documents have a role
similar to that of a tool or technology that enables certain kinds of
association, abstraction and/or simplification.[1075] Simplification is an
essential character of writing policy documents,[1076] but I agree with
Thomas Yarrow that this does not necessarily imply evasion or
disguise as certain 'erasures' are essential to enhance comprehension
and facilitate dialogue.[1077]

Unlike many other organisations, meetings are not as commonplace in the work of the BAC but they are important. Typically when a

---

1073 Don Brenneis. Performing Promise. In Annelise Riles (ed.), *Documents: Artefacts of Modern Knowledge*. Ann Arbor: The University of Michigan Press, 2006, pp 41-70, at 65.

1074 Annelise Riles, [Deadlines]: Removing the Brackets on Politics in Bureaucratic and Anthropological Analysis. In Annelise Riles (ed.), *Documents: Artefacts of Modern Knowledge*. Ann Arbor: The University of Michigan Press, 2006, pp. 71-92, at 87.

1075 Dorothy Smith, Texts, Facts and Femininity: Exploring the Relations of Ruling. London: Routledge, 1990.

1076 Raymond Apthorpe, Writing Development Policy and Policy Analysis Plain or Clear: On Language, Genre and Power. In Cris Shore and S Wright (eds.), *Anthropology of Policy: Critical Perspectives on Governance and Power*. London: Routledge, 1997.

1077 Thomas Yarrow, This is not the academic world of right and wrong: The obviation of truth through NGO documentary practice, *Cambridge Anthropology* (2006) 26: 50-59, at 57.

meeting is convened, there is an implicit understanding that either there is someone important to meet or there are important decisions to be made. During my time in the field, meetings have been convened to decide on various aspects of documents being prepared concerning issues in egg donation and/or human-animal combinations. As such, meetings are arguably 'tools' in the production of documents. More specifically, they are what Helen Schwartzman refers to as "communicative events". [1078] In combination with documents (like the Beige Book and anecdotal reports used in the Open Market Committee meetings of the Federal Reserve Board), [1079] meetings as communicative events give form and occasion to the para-ethnographic (discussed above).

Actor-Network-Theory

In *Science in Action*, Bruno Latour presents technology as, in essence, a 'black-box' constructed to secure the interests of a scientist and her or his enrolled allies, all of whom are intricately bound together by way of a network. [1080] Within this network, we find the contributions of not only human agents but also non-human actants. The explicit purpose of this exercise is to sensitise our research to stronger and weaker heterogeneous associations. [1081] More recently, he indicates that the way in which machines attribute roles and actions between humans and nonhumans may be understood by comparing machines

---

[1078] Helen B Schwartzman, *Ethnography in Organizations*. Newbury Park CA: Sage Publications, 1993, at 39-40.

[1079] Douglas R Holmes and George E Marcus, Fast Capitalism: Para-Ethnography and the Rise of the Symbolic Analyst. In Melissa S Fisher and Greg Downey (eds.), *Frontiers of Capital: Ethnographic Reflections on the New Economy*. Durham and London: Duke University Press, 2006, pp 33-57, at 37-38.

[1080] Bruno Latour, *Science in Action: How to Follow Scientists and Engineers through Society*. Cambridge MA: Harvard University Press, 1987, at 130-133. At its best, technology such as the thermometer becomes an "obligatory point of passage" that defies dissent to its prescriptions.

[1081] *Ibid*, at 127 and 240.

with texts, since the inscription of builders and users in a mechanism is very much the same as that of authors and readers in a story.[1082] In the design of a machine, engineers attempt to confine users within a particular frame or script through a process that Latour refers to as inscription, translation or delegation. The intended behaviour can be imposed on human users by nonhuman delegates through prescription, which is the moral and ethical dimension of the mechanism. The result is that the sum of morality (prescribed by nonhuman delegates) increases enormously with the population of nonhumans.[1083]

Two features of Latour's Actor-Network-Theory (ANT) are especially pertinent to my research. The first is anti-essentialism, particularly in not differentiating between science (as knowledge) and technology (as artefact), or to otherwise privilege science over other knowledge practices. It also blurs the divide between social facts (or positivism) and moral norms. Second, ANT advances a relational materiality, which postulates that all entities achieve significance in relation to others, thereby by-passing the distinction between agency and structure.[1084] Rather than personify things, Latour endeavours to denaturalise voice and give emphasis to mediation, material agency and facticity.[1085] In this research, I apply

---

[1082] Bruno Latour, Where are the Missing Masses? The Sociology of a Few Mundane Artefacts. In Wiebe Bijker and John Law (eds.), *Shaping technology/Building Society: Studies in Sociotechnical. Change* Cambridge MA: MIT Press, 1992, pp 225-259, at 236.

[1083] *Ibid*, at 247.

[1084] An account of the dehumanisation of agency is provided by Kapil Raj. See: Kapil Raj, When human travellers become instruments: The Indo-British exploration of Central Asia in the nineteenth century. In Marie-Noëlle Bourguet, Christian Licoppe and H Otto Sibum (eds.), *Instruments, Travel and Science: Itineraries of precision from the seventeenth to the twentieth century.* London and New York: Routledge, 2002, pp. 156-188.

[1085] Bruno Latour (translated by Catherine Porter), *Politics of Nature: How to Bring the Sciences into Democracy.* Cambridge MA: Harvard University Press, 2004, at 68.

ANT more generally, and in a manner that Mariana Valverde, Ron Levi and Dawn Moore explain as:[1086] "In keeping with ANT/STS methodology, our approach treats all uses and deployments of knowledge claims as equal, without making judgments about who should or should not be making these claims." Following Michel Foucault and Bruno Latour, they argue that "knowledges do not belong to anyone or to any site. Knowledges are always circulating, changing, being taken apart, and reassembled in new shapes by new actors."[1087] In a similar vein, Annelise Riles has applied ANT to analyse human rights activism in Fiji. She shows that by studying specific textual technique of bracketing phrases on which there have been no general agreement, these brackets have become an actor in their own right, particularly in enabling a document on women's right to be crafted.[1088] As Ron Levi and Mariana Valverde explan:[1089]

> Riles's point is *not* that the women do not have agency, but that if we only ask about agency, structure, and material resources, using conventional social science, we will miss seeing things that actually made a crucial difference in real life, such as, in this case, the little technology for governing people, words, and laws that is the UN parenthesis.

Returning to the subject of ethnography, Christine Hine observes that due perhaps to the displacement of human agency, "[a]ctor network theory has often not been overtly ethnographic, nor indeed has it dwelt particularly on any links with methodological traditions

---

[1086] Mariana Valverde, Ron Levi and Dawn Moore, Legal Knowledges of Risk. In Law Commission of Canada, *Law and Risk*. Vancouver and Toronto: University of British Columbia Press, 2005, pp 86-120, at 89.

[1087] *Ibid.*

[1088] Annelise Riles, *The Network Inside Out*. Ann Arber: University of Michigan Press, 2001.

[1089] Ron Levi and Mariana Valverde, Studying Law by Association: Bruno Latour Goes to the Conseil d'État, *Law & Social Inquiry* (2008) 33, 3: 805-825, at 812.

from social science or anthropology."[1090] Instead, STS scholars have innovatively developed ethnographic approaches so that the locality of science itself not only becomes a matter for study, but is widened beyond the laboratory to include social and cultural phenomena in multiple localities.[1091]

My choice of Latour's ANT was largely influenced by a growing sense that 'law' could not be neatly separated from the other knowledge fields, such as 'science', 'politics' and especially 'ethics' in my research into the establishment of a bioethical governance framework for human pluripotent stem cell research. More importantly, ANT does not regard the 'social' as a thing, but as "many connecting elements circulating inside tiny conduits."[1092] In his study of the production of legal knowledge, Latour gives emphasis to:

[1090] Christine Hine, Multi-sited Ethnography as Middle-Range Methodology for Contemporary STS. *Science, Technology, and Human Values* (2007) 32, 6: 652-671, at 660. Hine's perception may be rooted in the common perception that ANT is anti-normative given its overt emphasis of the descriptive. The correctness of such a view is contested. The ethnographic tradition is itself diverse, with applications that could include generating grounded theory, extending theoretical frames, challenging established wisdom and theorising from alternative data. See: Antony J Puddephatt, William Shaffir and Steven Kleinknecht, Exercises in reflexivity: situating theory in practice. In Antony J Puddephatt, William Shaffir and Steven W Kleinknecht (eds.), *Ethnographies revisited: constructing theory in the field*. London and New York: Routledge, 2009, pp 1-34.

[1091] Attila Bruni, Shadowing software and clinical records: On the ethnography of non-humans and heterogeneous contexts. *Organization* (2005) 12, 3: 357-378; John Law, *After method: Mess in social science research*. London: Routledge, 2004; David J Hess, Ethnography and the development of science and technology studies. In Paul Atkinson, Amanda Coffey, Sara Delamont; John Lofland, and Lyn Lofland (eds.), *Sage handbook of ethnography*, pp 234-245. Thousand Oaks, CA: Sage, 2001.

[1092] Bruno Latour, *Reassembling the Social: An Introduction to Actor-Network-Theory*. Oxford: Oxford University Press, 2007, at 5. More importantly, ANT "claims that it is possible to trace more sturdy relations and discover more revealing patterns by finding a way to register the links between unstable and shifting frames of reference rather than by trying to keep one frame stable". *Ibid*, at 24.

... law as a way of arranging the social world rather than as a field that is produced through external social causes[, principally by treating] law as a network of people and of things in which legality is not a field to be studied independently, but is instead a way in which the world is assembled, as attribute that is attached to events, people, documents, and other objects when they become part of the decision-making process in the Conseil d'État.[1093]

By focusing on the details relating to the progression of legal cases through the French Supreme Court of Appeal for cases on administrative law, 'law' is made through chains of networks and translations involving texts, people, architecture, concepts and office objects – none of which are completely 'internal' or 'external' to the phenomenon of 'law'.[1094] Latour describes 'law' as a hybrid or "factish", involving both material and ideological elements that cannot be entirely separated or purified.[1095] Legality is to be understood in turn by the relations among its constituting documents and other entities.[1096] In other words, Latour regards legal decision-making as critically the *mediation* of associations between a dossier of documents (which could include death certificates, receipts, reports of eyewitnesses) with library documents (such as statutes or past decisions). As Levi and Valverde explain, Latour's account of law is associational and mediatory, in that it is a 'documentary network' and is concerned with "import-export ... [and] seeks to stitch together bits of the outside world with the network of files".[1097]

[1093] Ron Levi and Mariana Valverde, Studying Law by Association: Bruno Latour Goes to the Conseil d'État, *Law & Social Inquiry* (2008) 33, 3: 805-825, at 806.

[1094] Bruno Latour, *La fabrique du droit: Une ethnographie du Conseil d'État* [The factory of law: an ethnography of the Conseil d'État]. Paris: La Découverte, 2002, at 79-81 and 103 to 104. See discussion by Levi and Valverde: *Ibid*, at 813-814.

[1095] Latour: *Ibid*, at 297.

[1096] *Ibid*, at 88-89.

[1097] Ron Levi and Mariana Valverde, Studying Law by Association: Bruno Latour Goes to the Conseil d'État, *Law & Social Inquiry* (2008) 33, 3: 805-825, at 818-819 (Emphasis in original). Levi and Valverde describe the Latourian approach as "a study of practice and of assemblage" that is "deeply empiricist, seeking to

A critical contribution from Latour's works is his emphasis that scientists as well as lawyers represent, through a variety of means that include staging or mediation, which has a distinctive agency. Lisa Disch observes that in amalgamating 'fact' (fait) and 'fetish' (fétiche) in the term 'faitiche', Latour attempts to highlight that "agency is not localized in any particular agent but that materializes when an activity that engages actors in an exchange of properties produces something that 'overtakes' them".[1098] Similarly, in defining a scientific experiment as a 'movement' of three distinct trials that entail a story, a situation (composed of apparatuses that isolate the properties of the entity and stage it) and a trial of peers, Latour is said to have presented an autoethnography of the laboratory; or a means to "talk about agency that is not seated in a subject but rather distributed throughout a system of representation or a field of action".[1099] A successful experiment is thereby also an indexical sign that is generative of ontological and epistemological content and encompasses representations that are political, symbolic and juridical all at once.[1100]

---

demonstrate the wide range of human and nonhuman actors required for law to remain in place" (at 822). For the purposes of this research, an important feature of the approach is that it enables the mentalities and rationalities of government as articulated in statutes, cases and briefs to be included, along with the wide range of nonhuman actants: *Ibid*.

1098 Lisa Disch, Faitiche-izing the People: What Representative Democracy Might Learn from Science Studies. In Bruce Braun and Sarah J Whatmore (eds.), *Political Matter: Technoscience, Democracy, and Public Life*. Minneapolis and London: University of Minnesota Press, 2010, pp 267-296, at 275. Disch adds that (*Ibid*; Emphasis in original): "Latour goes out of his way to define *faitiche* as a kind of movement or exchange – a passage or passing – rather than as a kind of thing ... autonomy is not a localized capacity but a distributed agency that comes from the exchange of properties among an author, an apparatus, and a phenomenon."

1099 *Ibid*, at 281.

1100 *Ibid*, at 282-283. Latour explains an experiment is "a text about a nontextual situation, later tested by others to decide whether or not it is simply a text. If the final trial is successful, then *it* is not just a text, there is indeed a real situation behind it, and both the actor and its authors are endowed with a new competence." In other words, the successful replication of an experimental outcome renders the experimental apparatuses as 'reliable witnesses' and the

In my research, ANT has been a means of understanding the role of law in bioethics, particularly in terms of the artefacts – both tangible and intangible – that enrol complex networks of other actors, values and practices. It has also been a means of explicating these artefacts as a complex site of power, relationships, potentialities and influences, as well as their found environment. In this respect, ANT has informed and influence my research in a way that it has in the work of scholars on the regulation of pharmaceutical products in Djibouti,[1101] tobacco and medicinal nicotine products,[1102] houses in multiple occupation,[1103] work life balance,[1104] among others.[1105] But unlike these studies, my research is not limited to being an account of law in ANT. In this respect, scholars like Kyle McGee has provided an instructive ANT account of law as a regime of enunciation, both within and outside of the courthouse, and animated through series of mediations by mundane things like legal documents, turnstiles and speed-bumps.[1106] Similar to these scholars, my research is intended to explicate on the form of law in terms of its rationales, ideas, materials, practices and networks. However, I go further in examining the role of these rationales, ideas, materials, practices and networks pre- and post-enunciation, where law is itself but a contributing form in the synergised space of bioethics.

---

scientist as a legitimate spokesperson for the experimented phenomenon. See Bruno Latour, *Pandora's Hope: Essays on the Reality of Science Studies*. Cambridge MA and London: Harvard University Press, 1999, at 123-124.

[1101] Emilie Cloatre and Robert Dingwall, "Embedded regulation": The migration of objects, scripts and governance, *Regulation & Governance* (2013) 7, 365-386.

[1102] Catriona Rooke, Emilie Cloatre and Robert Dingwall, The Regulation of Nicotine in the United Kingdom: How Nicotine Gum Came to Be a Medicine, but Not a Drug, *Journal of Law and Society* (2012) 39, 1: 39-57.

[1103] Dave Cowan and Helen Carr, Actor-network Theory, Implementation, and the Private Landlord, *Journal of Law and Society* (2008) 35, s1: 149-166.

[1104] Emily Grabham, Legal Form and Temporal Rationalities in UK Work-Life Balance Law, *Australian Feminist Studies* (2014) 29, 79: 67-84.

[1105] See for instance, essays in the collection: Emilie Cloatre and Martyn Pickersgill (eds.), *Knowledge, Technology and Law*. Abingdon and New York: Routledge, 2015.

[1106] Kyle McGee, *Bruno Latour: The Normativity of Networks*. London and New York: Routledge, 2014, at 147-181 especially.

Bibliography

N.B. For Laws (Conventions, Statutes, etc.) and Law Cases, please refer to Index.

Abbott, Alison. 'Ethical' stem-cell paper under attack, *Nature* (7 September 2006) 443: 12.

Academy of Medical Sciences. *Animals Containing Human Material*. London: Academy of Medical Sciences, July 2011.

———— *Inter-species embryos*. London: Academy of Medical Sciences, June 2007.

Adams, Maurice and John Griffiths. Against 'comparative method': explaining similarities and differences. In Maurice Adams and Jacco Bomhoff (eds.), *Practice and Theory in Comparative Law*. Cambridge: Cambridge University Press, 2012, pp 279-301.

Amos, Jonathan. 'Virgin conception' first for UK. *BBC News*, 9 September 2005.

Andorno, Roberto. Global bioethics at UNESCO: in defence of the Universal Declaration on Bioethics and Human Rights, *Journal of Medical Ethics* (2007) 33, 3: 150-154.

Annas, George J. *American bioethics: Crossing human rights and health law boundaries*. Oxford and New York: Oxford University Press, 2005.

Apthorpe, Raymond. Writing Development Policy and Policy Analysis Plain or Clear: On Language, Genre and Power. In Cris Shore and S Wright (eds.), *Anthropology of Policy: Critical Perspectives on Governance and Power*. London: Routledge, 1997, pp 43-58.

Baker, Robert. *Before Bioethics: A History of American Medical Ethics from the Colonial Period to the Bioethics Revolution*. New York: Oxford University Press, 2013.

Ballantyne, Angela and Sheryl De Lacey. Wanted – Egg donors for research: a research ethics approach to donor recruitment and compensation. *The International Journal of Feminist Approaches to Bioethics* (2008) 1, 145-164.

Barber, Karin. *The Anthropology of Texts, Persons and Publics: Oral and written culture in Africa and beyond*. Cambridge: Cambridge University Press, 2007.

Bartlett, Zane. Induced Pluripotent Stem Cell Experiments by Kazutoshi Takahashi and Shinya Yamanaka in 2006 and 2007. In *Embryo Project Encyclopedia*. Arizona: Arizona State University, 2015.

Bateson, Mary Catherine. The Double Bind: Pathology and Creativity, *Cybernetics and Human Knowledge* (2005) 12, 1-2: 11-21.

Baylis, Françoise and Jason Scott Robert. Part-Human Chimeras: Worrying the Facts, Probing the Ethics, *American Journal of Bioethics* (2007) 7, 5: 41-45.

Beauchamp, Tom L. Informed Consent: Its History, Meaning, and Present Challenges, *Cambridge Quarterly of Healthcare Ethics* (2011) 20: 515-523.

Beck, Anthony. Foucault and Law: The Collapse of Law's Empire *Oxford Journal of Legal Studies* (1996) 16: 489-502.

Beck, Ulrich. Cosmopolitan realism: on the distinction between cosmopolitanism in philosophy and the social science, *Global Networks* (2004) 4, 2: 131-156.

———— *Risk Society: Towards a New Modernity*. London: Sage Publications, 1992.

Beck, Ulrich; Anthony Giddens and Scott Lash. *Reflexive modernization: politics, tradition, and aesthetics in the modern social order*. Cambridge: Polity Press, 1994.

Berlin, Isaiah. *The Crooked Timber of Humanity*. Princeton: Princeton University Press, 1990.

Bernstein, Peter L. *Against the Gods: The Remarkable Story of Risk*. New York: John Wiley & Sons, 1998.

Bingham, Thomas H. *Widening Horizons: The Influence of Comparative Law and International Law on Domestic Law*. Cambridge: Cambridge University Press, 2010.

Bioethics Advisory Committee. *Ethical Guidelines for Human Biomedical Research*. Singapore: Bioethics Advisory Committee, 2015.

————— *Human-Animal Combinations in Stem Cell Research*. Singapore: Bioethics Advisory Committee, September 2010.

————— *Press Release: Human-Animal Combinations in Stem Cell Research*, 22 September 2010.

————— *Human-Animal Combinations for Biomedical Research: A Consultation Paper*. Singapore: Bioethics Advisory Committee, 8 January 2008.

————— *Donation of Human Eggs for Research*. Singapore: Bioethics Advisory Committee, 3 November 2008.

————— *Donation of Human Eggs for Research: A Consultation Paper*. Singapore: Bioethics Advisory Committee, 7 November 2007.

————— *Personal Information in Biomedical Research*. Singapore: Bioethics Advisory Committee, May 2007.

————— *Research Involving Human Subjects: Guidelines for IRBs*. Singapore: Bioethics Advisory Committee, November 2004.

————— *Ethical, Legal and Social Issues in Human Stem Cell Research, Reproductive and Therapeutic Cloning*. Singapore: Bioethics Advisory Committee, 21 June 2002.

————— *Human Tissue Research*. Singapore: Bioethics Advisory Committee, November 2002.

Black, Max. Models and Metaphors: *Studies in Language and Philosophy*. Ithaca and London: Cornell University Press, 1962.

Blichner, Lars Chr and Anders Molander. Mapping Juridification, *European Law Journal* (2008) 14, 1: 36-54.

Boisson de Chazournes, Laurence. New Technologies, the Precautionary Principle, and Public Participation. In Thérèse Murphy (ed.), *New Technologies and Human Rights*. Oxford: Oxford University Press, 2009, pp 161-194.

Bourdieu, Pierre (tr. Richard Nice). *The Logic of Practice*. Stanford CA: Stanford University Press, 1990.

————— (tr. Richard Terdiman). The Force of Law: Toward a Sociology of the Juridical Field, *Hastings Law Journal* (1987) 38: 805-853.

Boyer, Dominic. Thinking through the Anthropology of Experts, *Anthropology in Action* (2008) 15, 2: 38-46.

Brenneis, Don. Performing Promise. In Annelise Riles (ed.), *Documents: Artefacts of Modern Knowledge*. Ann Arbor: The University of Michigan Press, 2006, pp 41-70.

British Academy. *Carlton House Terrace*. London: British Academy, 2007.

Brownsword, Roger and Morag Goodwin. *Law and the Technologies of the Twenty-First Century*. Cambridge: Cambridge University Press, 2012.

Brownsword, Roger and Karen Yeung. Regulating Technologies: Tools, Targets and Thematics. In Roger Brownsword and Karen Yeung (eds.), *Regulating Technologies: Legal Futures, Regulatory Frames and Technological Fixes*. Oxford and Portland: Hart Publishing, 2008, pp 3-22.

Brooke, Michael QC and Ian Forrester QC. The Use of Comparative Law in A & Others v National Blood Authority. In Guy Canivet, Mads Andenas and Duncan Fairgrieve (eds.), *Comparative Law Before the Courts*. London: The British Institute of International and Comparative Law, 2004, pp 57-83.

Bruni, Attila. Shadowing software and clinical records: On the ethnography of non-humans and heterogeneous contexts. *Organization* (2005) 12, 3: 357-378

Bucchi, Massimiano and Federico Neresini. Science and Public Participation. In E J Hackett, O Amsterdamska, M Lynch and J Wajcman (eds.), *The Handbook of Science and Technology Studies*. Cambridge MA: MIT Press, 2008, pp 449-472.

Callon, Michel. Some Elements of a Sociology of Translation: Domestication of Scallops and the Fishermen of St. Brieuc Bay. In John Law (ed.), *Power, Action and Belief: A New Sociology of Knowledge?* London: Routledge & Kegan Paul, 1986, pp 196-229.

Canivet, Guy. The Use of Comparative Law Before the French Private Law Courts. In Guy Canivet, Mads Andenas and Duncan Fairgrieve (eds.), *Comparative Law Before the Courts*. London: The British Institute of International and Comparative Law, 2004, pp 181-193.

Cannell, Fenella. Concepts of Parenthood: the Warnock Report, the Gillick debate, and modern myths, *American Ethnologist* (1990) 17, 4: 667-686.

Capron, Alex M. American Law and the Governance of Research Ethics: Time for International Change *Singapore Academy of Law Journal* (2010) 22: 769-784.

———— What contributions have social science and the law made to the development of policy on bioethics? *Daedalus* (1999) 128, 4: 295-325.

Cardozo, Benjamin N. *The Growth of Law*. New Haven: Yale University Press, 1924.

Carruthers, Bruce G and Terence C Halliday. Negotiating Globalization: Global Scripts and Intermediation in the Construction of Asian Insolvency Regimes. *Law & Social Inquiry* (2006) 31, 3: 521-584.

Carson, Sandra A; David A Eschenbach, Geoffrey P Lomax, Valerie Montgomery Rice, Mark V Sauer, Robert N Taylor. Proposed oocyte donation guidelines for stem cell research, *Fertility and Sterility* (2010) 94, 7: 2503-2506

Carver, Terrell and Jernej Pikalo. Editors' introduction. In Terrell Carver and Jernej Pikalo (eds.), *Political Language and Metaphor: Interpreting and changing the world*. London and New York: Routledge, 2008, pp 1-12.

Caulfield, Timothy; Amy Zarzeczny, Jennifer McCormick, Tania Bubela, Christine Critchley, Edna Einsiedel, Jacques Galipeau, Shawn Harmon, Michael Huynh, Insoo Hyun, Judy Illes, Rosario M Isasi, Yann Joly, Graeme T Laurie, Geoffrey P Lomax, Holly Longstaff, Michael McDonald, Charles Murdoch, Ubaka Ogbogu, Jason Owen-Smith, Shaun Pattinson, Shainur Premji, Barbara von Tigerstrom, David E. Winickoff. The Stem Cell Research Environment, *Stem Cell Reviews and Reports* (2009) 5, 82-88.

Caulfield, Timothy; Kamenova K, Ogbogu U, Zarzeczny A, Baltz J, Benjaminy S, Cassar P A, Clark M, Rosario M Isasi, Bartha M Knoppers, Knowles L, Korbutt G, Lavery J V, Geoffrey P Lomax, Master Z, McDonald M, Preto N, Toews M. Research ethics and stem cells: Is it time to re-think current approaches to oversight? *EMBO reports* (2015) 16, 1: 2-6.

Chan, Sarah. A Bioethics for All Seasons, *Journal of Medical Ethics* (2015) 14: 17-21.

Chan, Leo Tak-hung. *The Discourse on Foxes and Ghosts: Ji Yun and Eighteenth-Century Literati Storytelling*. Hong Kong: Chinese University Press, 1998.

Channel News Asia. BAC recommends setting up a body to monitor stem cell research, 22 September 2010 (Singapore).

Chen, Huifen. Panel favours compensating women who donate eggs for research. *The Business Times*, 4 November 2008.

———— Payment for women's eggs being mulled. *The Business Times*, 8 November 2007.

Chen, Dung-sheng and Chia-Ling Wu. Introduction: Public Participation in Science and Technology in East Asia. *East Asian Science, Technology and Society: an International Journal* (2007) 1: 15-18.

Chen, Hua Biao [陈华彪], [人面兽身], Human Face Beast Body [联合早报], Combined Morning Paper, 1 July 2007.

Chia, Roland. Hybrids, Cybrids and Chimeras: *The Ethics of Interspecies Research*. Singapore: National Council of Churches of Singapore, 2012.

Chinese Medical Doctor Association [中国医师协会]. Can you accept human-animal combinations? [你能否接受人兽嵌合体?], 1 September 2008.

———— Birth of Human-Animal Hybrid Embryo [人兽混合胚胎问世] 3 April 2008.

Chua, Grace. Call for national body on stem cell research: It should review research involving human-animal combination of cells, *The Straits Times*, 23 September 2010.

Chua, Huiling. Bioethics Advisory Committee: Establish National Body to Control Human-Animal Stem Cell Research, *Joint Morning Newspaper*, 23 September 2010.

Clark, Jon and Lord Wedderburn. Juridification – a Universal Trend? In Gunther Teubner (ed.), *Juridification of Social Spheres: A Comparative Analysis in the Areas of Labor, Corporate Antitrust and Social Welfare Law*. Berlin: Walter de Gruyter & Co, 1987, pp 163-190.

Cloatre, Emilie and Martyn Pickersgill (eds.). *Knowledge, Technology and Law*. Abingdon and New York: Routledge, 2015.

Cloatre, Emilie and Robert Dingwall. "Embedded regulation": The migration of objects, scripts and governance, *Regulation & Governance* (2013) 7, 365-386.

Cochrane, Rexmond C. *The National Academy of Sciences: The First Hundred Years 1863-1963*. Washington DC: National Academy of Sciences, 1978.

Cockburn, Tom. Children and the feminist ethic of care, *Childhood – a Global Journal of Child Research* (2005) 12, 1: 71-89.

Coglianese, Cary. Engaging Business in the Regulation of Nanotechnology. In Christopher J Bosso (ed.), *Governing Uncertainty: Environmental Regulation in the Age of Nanotechnology*. Washington DC and London: RFF Press, 2010, pp 46-79.

Cohen, Cynthia B and Mary A Majumder. Future Directions for Oversight of Stem Cell Research in the United States, *Kennedy Institute of Ethics Journal* (2009) 19, 1: 79-103.

Cohen, Jean; Howard Jones Jr., Ian Cooke and Roger Kempers (eds.). IFFS Surveillance 07. *Fertility and Sterility* (2007) 87 Suppl. 1: S1-S67.

Cortina, Adela. Bioethics and Public Reason: A Report on Ethics and Public Discourse in Spain, *Cambridge Quarterly of Healthcare Ethics* (2009) 18: 241-250.

Couso, Javier; Alexandra Huneeus and Rachel Sieder, *Cultures of Legality: Judicialization and Political Activism in Latin America*. Cambridge: Cambridge University Press, 2010.

Colebatch, Hal K; Robert Hoppe and Mirka Noordegraaf. Understanding Policy Work. In Hal K Colebatch, Robert Hoppe and Mirko Noordegraaf (eds.), *Working for Policy*. Amsterdam: Amsterdam University Press, 2010, pp 11-25.

Collier, Stephen J and Aihwa Ong. Global Assemblages and Anthropological Problems. In Aihwa Ong and Stephen J Collier (eds.), *Global Assemblages: Technology, Politics, and Ethics as Anthropological Problems*. Singapore: Blackwell Publishing, 2005, pp 3-21.

Committee on Risk Perception and Communication, National Research Council. *Improving Risk Communication*. Washington, DC: National Academy Press, 1989.

Committee on the Institutional Means for the Assessment of Risk to Public Health, Commission on Life Sciences, and National Research Council. *Risk Assessment in the Federal Government: Managing the Process*. Washington DC: National Academy Press, 1983.

Congregation for the Doctrine of the Faith. *Dignitas Personae: On Certain Bioethical Questions*. Vatican City: Congregation for the Doctrine of the Faith, 2008.

Cotterrell, Roger. Comparatists and Sociology. In Pierre Legrand and Roderick Munday (eds.), *Comparative Legal Studies: Traditions and Transitions*. Cambridge: Cambridge University Press, 2003, pp 131-153.

Council for International Organizations of Medical Sciences (CIOMS), *International Ethical Guidelines for Biomedical Research Involving Human Subjects*, 2002 (updated).

Cowan, Dave and Helen Carr. Actor-network Theory, Implementation, and the Private Landlord, *Journal of Law and Society* (2008) 35, s1: 149-166.

Crichton, Michael. *Next.* New York: HarperCollins Publishers, 2006.

Cunliffe, Ann L and Jong S Jun. The Need for Reflexivity in Public Administration, *Administration & Society* (May 2005) 37, 2: 225-242.

Daley, George Q; Heather M Rooke and Nancy Witty. Global Forum Discusses Stem Cell Research Strategy, *Cell Stem Cell* (2007) 2: 435-436.

Daley, George Q; Insoo Hyun, Jane F Apperley, Roger A Barker, Nissim Benvenisty, Annelien L Bredenoord, Christopher K Breuer, Timothy Caulfield, Marcelle I Cedars, Joyce Frey-Vasconcells, Helen E Heslop, Ying Jin, Richard T Lee, Christopher McCabe, Megan Munsie, Charles E Murry, Steven Piantadosi, Mahendra Rao, Heather M Rooke, Douglas Sipp, Lorenz Studer, Jeremy Sugarman, Masayo Takahashi, Mark Zimmerman and Jonathan Kimmelman. Setting Global Standards for Stem Cell Research and Clinical Translation: The 2016 ISSCR Guidelines. *Stem Cell Reports* (2016) 6: 1-11.

Daley, George Q. Letter from the President, *Cell Stem Cell* (2008) 3: 151-152.

Danish Council of Ethics (with the Danish Ethical Council for Animals). *Man or Mouse: Ethical aspects of chimera research.* Copenhagen: Danish Council of Ethics, 2007.

Dannemann, Gerhard. Comparative Law: Study of Similarities or Differences? In Mathias Reimann and Reinhard Zimmermann (eds.), *The Oxford Handbook of Comparative Law.* Oxford and New York: Oxford University Press, 2006, pp 383-419.

Daston, Lorraine. The Glass Flowers. In Lorraine Daston (ed.), *Things That Talk: Object Lessons from Art and Science.* New York: Zone Books, 2004, pp 223-254.

Davis, J Clarence. Foreword: Nanotechnology, Risk, and Governance. In Christopher J Bosso (ed), *Governing Uncertainty: Environmental Regulation in the Age of Nanotechnology.* Washington DC and London: RFF Press, 2010, pp xii to xviii.

de Chávez Guerrero, Manuel H R (ed.). *12th World Congress of Bioethics: Inspire the Future to Move the World.* Mexico City: National Bioethics Commission of Mexico, 2015.

de Dampierre, Florence. *Chairs: A History.* New York: Abrams, 2006.

de S Cameron, Nigel M and A V Henderson. Brave New World at the General Assembly: The United Nations Declaration on Human Cloning. *Minnesota Journal of Law Science and Technology* (2008) 9: 145-238.

de S-O-l'E Lasser, Mitchel. *Judicial Transformations: The Rights Revolution in the Courts of Europe.* Oxford and New York: Oxford University Press, 2009.

de S-O-l'E Lasser, Mitchel. Transforming Deliberations. In Nick Huls, Maurice Adams and Jacco Bomhoff (eds.), *The Legitimacy of Highest Courts' Rulings: Judicial Deliberations and Beyond.* The Hague: TMC Asser Press, 2009, pp 33-53.

de S-O-l'E Lasser, Mitchel. *Judicial Deliberations: A Comparative Analysis of Judicial Transparency and Legitimacy.* New York and Oxford: Oxford University Press, 2004.

Dean, Mitchell. Risk calculable and incalculable. In Deborah Lupton (ed.), *Risk and Sociocultural Theory: New Directions and Perspectives.* Cambridge: Cambridge University Press, 1999, pp 131-159.

Deech, Ruth and Anna Smajdor. *From IVF to Immortality: Controversy in the Era of Reproductive Technology.* Oxford: Oxford University Press, 2007.

Deflem, Mathieu. The Legal Theory of Jürgen Habermas. In Reza Banakar and Max Travers (eds.), *Law and Social Theory.* Oxford: Hart Publishing, 2013, pp 75-90.

Degrazia, David. Human-Animal Chimeras: Human Dignity, Moral Status, and Species Prejudice, *Metaphilosophy* (2007) 38, 2-3: 309-329.

Department of Health, UK, *Review of the Human Fertilisation and Embryology Act: Proposals for revised legislation (including establishment of the Regulatory Authority for Tissue and Embryos).* London: Department of Health, December 2006.

————— *Stem Cell Research: Medical Progress with Responsibility.* London: Department of Health, June 2000.

Derrida, Jacques (tr. David Wills). The Animal That Therefore I Am (More to Follow), *Critical Inquiry* (2002) 28: 369-418.

————— Force of Law: The mystical foundation of authority. *Cardozo Law Review* (1990) 11: 920-1045.

Devolder, Katrien. *The Ethics of Embryonic Stem Cell Research*. Oxford: Oxford University Press, 2015.

Dickenson, Donna. *Property in the body: feminist perspectives*. Cambridge: Cambridge University Press, 2007.

Dickenson, Donna and Itziar A Idiakez. Ova Donation for stem cell research: an international perspective. *The International Journal of Feminist Approaches to Bioethics* (2007) 1, 125-144.

Disch, Lisa. 'Faitiche'-izing the People: What Representative Democracy Might Learn from Science Studies. In Bruce Braun and Sarah J Whatmore (eds.), *Political Matter: Technoscience, Democracy, and Public Life*. Minneapolis and London: University of Minnesota Press, 2010, pp 267-296.

Douglas, Heather E. *Science, Policy, and the Value-Free Ideal*. Pittsburgh: University of Pittsburgh Press, 2009.

Douglas, Mary. *How Institutions Think*. Syracuse: Syracuse University Press, 1986.

Douglas, Mary and Aaron Wildavsky. *Risk and Culture: An Essay on the Selection of Technical and Environmental Dangers*. University of California Press: Berkeley and Los Angeles, 1982.

Drori, Gili S; John W Meyer, Francisco O Ramirez, and Evan Schofer. *Science in the Modern World Polity: Institutionalization and Globalization*. Stanford, CA: Stanford University Press, 2003.

Durkheim, Emile (tr. Karen E Fields). *The Elementary Forms of Religious Life*. New York: The Free Press, 1995 [1912].

Düwell, Marcus. *Bioethics: Methods, Theories, Domains*. London and New York: Routledge, 2013.

Dworkin, Ronald. *Law's Empire*. Cambridge MA: Harvard University Press, 1986.

Edwards, Jeanette; Penny Harvey and Peter Wade. *Anthropology and Science: Epistemologies in Practice*. Oxford: Berg, 2007.

Eisner, Marc Allen. Institutional Evolution or Intelligent Design? Constructing a Regulatory Regime for Nanotechnology. In Christopher J Bosso (ed.), *Governing Uncertainty: Environmental Regulation in the Age of Nanotechnology*. Washington DC and London: RFF Press, 2010, pp 28-45.

Elliott, John M; Calvin W L Ho and Sylvia Lim. *Bioethics in Singapore: the Ethical Microcosm*. Singapore: WorldScientific, 2010.

Elliott, Carl. *A philosophical disease: Bioethics, culture and identity*. New York: Routledge, 1999.

Emanuel, Ezekiel. The Evolving Norms of Medical Ethics. In Ronald M Green, Aine Donovan and Steven A Jauss (eds.), *Global Bioethics: Issues of Conscience for the Twenty-First Century*. Oxford: Clarendon Press, 2008, pp 53-76.

Errera, Roger. The Use of Comparative Law Before the French Administrative Law Courts. In Guy Canivet, Mads Andenas and Duncan Fairgrieve (eds.), *Comparative Law Before the Courts*. London: The British Institute of International and Comparative Law, 2004, pp 153-163.

European Society on Human Reproduction and Embryology Task Force on Ethics and Law. Oocyte donation for non-reproductive purposes. *Human Reproduction* (2007) 22: 1210-1213.

Evanoff, Richard. *Bioregionalism and Global Ethics: A Transnational Approach to Achieving Ecological Sustainability, Social Justice, and Human Well-being*. New York and London: Routledge, 2011.

Evans, John H. *The History and Future of Bioethics: a Sociological View*. Oxford and New York: Oxford University Press, 2012.

Evens, Terry M S. *Anthropology as Ethics: Nondualism and the Conduct of Sacrifice*. New York and Oxford: Berghahn Books, 2009.

Everson, Michelle and Ellen Vos. The scientification of politics and the politicisation of science. In Michelle Everson and Ellen Vos (eds.), *Uncertain Risks Regulated*. Abingdon and New York: Routledge, 2009, pp 1-17.

Ewald, François. Norms, Discipline, and the Law, *Representations* (1990) 30:138-161.

Falk Moore, Sally. Political Struggles in Legal Arenas: Some African Instances. In Max Kirsch (ed.), *Inclusion and Exclusion in the Global Arena*. New York: Routledge, 2006, pp 269-286.

———— *Law and Anthropology: A Reader*. Cornwall: Blackwell Publishing, 2005.

Ferguson, Niall. *The Ascent of Money: A Financial History of the World*. New York: Penguin Books, 2008.

Fischer, Frank. *Reframing Public Policy: Discursive Politics and Deliberative* *Practices*. New York: Oxford University Press, 2003.

Fiss, Peer C and Paul M Hirsch. The Discourse of Globalization: Framing and Sensemaking of an Emerging Concept, American *Sociological Review* (2005) 70, 1: 29-52.

Fortun, Kim. *Advocacy after Bhopal: Environmentalism, Disaster, New Global Orders*. Chicago and London: University of Chicago Press, 2001.

Foucault, Michel (tr. David Macey). *'Society Must Be Defended': Lectures at the Collège de France, 1975-76*. London: Allen Lane, 2003.

——————— Ethics: Subjectivity and Truth. In Paul Rabinow (ed.), *Essential Works of Michel Foucault, 1954-1984*. The New Press: New Press: 1997.

——————— Governmentality. In Graham Burchell, Colin Gordon and Peter Miller (eds.), *The Foucault Effect: Studies in Governmentality*. Hertfordshire: Harvester Wheatsheaf, 1991, pp 87-104.

——————— *History of Sexuality* (Volume 1). New York: Vintage Books, 1990.

——————— (tr. Alan Sheridan). *Discipline and Punish: The Birth of the Prison*. New York: Vintage, 1995.

——————— (tr. Colin Gordon *et al*.). *Power/Knowledge: Selected Interviews and Other Writings 1972-1977*. Brighton: Harvester Press, 1980.

——————— The subject and power. In Hubert Dreyfus and Paul Rabinow (eds.), *Michel Foucault: Beyond Structuralism and Hermeneutics*. Chicago: Chicago University Press, 1982, pp 208-226.

——————— (tr. Robert Hurley). *The Will to Knowledge: The History of Sexuality, Vol. 1*. Harmondsworth: Penguin, 1979.

Fox, Renée C and Judith P Swazey, *Observing Bioethics*. New York: Oxford University Press, 2008.

Franklin, Sarah and Celia Roberts. *Born and Made: An Ethnography of Preimplantation Genetic Diagnosis*. Princeton, NJ: Princeton University Press, 2006.

Franklin, Sarah. Stem cells r us: emergent life forms and the global biological. In Aihwa Ong and Stephen J Collier, *Global Assemblages: Technology, Politics and Ethics as Anthropological Problems*. Singapore: Blackwell Publishing, 2006, pp 59-78.

Freedland, Mark. Introduction: Comparative and International Law in the Courts. In Guy Canivet, Mads Andenas and Duncan Fairgrieve (eds.),

Comparative Law Before the Courts. London: The British Institute of International and Comparative Law, 2004, pp xv-xxvi.

Freeman, Richard. Epistemological Bricolage: How Practitioners Make Sense of Learning, *Administration & Society* (July 2007) 39, 4: 476-496.

Fukuyama, Francis. *The Origins of Political Order: From Prehuman Times to the French Revolution*. New York: Farrar, Straus and Giroux, 2011.

Fuller, Lon L. *The Morality of Law*. New Haven: Yale University Press, 1969.

Funnell, Warwick; Robert Jupe and Jane Andrew. *In Government We Trust: Market Failure and the Delusions of Privatisation*. London: Pluto Press, 2009.

Gadamer, Hans-Georg (tr. & rev. Joel Weinsheimer and Donald G Marshall). *Truth and Method*. London and New York: Continuum, 2004.

Gatter, Robert. Human Subjects Research and Conflicts of Interest – Walking the Talk of Trust in Human Subjects Research: The Challenge of Regulating Financial Conflicts of Interest, *Emory Law Journal* (2003) 52: 327-401.

Gazzaniga, Michael S. Human: *The science behind what makes your brain unique*. New York: HarperCollins Publishing, 2008.

Geesink, Ingrid; Barbara Prainsack and Sarah Franklin. Stem Cell Stories 1998-2008, *Science as Culture* (2008) 17, 1: 1-11.

Gelfert, Axel. Before Biopolis: Representations of the Biotechnology Discourse in Singapore, *East Asian Science, Technology and Society: and International Journal* (2013) 7, 1: 103-123.

Geoff Watts (ed.). *Hype, Hope and hybrids: Science, policy and media perspectives of the Human Fertilisation and Embryology Bill*. London: The Academy of Medical Sciences, Medical Research Council, Science Media Centre and Wellcome Trust, 2009.

German Ethics Council. *Human-animal mixtures in research: Opinion*. Berlin: German Ethics Council, 2011.

Geron. *Geron Initiates Clinical Trial of Human Embryonic Stem Cell-Based Therapy*, Press Release, 11 October 2010.

Giddens, Anthony. *The Third Way and its Critics*. Cambridge: Polity Press, 2000.

——— *Modernity and Self-Identity: Self and Society in the Late Modern Age*. Cambridge: Polity Press, 1991.

————— *The Consequences of Modernity*. Stanford: Stanford University Press, 1990.

Gillott, John. *Bioscience, Governance and Politics*. Basingstoke: Palgrave Macmillan, 2014.

Glenn, H Patrick. *Legal Traditions of the World: Sustainable Diversity in Law*. Oxford and NY: Oxford University Press, 2007 (3rd ed.).

Golder, Ben and Peter Fitzpatrick. *Foucault's Law*. London and New York: Routledge, 2009.

Goody, Jack. Globalization and the Domestic Group. In Max Kirsch (ed.), *Inclusion and Exclusion in the Global Arena*. New York: Routledge, 2006, pp 31-41.

Gordley, James. The universalist heritage. In Pierre Legrand and Roderick Munday (eds.), *Comparative Legal Studies: Traditions and Transitions*. Cambridge: Cambridge University Press, 2003, pp 31-45.

Gostin, Lawrence O. *Global Health Law*. Cambridge MA: Harvard University Press, 2014.

Gottweis, Herbert; Brian Salter and Catherine Waldby. *The Global Politics of Human Embryonic Stem Cell Science: Regenerative Medicine in Transition*. Basingstoke: Palgrave Macmillan, 2009.

Grabham, Emily. Legal Form and Temporal Rationalities in UK Work-Life Balance Law, *Australian Feminist Studies* (2014) 29, 79: 67-84.

Greely, Henry T; Mildred K Cho, Linda F Hogle and Debra M Satz. Thinking About the Human Neuron Mouse. *The American Journal of Bioethics* (2007) 7, 5: 27-40.

Greely, Henry T. Defining Chimeras ... and Chimeric Concerns. *The American Journal of Bioethics* (2003) 3, 3: 17-20.

Greene, Mark *et al*. Moral Issues of Human-Non-Human Primate Neural Grafting, *Science* (2005) 309: 385-386.

Greenhouse, Carol J. Fieldwork on Law. *Annual Review of Law and Social Sciences* (2006) 2: 187-210.

Gregg, Benjamin. *Coping in Politics with Indeterminate Norms: A Theory of Enlightened Localism*. New York: State University of New York Press, 2003.

Guo X F and Li T B [郭秀芳与李腾宝]. Human-Animal Strange Research, Raises All Kinds of Issues: Meat with Human Cells, do you dare eat?

[人兽怪研究, 引发各种问题: 带人细胞的肉, 你敢吃吗?], New People's Night Paper [新民晚报], 8 January 2008.

Gusterson, Hugh. Nuclear futures: anticipatory knowledge, expert judgment, and the lack that cannot be filled. *Science and Public Policy* (October 2008) 35, 8: 551-560.

Guston, David H. Understanding 'anticipatory governance', *Social Studies of Science* (2014) 44, 2: 218-242.

Habermas, Jürgen (tr. William Regh). *Between Facts and Norms: Contributions to a Discourse Theory of Law and Democracy.* Cambridge MA: MIT Press, 1998.

———— *The Structural Transformation of the Public Sphere: An Inquiry into a Category of Bourgeois Society.* Cambridge MA: MIT Press, 1991.

———— *The Theory of Communicative Action* (in two volumes). Boston: Beacon Press, 1987.

Hackett, Jamie A and Azim M Surani. Regulatory principles of pluripotency: from the ground state up, *Cell Stem Cell* (2014) 15, 416-430.

Haggerty, Kevin D. From Risk to Precaution: The Rationalities of Personal Crime Prevention. In Richard V Ericson and Aaron Doyle (eds.), *Risk and Morality.* Toronto, Buffalo and London: University of Toronto Press, 2003, pp 193-214.

Hajer, Maarten A. *Authoritative governance: Policy-making in the Age of Mediatization.* New York: Oxford University Press, 2009.

Halliday, Terence C and Bruce G Carruthers. The Recursivity of Law: Global Norm Making and National Lawmaking in the Globalization of Corporate Insolvency Regimes, *American Journal of Sociology* (January 2007) 12, 4: 1135-1202.

Halliday, Terence C. Recursivity of Global Normmaking: A Sociolegal Agenda, *Annual Review of Law and Social Science* (2009) 5: 263-289.

Han, Fook Kwang; Zuraidah Ibrahim, Chua Mui Hoong, Lydia Lim, Ignatius Low, Rachel Lin and Robin Chan. *Lee Kuan Yew: Hard Truths to Keep Singapore Going.* Singapore: Straits Times Press, 2011.

Handler, Sarah. *Ming Furniture: In the Light of Chinese Architecture.* Berkeley and Toronto: Ten Speed Press, 2005.

Haran, Joan; Jenny Kitzinger, Maureen McNeil and Kate O'Riordan. *Human Cloning in the Media: From science fiction to science practice.* London and New York: Routledge, 2008, pp 95-120.

Haraway, Donna. *The Haraway Reader*. New York and London: Routledge, 2004.

Harmon, Shawn H E and Graeme T Laurie. *Yearworth v. North Bristol NHS Trust*: Property, Principles, Precedents and Paradigms, *Cambridge Law Journal* (2010) 69, 3: 476-493.

Harper, Richard. *Inside the IMF: An Ethnography of Documents, Technology and Organisational Action*. London: Academic Press, 1998.

Hart, H L A. *The Concept of Law*. Oxford: Clarendon, 1961.

Hauskeller, Michael. Making Sense of What We Are: A Mythological Approach to Human Nature, *Philosophy* (2009) 84: 95-109.

Heelas, Paul and Paul Morris. *The Values of the Enterprise Culture: the Moral Debates*. London and New York: Routledge, 1992.

Hegel, Georg W F (ed. Thomas Malcolm Knox). *Hegel's Philosophy of Right*. Oxford: Oxford University Press, [1820] 2015.

Heger Boyle, Elizabeth; Barbara J McMorris and Mayra Gomez. Local Conformity to International Norms, *International Sociology* (2002) 17, 1: 5-33.

Heimer, Carol A. Conceiving Children: How Documents Support Case versus Biographical Analyses. In Annelise Riles (ed.), *Documents: Artefacts of Modern Knowledge*. Ann Arbor: University of Michigan Press, 2006, pp 95-126.

Hermerén, Göran. Ethical considerations in chimera research, *Development* (2015) 142: 3-5.

Hess, David J. Ethnography and the development of science and technology studies. In Paul Atkinson, Amanda Coffey, Sara Delamont, John Lofland, and Lyn Lofland (eds.), *Sage handbook of ethnography*. Thousand Oaks, CA: Sage, 2001, pp 234-245.

Hickman, Tom R. The Reasonableness Principle: Reassessing its Place in the Public Sphere, *Cambridge Law Journal* (2004) 63, 1: 166-198.

Hilgartner, Stephen. *Science on Stage: Expert Advice as Public Drama*. Stanford: Stanford University Press, 2000.

————— The Social Construction of Risk Objects: or, How to Pry Open Networks of Risk. In James F Short and Lee Clarke (eds.), *Organizations, Uncertainties, and Risk*. Boulder, CO: Westview Press, 1992, pp 39-53.

Hine, Christine. Multi-sited Ethnography as Middle-Range Methodology for Contemporary STS. *Science, Technology, and Human Values* (2007) 32, 6: 652-671.

Ho, Calvin W L; Andreas Reis and Abha Saxena. Vulnerability in International Policy Discussion on Research involving Children, *Asian Bioethics Review* (2015) 7, 2: 230-249.

Ho, Calvin W L; Benjamin J Capps and Teck Chuan Voo. Stem Cell Science and its Public: The Case of Singapore, *East Asian Science, Technology and Society: An International Journal* (2010) 4: 7-29.

Ho, Calvin W L. Governing Cloning: United Nations' Debates and the Institutional Context of Standards. In Benjamin J Capps and Alastair V Campbell (eds.), *Contested Cells: Global Perspectives on the Stem Cell Debate*. London: Imperial College Press, 2010, pp 121-154.

Hoff, Shannon. *The Laws of the Spirit: A Hegelian Theory of Justice*. Buffalo: SUNY Press, 2014.

Holden, Kerry and David Demeritt. Democratising science? The politics of promoting biomedicine in Singapore's developmental state. *Environment and Planning D: Society and Space* (2008) 26, 68-86.

Holm, Søren and T Takala. High hopes and automatic escalators: a critique of some new arguments in bioethics, *Journal of Medical Ethics* (2007) 33, 1: 1-4.

Holmes, Douglas R and George E Marcus. Cultures of Expertise and the Management of Globalization: Toward the Re-Functioning of Ethnography. In Aihwa Ong and Stephen J Collier (eds.), *Global Assemblages: Technology, Politics and Ethics as Anthropological Problems*. Singapore: Blackwell Publishing, 2005, pp 235-252.

————— Fast Capitalism: Para-Ethnography and the Rise of the Symbolic Analyst. In Melissa S Fisher and Greg Downey (eds.), *Frontiers of Capital: Ethnographic Reflections on the New Economy*. Durham and London: Duke University Press, 2006, pp 33-57.

Hommels, Anique; Jessica Mesman and Wiebe E Bijker (eds.). *Vulnerability in Technological Cultures: New Directions in Research and Governance*. Cambridge MA: MIT Press, 2014.

Hong, Sungook. The Hwang Scandal that "shook the world of science", *East Asian Science, Technology and Society: an International Journal* (2008) 2: 1-7.

House of Commons Science and Technology Select Committee, UK. *Reproductive Technologies and the Law*. London: HMSO, 2005.

House of Lords Select Committee, UK. *Stem Cell Research*. London: HMSO, 2002.

Howard, Judith A. Social Psychology of Identities, *Annual Review of Sociology* (2000) 26: 367-393.

Huang, Claire Jingyi. Bioethics advisory panel proposes national body to monitor stem-cell research: one of 5 recommendations following 2-year consultation exercise, *TODAY*, 23 September 2010.

Human Fertilisation and Embryology Authority, UK. *Hybrids and Chimeras: A report on the findings of the consultation*. London: Human Fertilisation and Embryology Authority, October 2007.

———— *Press Statement*, 26 April 2007.

———— *Code of Practice*. London: Human Fertilisation and Embryology Authority, 2009 (October 2015, 8th ed.).

Hunt, Alan. Risk and Moralization in Everyday Life. In Richard V Ericson and Aaron Doyle (eds.), *Risk and Morality*. Toronto, Buffalo and London: University of Toronto Press, 2003, pp 165-192.

———— Foucault expulsion of law – toward a retrieval, *Law and Social Inquiry* (1992) 17, 1: 1-38.

Hunt, Alan and Gary Wickham. *Foucault and Law: Towards a Sociology of Law as Governance*. Pluto Press: Finland, 1994.

Hyland, Richard. *Gifts: a study in comparative law*. New York: Oxford University Press, 2009.

Hyun, Insoo. From naïve pluripotency to chimeras: a new ethical challenge? *Development* (2015) 142: 6-8.

———— *Bioethics and the Future of Stem Cell Research*. Cambridge and New York: Cambridge University Press, 2013.

Hyun, Insoo; Amy Wilkerson and Josephine Johnston. Embryology Policy: Revisit the 14-day rule, *Nature* (2016) 533, 7602: 169-171.

India (Government of; Ministry of Health and Family Welfare) and National Academy of Medical Sciences (Indian Council of Medical Research). *National Guidelines for Accreditation, Supervision and Regulation of ART Clinics in India*. New Delhi: S Narayan & Sons, 2005.

International Federation of Fertility Societies. *IFFS Surveillance 2013*. Mount Royal NJ: International Federation of Fertility Societies, October 2013.

Indian Council of Medical Research, Department of Health Research and Department of Biotechnology, *Guidelines for Stem Cell Research*, 2013.

International Risk Governance Council. *Risk Governance: Towards an Integrative Approach*. Geneva: International Risk Governance Council, September 2005.

International Society for Stem Cell Research. *Guidelines for Stem Cell Science and Clinical Translation*, 2016.

————— *Position* Statement on the Provision and Procurement of Human Eggs for Stem Cell Research, *Cell Stem Cell* (2013) 12: 285-291.

————— *Press Release: ISSCR Comments on Draft Guidelines for Embryonic Stem Cell Funding*, 22 May 2009.

————— Ethics Report on Interspecies Somatic Cell Nuclear Transfer Research, *Cell Stem Cell* (2009) 5, 1: 27-30.

————— *Press Release: Letter to German Government supporting changes to Stem Cell Act*, 2002, 7 March 2008.

————— Ethical Standards for Human-to-Animal Chimera Experiments in Stem Cell Research, *Cell Stem Cell* (2007) 1, 4: 159-163.

————— *Guidelines for the Conduct of Human Embryonic Stem Cell Research*, 2006.

Institute of Medicine and National Research Council, Linda Giudice, Eileen Santa and Robert Pool (eds.). *Assessing the Medical Risks of Human Oocyte Donation for Stem Cell Research*. Washington DC: National Academies Press, 2007.

Isasi, Rosario M and Bartha M Knoppers. Mind the Gap: Policy Approaches to Embryonic Stem Cell and Cloning Research in 50 Countries, *European Journal of Health Law* (2006) 13: 9-26

Isasi, Rosario M and Bartha M Knoppers. Beyond the permissibility of embryonic and stem cell research: substantive requirements and procedural safeguards, *Human Reproduction* (2006) 21, 10: 2474-2481.

Ivison, Duncan. The Technical and the Political: Discourses of Race, Reasons of State *Social and Legal Studies* (1998) 7: 589-594.

Jacob, Marie-Andrée and Annelise Riles. The New Bureaucracies of Virtue, *Political and Legal Anthropology Review* (2007) 30, 2: 181-191.

Jacob, Marie-Andrée. Form-made Persons: Consent forms as Consent's Blind-Spot, *Political and Legal Anthropology Review* (2007) 30, 2: 248-268.

Jasanoff, Sheila. Making Order: Law and Science in Action. In Edward J Hackett, Olga Amsterdamska, Michael E Lynch, Judy Wajcman, Wiebe E Bijker, *Handbook of Science and Technology Studies*. Cambridge MA: MIT Press, 2007 (3rd ed), pp 761-789.

————— Law's Knowledge: Science for Justice in Legal Settings, *American Journal of Public Health* (2005) 95, S1: S49-S58.

————— *Designs on Nature: Science and Democracy in Europe and the United States*. Princeton: Princeton University Press, 2005.

Jensen, Eric A. *The Therapeutic Cloning Debate: Global Science and Journalism in the Public Sphere*. Farnham: Ashgate, 2014.

Jenson, Jane and Boaventura de Sousa Santos. Introduction: Case Studies and Common Trends in Globalizations. In Jane Jenson and Boaventura de Sousa Santos (eds.). *Globalizing Institutions: Case Studies in Regulation and Innovation*. Aldershot: Ashgate, 2000, pp 9-26.

Jones, Dan. Moral psychology: the depths of disgust, *Nature* (14 June 2007) 447, 7146: 768-771.

Jones, David A. What does the British public think about human-animal hybrid embryos? *Journal of Medical Ethics* (2009) 35, 3: 168-170.

Jones, Howard Jr.; Ian Cooke, Roger Kempers, Peter Brinsden and Doug Saunders (eds.). *IFFS Surveillance 2010*. Mount Royal NJ: International Federation of Fertility Societies, September 2010.

Jonsen, Albert R. *The Birth of Bioethics*. New York: Oxford University Press, 2003.

Kaan, Terry. At the Beginning of Life, *Singapore Academy of Law Journal* (2010) 22: 883-918

Kamm, Frances M. *Bioethical Prescriptions: To Create, End, Choose, and Improve Lives*. Oxford and New York: Oxford University Press, 2013.

Kant, Immanuel (tr. M Campbell Smith). *Perpetual Peace: a philosophical essay*. London: G Allen & Unwin, [1795] 1917.

Karpowicz, Phillip; Cynthia B Cohen and Derek van der Kooy. It is ethical to transplant human stem cells into nonhuman embryos, *Nature Medicine* (2004) 10, 4: 331-335.

Kass, Leon R. The Wisdom of Repugnance, *New Republic* (2 June 1997) 216, 22: 17-26.

Kawar, Leila. Commanding Legality: The Juridification of Immigration Policy Making in France, *Journal of Law and Courts* (Spring 2014), 2, 1: 93-116.

Keller, William W and Richard J Samuels. Innovation and the Asian economies. In William W Keller and Richard J Samuels (eds.), *Crisis and Innovation in Asian Technology*. Cambridge: Cambridge University Press, 2003, pp 1-22.

Kelman, Mark. *A Guide to Critical Legal Studies*. Cambridge MA: Harvard University Press, 1987.

Kelsen, Hans (tr. Anders Wedberg). *General Theory of Law and State*. Cambridge MA: Harvard University Press, 1945.

————— (tr. Max Knight). *Pure Theory of Law*. Berkeley and Los Angeles: University of California Press, 1967.

————— (tr. Michael Hartney). *General Theory of Norms*. Oxford: Clarendon Press, 1991.

————— *What is Justice? Justice, Law and Politics in the Mirror of Science*. Berkeley, Los Angeles and London: University of California Press, 1971.

Kemshall, Hazel. *Risk, Social Policy and Welfare*. Buckingham: Open University Press, 2002.

Kennedy, David. The methods and the politics. In Pierre Legrand and Roderick Munday (eds.), *Comparative Legal Studies: Traditions and Transitions*. Cambridge: Cambridge University Press, 2003, pp 345-433.

Kim, Sungmoon. Public Reason Confucianism: A Construction, *American Political Science Review* (2015) 109, 1: 187-200.

Kim, Leo. Explaining the Hwang scandal: national scientific culture and its global relevance, *Science as Culture* (2008) 17: 397-415.

Kim, Tae-Ho. How could a scientist become a national celebrity: Nationalism and Hwang Woo-Suk scandal, *East Asian Science, Technology and Society: An International Journal* (2008) 2: 27-45.

Kitcher, Philip. *Preludes to Pragmatism: Toward a Reconstruction of Philosophy*. Oxford: Oxford University Press, 2012.

Knoppers, Bartha M. Does policy grow on trees? *BMC Medical Ethics* (2014) 15: 87.

Knoppers, Bartha M; Emily Kirby and Rosario M Isasi. Genetics and Stem Cell Research: Models of International Policy-making. In John M Elliott, Calvin W L Ho and Sylvia S N Lim (eds.), *Bioethics in Singapore: The Ethical Microcosm*. Singapore: World Scientific, 2010, pp 133-163.

Kohli, Atul. *State-Directed Development: Political Power and Industrialization in the Global Periphery*. New York: Cambridge University Press, 2004.

Kono, Tomohiro; Yayoi Obata, Quiong Wu, Katsutoshi Niwa, Yukiko Ono, Yuji Yamamoto, Eun Sung Park, Jeong-Sun Seo and Hidehiko Ogawa. Birth of Parthenogenetic mice that can develop to adulthood, *Nature* (22 April 2004) 428, 6985: 860-864.

Kurkchiyan, Marina. Russian Legal Culture: An Analysis of Adaptive Response to an Institutional Transplant, *Law & Social Inquiry* (2009) 34, 2: 337-364.

Lakoff, Andrew and Stephen J Collier. Infrastructure and Event: The Political Technology of Preparedness. In Bruce Braun and Sarah J Whatmore (eds.), *Political Matter: Technoscience, Democracy, and Public Life*. Minneapolis and London: University of Minnesota Press, 2010, pp 243-266.

Landry, Donald W and Howard A Zucker. Embryonic death and the creation of human embryonic stem cells, *Journal of Clinical Investigations* (2004) 114: 1184-1186.

Latour, Bruno (tr. Catherine Porter). *An Inquiry into Modes of Existence: An Anthropology of the Moderns*. Cambridge MA: Harvard University Press, 2013.

————— Networks, Societies, Spheres: Reflections of an Actor-Network Theorist, *International Journal of Communication* (2011) 5: 796-810.

————— *Reassembling the Social: An Introduction to Actor-Network-Theory*. Oxford: Oxford University Press, 2007.

————— (tr. Catherine Porter). *Politics of Nature: How to Bring the Sciences into Democracy*. Cambridge MA: Harvard University Press, 2004.

————— Scientific Objects and Legal Objectivity. In Alain Pottage and Martha Mundy (eds.), *Law, Anthropology, and the Constitution of the Social: Making Persons and Things*. Cambridge: Cambridge University Press, 2004, pp 73-114.

————— *La fabrique du droit: Une ethnographie du Conseil d'État*. Paris: La Découverte, 2002.

————— *Pandora's Hope: Essays on the Reality of Science Studies*. Cambridge MA and London: Harvard University Press, 1999.

————— *Science in Action: How to Follow Scientists and Engineers through Society*. Cambridge MA: Harvard University Press, 1987.

————— *We Have Never Been Modern*. New York and London: Harvester Wheatsheaf, 1993 [1991].

————— Where are the Missing Masses? The Sociology of a Few Mundane Artefacts. In Wiebe Bijker and John Law (eds.), *Shaping technology/ Building Society: Studies in Sociotechnical Change.* Cambridge MA: MIT Press, 1992, pp 225-259.

Latour, Bruno and John Law. *The Pasteurization of France.* Cambridge MA: Harvard University Press, 1988.

Laurie, Graeme T; Shawn H E Harmon and Fabiana Arzuaga. Foresighting Futures: Law, New Technologies, and the Challenges of Regulating for Uncertainty, *Law, Innovation and Technology* (2012) 4, 1: 1-33.

Law, John. *After method: Mess in social science research.* London: Routledge, 2004

Lawlor, Leonard. A Note on the Relation between Étienne Souriau's L'Instauration philosophique and Deleuze and Guattari's What is Philosophy? (2011) *Deleuze Studies* 5, 3: 400-406.

Leach, Melissa; Ian Scoones and Brian Wynne. Introduction: science, citizenship and globalization. In Melissa Leach, Ian Scoones and Brian Wynne (eds.), *Science and citizens: Globalization and the challenge of engagement,* London and New York: Zed Books, 2007, pp 3-14.

Leaf, Murray J. Ethnography and Pragmatism. In Alfonso Morales (ed.), *Renascent Pragmatism: Studies in Law and Social Science.* Cornwall: Ashgate Publishing, 2003, pp 92-117.

Lee, Lisa M and Frances A McCarty. Growth in U.S. Postsecondary Bioethics Degrees, *Hastings Center Report* (2016) 46, 2: 19-21.

Lee, Robert and Derek Morgan. *Human Fertilisation & Embryology: regulating the reproductive revolution.* London: Blackstone Press, 2001.

Leem, So Yeon and Jin Hee Park. Rethinking women and their bodies in the age of biotechnology: feminist commentaries on the Hwang Affair, *East Asian Science, Technology and Society: an International Journal* (2008) 2: 9-26.

Legrand, Pierre. Alterity: About Rules, For Example. In Peter Birks and Arianna Pretto (eds.), *Themes in Comparative Law: In Honour of Bernard Rudden.* Oxford and New York: Oxford University Press, 2002, pp 21-33.

————— European Legal Systems are not Converging, *International and Comparative Law Quarterly* (1996) 45: 52.

————— The same and the different. In Pierre Legrand and Roderick Munday (eds.), *Comparative Legal Studies: Traditions and Transitions.* Cambridge: Cambridge University Press, 2003, pp 240-311.

Lessig, Lawrence. The Law of the Horse: What Cyberlaw Might Teach, *Harvard Law Review* (1999) 113: 501.

Levi, Ron and Mariana Valverde. Studying Law by Association: Bruno Latour Goes to the Conseil d'État, *Law & Social Inquiry* (2008) 33, 3: 805-825.

Levine, Amy. Book Review – Advocacy After Bhopal: Environmentalism, Disaster, New Global Order, *Political and Legal Anthropology Review* (2003) 26, 2: 171-175.

Lewis, Graham. Regenerative Medicine at a Global Level: Current Patterns and Global Trends. In Andrew Webster (ed.), *The Global Dynamics of Regenerative Medicine: A Social Science Critique.* Basingstoke and New York: Palgrave Macmillan, 2013, pp 18-57.

Link, Albert N and Jamie R Link. *Government as Entrepreneur.* New York: Oxford University Press, 2009.

Liu, Jennifer. Asian Regeneration? Technohybridity in Taiwan's biotech? *East Asian Science Technology and Society International Journal* (2012) 6, 3: 401-414.

Loick, Daniel. Juridification and politics: From the dilemma of juridification to the paradoxes of rights, *Philosophy and Social Criticism* (2014) 40, 8: 757-778.

Lomax, Geoffrey P; Zach W Hall and Bernard Lo. Responsible Oversight of Human Stem Cell Research: The California Institute of Regenerative Medicine's Medical and Ethical Standards, *PLoS Medicine* (2007) 4, 5: 0803-0805.

Lomax, Geoffrey P. Rejuvenated Federalism: State-Based Stem Cell Research Policy. In Benjamin J Capps and Alastair V Campbell (eds.), *Contested Cells: Global Perspectives on the Stem Cell Debate.* London: Imperial College Press, 2010, pp 359-375.

López, José Julián and Janet Lunau. ELSIfication in Canada: Legal Modes of Reasoning, *Science as Culture* (March 2012) 21, 1: 77-99.

Lowrance, William W. *Of Acceptable Risk: Science and the Determination of Safety.* Los Altos: W Kaufmann, 1976.

Luhmann, Niklas (tr. E King and M Albrow). *A sociological theory of law.* London: Routledge and Kegan Paul, 1985.

Luo, Serene. Human egg donation: No payment for pain, risks. *The Straits Times*, 6 November 2008.

Lupton, Deborah. *Risk.* London and New York: Routledge, 1999.

Mackellar, Calum and David Albert Jones. *Chimera's Children: Ethical, philosophical and religious perspectives on human-nonhuman experimentation.* London and New York: Continuum, 2012.

Mackenzie, Catherine; Wendy Rogers and Susan Dodds (eds.). *Vulnerability: New Essays in Ethics and Feminist Philosophy.* Oxford: Oxford University Press, 2013

Mahajan, Manjari. Designing epidemics: models, policy-making, and global foreknowledge in India's AIDS epidemic, *Science and Public Policy* (October 2008) 35, 8: 585-596.

MacLaren, Kim. Emotional Metamorphoses: The Role of Others in Becoming a Subject. In Sue Campbell, Letitia Meynell and Susan Sherwin (eds.), *Embodiment and Agency.* University Park PA: The Pennsylvania State University, 2009, pp 25-45.

Majumder, Mary A and Cynthia B Cohen. Future Directions for Oversight of Stem Cell Research in the United States: An Update, *Kennedy Institute of Ethics Journal* (2009) 19, 2: 195-200.

Malkki, Liisa H. Tradition and Improvisation in Ethnographic Field Research. In Allaine Cerwonka and Liisa H Malkki (eds.), *Improvising Theory: Process and Temporality in Ethnographic Fieldwork.* Chicago: University of Chicago Press, 2007, pp 162-187.

Maoz, Zeev. *Networks of Nations: The Evolution, Structure, and Impact of International Networks, 1816-2001.* New York: Cambridge University Press, 2011.

Marcus, George E. *Ethnography Through Thick and Thin.* Princeton NJ: Princeton University Press, 1998.

Marmor, Andrei. The Pure Theory of Law, *The Stanford Encyclopedia of Philosophy* (Spring 2016 Edition), Edward N. Zalta (ed.). Available at: http://plato.stanford.edu/archives/spr2016/entries/lawphil-theory/.

Marres, Noortje. Front-staging Nonhumans: Publicity as a Constraint on the Political Activity of Things. In Bruce Braun and Sarah J Whatmore (eds.), *Political Matter: Technoscience, Democracy, and Public Life.* Minneapolis and London: University of Minnesota Press, 2010, pp 177-209.

——————— The issues deserve more credit: pragmatist contributions to the study of public involvement in controversy. *Social Studies of Science* (2007) 37, 759-780.

McLaren, Anne. Free-Range Eggs? *Science* (2007) 316: 339.

McGee, Kyle. *Bruno Latour: The Normativity of Networks*. London and New York: Routledge, 2014.

Merry, Sally Engle. *Human Rights and Gender Violence: Translating International Law into Local Justice*. Chicago: University of Chicago Press, 2005.

——————— New Legal Realism and the Ethnography of Transnational Law, *Law & Social Inquiry* (2006) 31, 4: 975-995.

Merton, Robert K (ed. Norman W Storer). *The Sociology of Science: theoretical and empirical investigations*. Chicago: University of Chicago Press, 1973.

Meuwese, Anne and Mila Versteeg. Quantitative methods for comparative constitutional law. In Maurice Adams and Jacco Bomhoff (eds.), *Practice and Theory in Comparative Law*. Cambridge: Cambridge University Press, 2012, pp 230-257.

Michaels, Ralf. The Functional Method of Comparative Law. In Mathias Reimann and Reinhard Zimmermann (eds.), *The Oxford Handbook of Comparative Law*. Oxford and New York: Oxford University Press, 2006, pp 339-382.

Miller, Frances H. Medical Errors, New Drug Approval, and Patient Safety. In Jonathan B Wiener, Michael D Rogers, James K Hammitt and Peter H Sand (eds.), *The Reality of Precaution: Comparing Risk Regulation in the United States and Europe*. Washington DC and London: RFF Press, 2011, pp 257-284.

Miller, Clark. Civic Epistemologies: Constituting Knowledge and Order in Political Communities, *Sociology Compass* (2008) 2, 6: 1896-1919.

Miller, Clark A and Ira Bennett. Thinking longer term about technology: is there value in science fiction-inspired approaches to constructing futures? *Science and Public Policy* (October 2008) 35, 8: 567-606.

Ministry of Education, Culture, Sports, Science and Technology of Japan. *Guidelines for Distribution and Utilization of Human Embryonic Stem Cells*, 2014.

——————— *Guidelines for the Derivation of Human Embryonic Stem Cells*, 2014.

─────── [文部科学省], Background discussion on the purposes and uses of human cloned embryos [人クローン胚の研究目的の作成・利用の あり方に関する検討経緯等について]. Available at www.mext.go.jp.

─────── [文部科学省], Notice on Bioethics and Safety Considerations [生命倫理及び安全対策に係る留意事項]. Available at www.mext.go.jp.

Ministry of Health, Singapore. *Licensing Terms and Conditions for Assisted Reproduction Centres*, 2011.

─────── *Press Release: MOH accepts Bioethics Advisory Committee's recommendations on Human-Animal Combinations in Stem Cell Research*, 27 September 2010.

─────── *Allow for genuine research, leave out the yucky stuff,* Blog post 23 September 2010; The Straits Times: 24 September 2010.

─────── *Directive 1A/2006: BAC Recommendations for Biomedical Research*, 18 January 2006.

─────── *Operational Guidelines for Institutional Review Boards*. Singapore: Ministry of Health (Biomedical Research Regulation Division), December 2007.

Mitnick, Eric J. Rights, *Groups and Self-Invention: Group-differentiated Rights in Liberal Theory*. Cornwall: Ashgate Publishing, 2006.

Miyazaki, Hirokazu. Between arbitrage and speculation: an economy of belief and doubt. *Economy and Society* (August 2007) 36, 3: 396-415.

Mizuno, Hiroshi; Hidenori Akutsu, and Kazuto Kato. Ethical acceptability of research on human-animal chimeric embryos: summary of opinions by the Japanese Expert Panel on Bioethics, *Life Sciences, Society and Policy* (2015) 11: 15-21.

Moeran, Brian. From participant observation to observant participation. In Sierk Ybema, Dvora Yanow, Harry Wels and Frans Kamsteeg (eds.), *Organizational Ethnography: Studying the Complexities of Everyday Life*. Chennai India: Sage Publications, 2009, pp 137-155.

Montgomery, Jonathan. Bioethics as a Governance Practice, *Health Care Analysis* (2016) 24, 1: 3-23.

Morales, Alfonso. Forward – Pragmatism as a Discipline: (Re)Introducing Pragmatist Philosophy to Law and Social Science. In Alfonso Morales (ed.), *Renascent Pragmatism: Studies in Law and Social Science*. Cornwall: Ashgate Publishing, 2003, pp xi-xxiv.

Morrison, Margaret and Mary S Morgan. Models as mediating instruments. In Mary S Morgan and Margaret Morrison (eds.), *Models as Mediators: Perspectives on Natural and Social Science*. Cambridge: Cambridge University Press, 1999, pp 10-37.

Mottier, Veronique. Metaphors, mini-narratives and Foucauldian discourse theory. In Terrell Carver and Jernej Pikalo (eds.), *Political Language and Metaphor: Interpreting and changing the world*. London and New York: Routledge, 2008, pp 182-194.

Mulkay, Michael. *The Embryo Research Debate: Science and the Politics of Reproduction*. Cambridge: Cambridge University Press, 1997.

Nash, June C. *Practicing Ethnography in a Globalizing World*. New York: Alta Mira Press, 2007.

National Academy of Sciences. *Final report of the National Academies' human embryonic stem cell research advisory committee and 2010 amendment to the National Academies' guidelines for human embryonic stem cell research amended as of May 2010*. Washington DC: National Academies Press, 2010.

——————— *Guidelines for Human Embryonic Stem Cell Research*. Washington DC: National Academies Press, 2005 (amended 2007 and 2008).

——————— *2007 Amendments to the National Academies' Guidelines for Human Embryonic Stem Cell Research*. Washington, DC: National Academies Press, 2007.

——————— *2008 Amendments to the National Academies' Guidelines for Human Embryonic Stem Cell Research*. Washington, DC: National Academies Press, 2008.

——————— *Assessing the Medical Risks of Human Oocyte Donation for Stem Cell Research: Workshop Report*. Washington DC, 2007.

National Advisory Committee on Laboratory Animal Research, *Guidelines on the Care and Use of Animal for Scientific Purposes in Singapore*. Singapore: National Advisory Committee on Laboratory Animal Research, 2004.

National Bioethics Advisory Commission. *Ethical Issues in Human Stem Cell Research*. Rockville, MD: U.S. Government Printing Office, 1999.

National Commission for the Protection of Human Subjects of Biomedical and Behavioral Research, *The Belmont Report: Ethical Principles and Guidelines for the protection of human subjects of research*, 18 April 1979.

National Institutes of Health. *Guidelines for Human Stem Cell Research*, 74 Fed. Reg. 32, 170 (July 7, 2009).

———— *Guidelines on Human Stem Cell Research*, 2009.

———— *NIH Research Involving Introduction of Human Pluripotent Cells into Non-Human Vertebrate Animal Pre-Gastrulation Embryos*, NOT-OD-15-158, 23 September 2015.

———— *Notice of Criteria for Federal Funding of Research on Existing Human Embryonic Stem Cells and Establishment of NIH Human Embryonic Stem Cell Registry*. 7 November 2001.

———— *Stem Cells: A Primer issued by the US National Institutes of Health*. Washington DC: National Institutes of Health. May 2000.

National Medical Ethics Committee, Singapore. *Ethical Guidelines on Research Involving Human Subjects*. Singapore: Ministry of Health, August 1997.

National Research Council. *Understanding Risk: Informing Decisions in a Democratic Society*. Washington DC: National Academy Press, 1996.

Nelson, Nicole; Anna Geltzer and Stephen Hilgartner. Introduction: the anticipatory state: making policy-relevant knowledge about the future, *Science and Public Policy* (October 2008) 35, 8: 546-550.

Niederveen Pieterse, Jan. *Globalization and Culture: Global Melange*. Lanham: Rowman and Littlefield, 2004.

Noske, Catherine. Towards an Existential Pluralism: Reading through the Philosophy of Etienne Souriau, *Cultural Studies Review* (2015) 21, 1: 34-57.

Nuremberg Military Tribunal. *Trials of War Criminals before the Nuremberg Military Tribunals under Control Council Law No 10, Vol 2*. Washington, DC: US Government Printing Office, 1949, pp 181-182.

Nuyen A T. *Stem Cell Research and Interspecies Fusion: Some Philosophical Issues*, 2007. Position Paper available at http://www.bioethics-singapore.org.

O'Neill, Onora. Changing Constructions. In Thom Brooks and Martha C Nussbaum, *Rawls's Political Liberalism*. New York: Columbia University Press, 2015, pp 57-72.

———— *Autonomy and Trust in Bioethics*. Cambridge: Cambridge University Press, 2008.

Ong, Aihwa. An Analytics of Biotechnology and Ethics at Multiple Scales. In Aihwa Ong and Nancy N Chen (eds.), *Asian Biotech: Ethics and*

Communities of Fate. Durham and London: Duke University Press, 2010, pp 1-51.

OECD. *OECD Regulatory Policy Outlook 2015*. Paris: OECD Publishing, 2015.

———— *Better Regulation in Europe – The EU 15 project*, at: http://www.oecd.org/gov/regref/eu15

Pacholczyk, Tadeusz. The Wisdom of the Church is in her Silence, Too, *National Catholic Register*, 10 August 2003.

Pauer-Studer, Herlinde. Public Reason and Bioethics, *Medscape General Medicine* (2006) 8, 4: 13-21.

Peczenik, Aleksander. Justice in legal doctrine. In Guenther Doeker-Mach and Klaus A Ziegert (eds.), *Law, Legal Culture and Politics in the Twenty First Century*. Stuttgart: Franz Steiner Verlag, 2004, pp 197-211.

Piotrowska, Monika. Transferring Morality to Human-Nonhuman Chimeras, *American Journal of Bioethics* (2014) 14, 2: 4-12.

Polkinghorne, John. *Belief in God in an Age of Science*. New Haven and London: Yale University Press, 1998.

Posner, Richard. *Law, Pragmatism and Democracy*. Cambridge MA: Harvard University Press, 2003.

Pottage, Alain. Introduction: The Fabrication of Persons and Things. In Alain Pottage and Martha Mundy (eds.), *Law, Anthropology, and the Constitution of the Social: Making Persons and Things*. Cambridge: Cambridge University Press, 2004, pp 1-39.

Power, Michael. *The Risk Management of Everything: Rethinking the politics of uncertainty*. London: Demas, 2004.

———— Risk Management and the Responsible Organization. In Richard V Ericson and Aaron Doyle (eds.), *Risk and Morality*. Toronto, Buffalo and London: University of Toronto Press, 2003, pp 145-164.

Presidential/Congressional Commission on Risk Assessment and Risk Management. *Risk Assessment and Risk Management in Regulatory Decision-Making*. Washington DC: The Presidential/Congressional Commission on Risk Assessment and Risk Management, Final Report, Vol. 2, 1997.

Puddephatt, Antony J; William Shaffir and Steven Kleinknecht. Exercises in reflexivity: situating theory in practice. In Antony J Puddephatt, William Shaffir and Steven W Kleinknecht (eds.), *Ethnographies revisited:*

constructing theory in the field. London and New York: Routledge, 2009, pp 1-34.

Radin, Margaret Jane. *Contested Commodities.* Cambridge MA and London: Harvard University Press, 1996.

Raj, Kapil. When human travellers become instruments: The Indo-British exploration of Central Asia in the nineteenth century. In Marie-Noëlle Bourguet, Christian Licoppe and H Otto Sibum (eds.), *Instruments, Travel and Science: Itineraries of precision from the seventeenth to the twentieth century.* London and New York: Routledge, 2002, pp 156-188.

Rawls, John. *Political Liberalism.* New York: Columbia University Press, 1996.

———— *The Laws of Peoples.* Cambridge MA: Harvard University Press, 1999.

———— (ed. Samuel Freeman). *Collected Papers.* Cambridge MA: Harvard University Press, 1999.

Reynaert, Didier; Maria Bouverne-De Bie and Stijn Vandevelde. Between 'believers' and 'opponents': Critical discussions on children's rights, *International Journal of Children's Rights* (2012) 20: 155-168.

Riles, Annelise. [Deadlines]: Removing the Brackets on Politics in Bureaucratic and Anthropological Analysis. In Annelise Riles (ed.), *Documents: Artefacts of Modern Knowledge.* Ann Arbor: University of Michigan Press, 2006, pp 71-92.

———— Collateral Expertise: Legal Knowledge in the Global Financial Markets. *Current Anthropology* (December 2010) 51, 6: 795-818.

———— *Collateral Knowledge: Legal Reason in the Global Financial Market.* Chicago: University of Chicago Press, 2011.

———— Comparative Law and Socio-Legal Studies. In Mathias Reimann and Reinhard Zimmermann (eds.), *The Oxford Handbook of Comparative Law.* Oxford and New York: Oxford University Press, 2006, pp 775-813.

———— Encountering Amateurism: John Henry Wigmore and the Uses of American Formalism. In Annelise Riles (ed.), *Re-thinking the Masters of Comparative Law.* Oxford and Portland: Hart Publishing, 2001, pp 94-126.

———— Introduction: The Projects of Comparison. In Annelise Riles (ed.), *Re-thinking the Masters of Comparative Law.* Oxford and Portland: Hart Publishing, 2001, pp 1-18.

————— Property as Legal Knowledge: Means and Ends (2004) *Journal of the Royal Anthropological Institute* 10: 775-795.

————— Real time: Unwinding technocratic and anthropological knowledge. *American Ethnologist* (2004) 31, 3: 392-405.

————— Real Time: Unwinding Technocratic and Anthropological Knowledge. In Melissa S Fisher and Greg Downey (eds.), *Frontiers of Capital: Ethnographic Reflections on the New Economy*. Durham and London: Duke University Press, 2006, pp 86-107.

————— A New Agenda for the Cultural Study of Law: Taking on the Technicalities, *Buffalo Law Review* (2005) 53: 973-1033.

————— Representing In-Between: Law, Anthropology and the Rhetoric of Interdisciplinarity. *University of Illinois Law Review* (1994): 597-653.

————— *The Network Inside Out*. Ann Arbor: University of Michigan Press, 2001.

————— Wigmore's Treasure Box: Comparative Law in the Era of Information. *Harvard International Law Journal* (1999) 40, 1: 221-283.

Rivière, Peter. Unscrambling Parenthood, *Anthropology Today* (1985) 1, 4: 2-7.

Robben, Antonius C G M. Reflexive Ethnography. In Antonius C G M Robben and Jeffrey A Sluka (eds.), *Ethnographic Fieldwork: An Anthropological Reader*. Singapore: Blackwell, 2007, pp 443-446.

Robert, Jason Scott and Françoise Baylis. Crossing Species Boundaries, *American Journal of Bioethics* (2003) 3, 3: 1-13.

Roberts, Celia and Karen Throsby. Paid to share: IVF patients, eggs and stem cell research *Social Science & Medicine* (2008) 66: 159-169.

Robinson, William I. Globalization and the sociology of Immanuel Wallerstein: A critical appraisal. *International Sociology* (2011) 26, 6: 723-745.

Rooke, Catriona; Emilie Cloatre and Robert Dingwall. The Regulation of Nicotine in the United Kingdom: How Nicotine Gum Came to Be a Medicine, but Not a Drug, *Journal of Law and Society* (2012) 39, 1: 39-57.

Rose, Nikolas. *Powers of Freedom: Reframing Political Thought*. Cambridge: Cambridge University Press, 1999.

Rose, Nikolas; Pat O'Malley and Mariana Valverde. Governmentality. *Annual Review of Law and Social Sciences* (2006) 2: 83-104.

Rose, Nikolas and Mariana Valverde. Governed by Law? *Social and Legal Studies* (1998) 7: 541-551.

Rothenberg, Karen H and Michael R Ulrich. NIH Guidelines on Human Embryonic Stem Cell Research in Context: Clarity of Confusion, *World Stem Cell Report 2010*, pp 89-98.

Rothman, David J. *Strangers at the bedside: a history of how law and bioethics transformed medical decision making*. New York: BasicBooks, 1991.

Roussel, Violaine. New Moralities of Risk and Political Responsibility. In Richard V Ericson and Aaron Doyle (eds.), *Risk and Morality*. Toronto, Buffalo and London: University of Toronto Press, 2003, pp 117-144.

Rubin, Beatrix P. Therapeutic Promise in the Discourse of Human Embryonic Stem Cell Research, *Science as Culture* (2008) 17, 1: 13-27.

Russo, Lucio. *The Forgotten Revolution: How Science was Born in 300 BC and Why it had to be Reborn*. New York: Springer, 2003.

Rynning, Elizabeth. Legal tools and strategies for the regulation of chimbrids, In Jochen Taupitz and Marion Weschka (eds.), *CHIMBRIDS – Chimeras and Hybrids in Comparative European and International Research*. Heidelberg: Springer, 2009, pp 79-87.

Saletan, William. The Thing Is: At the bioethics council, human nature denies human nature. *Slate*, 7 March 2005.

Samshul Jangarodin, Oleh. Penubuhan badan semak dan pantau kerja penyelidikan sel induk disaran [Proposed establishment of monitoring body for stem cell research], *Berita Harian* [Daily News], 23 September 2010.

Samuel, Geoffrey. Comparative Law and the Legal Mind. In Peter Birks and Arianna Pretto (eds.), *Themes in Comparative Law: In Honour of Bernard Rudden*. Oxford and New York: Oxford University Press, 2002, pp 35-47.

Sandulli, Aldo. The Use of Comparative Law Before the Italian Public Law Courts. In Guy Canivet, Mads Andenas and Duncan Fairgrieve (eds.), *Comparative Law Before the Courts*. London: The British Institute of International and Comparative Law, 2004, pp 165-178.

Schelling, Thomas. *The Strategy of Conflict*. Cambridge: Harvard University Press, 1960.

Schwartzman, Helen B. *Ethnography in Organizations*. Newbury Park CA: Sage Publications, 1993.

Schwegler, Tara A. Take it from the top (down)? Rethinking neoliberalism and political hierarchy in Mexico, *American Ethnologist* (November 2008) 35, 4: 682-700.

Shepherd, Elizabeth. *Human Fertilisation and Embryology Bill [HL], HL Bill 6, 2007-08*. London: House of Lords Library Notes, 2007.

Shim, Jae-Mahn; Gerard Bodeker and Gemma Burford. Institutional heterogeneity in globalization: Co-development of western-allopathic medicine and traditional-alternative medicine, *International Sociology* (2011) 26, 6: 769-788.

Shore, Cris. Introduction. In Stephen Nugent and Cris Shore, *Elite Cultures: Anthropological Perspectives*. London and New York: Routledge, 2002.

Silbey, Susan S and Patricia Ewick. The Double Life of Reason and Law, *University of Miami Law Review* (2003) 57: 497-512.

Silverstein, Gordon. Law's Allure in American Politics and Policy: What It Is, What It is Not, and What it might yet to be, *Law & Social Inquiry* (Fall 2010) 35, 4: 1077-1097.

Simmons, Laurence. Shame, Levinas's Dog, Derrida's Cat (and Some Fish). In Laurence Simmons and Philip Armstrong (eds.), *Knowing Animals*. Leiden: Brill, 2007, pp 27-42.

Sinding, Aasen; Henriette, Siri Gloppen, Anne-Mette Magnussen and Even Nilssen. Introduction. In Henriette Sinding Aasen, Siri Gloppen, Anne-Mette Magnussen and Even Nilssen, *Juridification and social citizenship in the welfare state*. Cheltenham: Edward Elgar, 2014, pp 1-20.

Singapore Medical Council, *Ethical Code and Ethical Guidelines of the Singapore Medical Council*. Singapore: Singapore Medical Council, 2002.

Singh Grewal, David. *Network Power: The Social Dynamics of Globalization*. New Haven and London: Yale University Press, 2008.

Sleeboom-Faulkner, Margaret. Debates on human embryonic stem cell research in Japan: minority voices and their political amplifiers, *Science as Culture* (2008) 17: 85-97.

Smith, Christian. *What is a Person? Rethinking Humanity, Social Life, and the Moral Good from the Person Up*. Chicago and London: University of Chicago Press, 2010.

Smith, Dorothy. *Texts, Facts and Femininity: Exploring the Relations of Ruling*. London: Routledge, 1990.

Sperling, Stefan. *Reasons of Conscience: The Bioethics Debate in Germany.* Chicago: University of Chicago Press, 2013.

Star, Susan Leigh. This is Not a Boundary Object: Reflections on the Origin of a Concept, *Science, Technology, & Human Values* (2010) 35, 5: 601-617.

Stark, Laura. *Behind Closed Doors: IRBs and the Making of Ethical Research.* Chicago and London: University of Chicago Press, 2012.

Stem Cell Toolkit (UK): http://www.sc-toolkit.ac.uk/home.cfm

Stengers, Isabelle and Bruno Latour. The Sphinx of the Work. In Étienne Souriau (tr. Erik Beranek and Tim Howles), *The Different Modes of Existence.* Minneapolis: Univocal, 2015.

Stenvoll, Dag. Slippery slopes in political discourse. In Terrell Carver and Jernej Pikalo (eds.), *Political Language and Metaphor: Interpreting and changing the world.* London and New York: Routledge, 2008, pp 28-40.

Stevens, Tina M L. *Bioethics in America.* Baltimore: Johns Hopkins University Press, 2000.

Stolleis, Michael. The Legitimation of Law through God, Tradition, Will, Nature and Constitution. In Larraine Daston and Michael Stolleis (eds.), *Natural Law and Laws of Nature in Early Modern Europe: Jurisprudence, Theology, Moral and Natural Philosophy.* Cornwall: Ashgate Publishing, 2008.

Strathern, Marilyn. Accountability ... and ethnography. In Marilyn Strathern (ed.), *Audit Cultures: Anthropological studies in accountability, ethics and the academy.* London: Routledge, 2000, pp 279-304.

———— *After Nature: English Kinship in the Late Twentieth Century.* Cambridge: Cambridge University Press, 1992.

———— *Partial Connections.* Savage ML: Rowman & Littlefield Publishers, 1991.

Sunstein, Cass. Health-Health Tradeoffs. In Cass Sunstein (ed.), *Risk and Reason.* Cambridge: Cambridge University Press, 2002, pp 133-152.

Takahashi, K *et al.* Induction of Pluripotent Stem Cells from Adult Human Fibroblasts by Defined Factors, *Cell* (2007) 131, 5: 1-12.

Tan, Tania. Forum on ethics of mixing human, animal genes, *The Straits Times,* 14 August 2008.

Taupitz, Jochen and Marion Weschka (eds.). *CHIMBRIDS – Chimeras and Hybrids in Comparative European and International Research.* Heidelberg: Springer, 2009.

Testa, Giuseppe. Stem Cells through Stem Beliefs: The Co-Production of Biotechnological Pluralism, *Science as Culture* (2008) 17, 4: 435-448.

Teubner, Gunther. And God Laughed ... Indeterminacy, Self-Reference and Paradox in Law, *German Law Journal* (2011) 12: 376-406.

——— Juridification – Concepts, Aspects, Limits, Solutions. In Gunther Teubner (ed.), *Juridification of Social Spheres: A Comparative Analysis in the Areas of Labor, Corporate Antitrust and Social Welfare Law*. Berlin: Walter de Gruyter & Co, 1987, pp 3-48.

Thomas, William I and Dorothy S Thomas. *The child in America: Behaviour problems and programs*. New York: Knopf, 1928.

Thomas, Yan. Res Religiosae: on the categories of religion and commerce in Roman law. In Alain Pottage and Martha Mundy (eds.), *Law, Anthropology, and the Constitution of the Social: Making Persons and Things*. Cambridge: Cambridge University Press, 2004, pp 40-72.

Thompson, Charis. *Good Science: The Ethical Choreography of Stem Cell Research*. Cambridge MA and London: MIT Press, 2013.

——— Asian Regeneration? Nationalism and Internationalism in Stem Cell Research in South Korea and Singapore. In Aihwa Ong and Nancy N Chen (eds.), *Asian Biotech: Ethics and Communities of Fate*. Durham and London: Duke University Press, 2010, pp 95-117.

——— Why we should, in fact, pay for egg donation. *Regenerative Medicine* (2007) 2: 203-209.

Timmer, Andria D. Constructing the "Needy Subject": NGO Discourses of Roma Need, *Political and Legal Anthropology Review* (November 2010) 33, 2: 264-281.

Tonybee, Polly. Religion doesn't rule in this clash of moral universes, *The Guardian*, 25 March 2008.

Tulloch, John and Deborah Lupton. *Risk and Everyday Life*. London, Thousand Oaks and New Delhi: Sage, 2003.

UK Home Office, *Guidance on the use of Human Material in Animals. Advice Note 01/16*, January 2016.

Underhill, James W. *Creating Worldviews: Metaphor, Ideology and Language*. Edinburgh: Edinburg University Press, 2011.

United Nations Educational, Scientific and Cultural Organization. *Declaration on Race and Racial Prejudice* 1982.

————— *Universal Declaration on the Human Genome and Human Rights* 1998.

United Nations General Assembly, Sixth Committee Working Group. *Report of the Working Group Established Pursuant to General Assembly Decision 59/547 to Finalize the Text of a United Nations Declaration on Human Cloning.* U.N. Doc. A/C.6/59/L.27/Rev.1. 23 Feb, 2005.

United Nations General Assembly, *Declaration on Human Cloning,* A/Res/59/280, 23 March 2005.

————— *Rio Declaration on Environment and Development,* UN Doc. A/CONF.151/26, vol I, annex I, 1992.

————— *International Convention on Economic, Social and Cultural Rights,* 1966,

————— *Universal Declaration of Human Rights,* 1948.

Valverde, Mariana; Ron Levi and Dawn Moore. Legal Knowledges of Risk. In Law Commission of Canada, *Law and Risk.* Vancouver and Toronto: University of British Columbia Press, 2005, pp 86-120.

Valverde, Mariana. *Law and Order: Images, Meanings, Myths.* New Brunswick: Rutgers University Press, 2006.

Vastag, Brian. Private Efforts Pick Up Stem Cell Slack, *Journal of the American Medical Association* (2004) 291, 17: 2059.

van der Steen, Martijn. Ageing or silvering? Political debate about ageing in the Netherlands, *Science and Public Policy* (October 2008) 35, 8: 575-583.

von Bernstorff, Jochen and Thomas Dunlap. *The Public International Law Theory of Hans Kelsen: Believing in Universal Law.* Cambridge: Cambridge University Press, 2010.

Vis, Barbara. *Politics of Risk-taking: Welfare State Reform in Advanced Democracies.* Amsterdam: Amsterdam University Press, 2011.

Vogel, Kathleen M. 'Iraqi Winnebagos™ of death': imagined and realized futures of US bioweapons threat assessments, *Science and Public Policy* (October 2008) 35, 8: 561-573.

Wacquant, Loïc. Habitus as Topic and Tool: Reflections on becoming a prizefighter. In Antony J Puddephatt, William Shaffir and Steven W Kleinknecht (eds.), *Ethnographies revisited: constructing theory in the field.* London and New York: Routledge, 2009, pp 137-151.

Wallerstein, Immanuel. *The Modern World-System I: Capitalist Agriculture and the Origins of the European World-Economy in the Sixteenth Century.* New York: Academic Press, 1974.

Waring, Duff R and Trudo Lemmens. Integrating Values in Risk Analysis of Biomedical Research: The Case for Regulatory and Law Reform. In Law Commission of Canada, *Law and Risk.* Vancouver and Toronto: University of British Columbia Press, 2005, pp 156-200.

Warnock, Mary (Chairperson). *Report of the Committee of Inquiry into Human Fertilisation and Embryology.* London: H.M.S.O., Cmd. 9314, 1984.

Warnock, Mary. *Making Babies: Is there a right to have children?* Oxford: Oxford University Press, 2002.

—————— *Nature and Mortality: recollections of a philosopher in public life.* London and New York: Continuum, 2003.

Weale, Albert. New Modes of Governance, Political Accountability and Public Reason, *Government and Opposition* (2011) 46, 1: 58-80.

Weber, Max. *The Protestant Ethic and the Spirit of Capitalism.* New York and London: Routledge, 2005.

—————— Science as a vocation. In Wolfgang Schirmacher, *German Essays on Science in the 20th century.* New York: Continuum, 1996.

—————— (eds. Guenther Roth and Claus Wittich). *Economy and Society: An Outline of Interpretive Sociology* (in two volumes). Berkeley, Los Angeles and London: University of California Press, [1922] 1978.

—————— Science as a vocation. In H H Gerth and C W Mills (eds.), *From Max Weber.* London: Routledge, 1948, pp 129-156.

—————— Religious rejections of the world and their directions. In H H Gerth and C W Mills (eds.), *From Max Weber.* London: Routledge, 1948, pp 323-359.

Webster, Andrew. Introduction: The Boundaries and Mobilities of Regenerative Medicine. In Andrew Webster (ed.), *The Global Dynamics of Regenerative Medicine: A Social Science Critique.* Basingstoke and New York: Palgrave Macmillan, 2013, pp 1-17.

White, Ahmed. Max Weber and the Uncertainties of Categorical Comparative Law. In Annelise Riles (ed.), *Re-thinking the Masters of Comparative Law.* Oxford and Portland: Hart Publishing, 2001, pp 40-57.

Whitman, James Q. The Neo-Romantic Turn. In Mathias Reimann and Reinhard Zimmermann (eds.), *The Oxford Handbook of Comparative Law*. Oxford and New York: Oxford University Press, 2006, pp 312-344.

Wiener, Jonathan. The Rhetoric of Precaution. In Jonathan B Wiener, Michael D Rogers, James K Hammitt and Peter H Sand (eds.), *The Reality of Precaution: Comparing Risk Regulation in the United States and Europe*. Washington DC and London: RFF Press, 2011, pp 3-35.

———— The Real Pattern of Precaution. In Jonathan B Wiener, Michael D Rogers, James K Hammitt and Peter H Sand (eds.), *The Reality of Precaution: Comparing Risk Regulation in the United States and Europe*. Washington DC and London: RFF Press, 2011, pp 519-565.

Wilden, Anthony and Tim Wilson. The Double Bind: Logic, Magic and Economics. In Carlos Sluzki and Donald Ransom (eds.), *Double Bind: The Foundation of the Communicational Approach to the Family*. New York: Grune and Stratton, 1976, pp 263-286.

Wilkinson, Iain. *Risk, Vulnerability and Everyday Life*. London and New York: Routledge, 2010.

Wilson, Duncan. *The Making of British Bioethics*. Manchester: Manchester University Press, 2014.

Winston, Robert. *A Child Against All Odds*. Reading: Bantam Books, 2008.

Wittgenstein, Ludwig (ed. Rush Rhees and tr. A C Miles). *Remarks on Frazer's Golden Bough*. Swansea: The Brynmill Press, 1979.

Witty, Nancy. Strategic Planning: Progress and Potential, *Cell Stem Cell* (2007) 1: 383-386.

Wong, Joseph. *Betting on Biotech: Innovation and the Limits of Asia's Developmental State*. Ithaca and London: Cornell University Press, 2011.

World Medical Association. *Declaration of Helsinki – Ethical Principles for Medical Research Involving Human Subjects*, October 2013 (as amended).

Wynne, Brian. Public Participation in Science and Technology: Performing and Obscuring a Political-Conceptual Category Mistake. *East Asian Science, Technology and Society: an International Journal* (2007) 1: 99-110.

Xie Y Y [谢燕燕]. Bioethics Advisory Committee Consults the Public: Can you accept human-animal combinations, Combined Morning Paper [生物道德资询委员会征询公众:你是否接受人兽嵌合体, Combined Night Paper [联合早报], 9 January 2008.

Xu X Y [许翔宇]. Human-Animal Combinations? Bioethics Advisory Committee Seeks Public Opinion [人兽混合体? 生物道德资询委员会征询公众意见], Combined Night Paper [联合晚报], 8 January 2008.

Xu, Xiang Yu. Mouse with Consciousness, Pig with Feelings: Human-Animal Combinations; There will be Chaos in the World, *Joint Evening Newspaper*, 22 September 2010.

Yablon, Charles M. Are Judges Liars? A Wittgensteinian Critique of Law's Empire *Canadian Journal of Law and Jurisprudence* (1990) 3: 123.

Yanow, Dvora. Cognition meets action: Metaphors as models of and models for. In Terrell Carver and Jernej Pikalo (eds.), *Political Language and Metaphor: Interpreting and changing the world*. London and New York: Routledge, 2008, pp 225-238.

Yarrow, Thomas. This is not the academic world of right and wrong: The obviation of truth through NGO documentary practice, *Cambridge Anthropology* (2006) 26: 50-59.

Ybema, Sierk; Dvora Yanow, Harry Wels and Frans Kamsteeg. Studying everyday organizational life. In Sierk Ybema, Dvora Yanow, Harry Wels and Frans Kamsteeg (eds.), *Organizational Ethnography: Studying the Complexities of Everyday Life*. Chennai India: Sage Publications, 2009, pp 1-20.

Yu, J; Vodyanik M A, Smuga-Otto K, Antosiewicz-Bourget J, Frane J L, Tian S, Nie J, Jonsdottir G A, Ruotti V, Stewart R, Slukvin I I, Thomson J A. Induced Pluripotent Stem Cell Lines Derived from Human Somatic Cells, *Science* (21 December 2007) 318, 5858: 1917-1920.

Zweigert, Konrad and Hein Kötz (tr. Tony Weir). *An Introduction to Comparative Law*. Oxford: Clarendon Press, 1998 (revised 3rd ed.).

Index